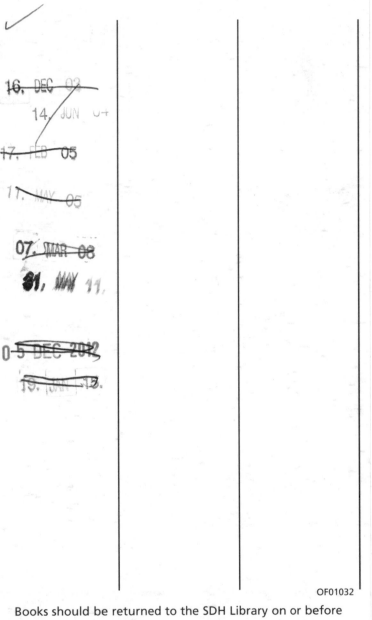

An Atlas of
Gastroenterology

A Guide to Diagnosis and Differential Diagnosis

THE ENCYCLOPEDIA OF VISUAL MEDICINE SERIES

An Atlas of
GASTROENTEROLOGY

A Guide to Diagnosis and Differential Diagnosis

Cyrus R. Kapadia, MD
Professor of Medicine and Director of the Internal Medicine Residency Training Program,
Department of Internal Medicine, Section of Digestive Diseases,
Yale University School of Medicine, CT

Caroline R. Taylor, MD
Associate Professor, Department of Diagnostic Radiology,
Yale University School of Medicine;
Chief, Diagnostic Imaging, VA Connecticut Health Care System, CT

and

James M. Crawford, MD, PhD
Professor and Chair, Department of Pathology,
Immunology and Laboratory Medicine,
University of Florida College of Medicine, FL

The Parthenon Publishing Group
International Publishers in Medicine, Science & Technology

A CRC PRESS COMPANY
BOCA RATON   LONDON   NEW YORK   WASHINGTON, D.C.

Library of Congress Cataloging-in-Publication Data
Kapadia, Cyrus R.
   An atlas of gastroenterology / Cyrus R. Kapadia, Caroline
Taylor and James M. Crawford.
      p. ; cm. – (The encyclopedia of visual medicine series)
   Includes bibliographical references and index.
   ISBN 1-85070-581-X (alk. paper)
     1. Gastrointestinal system--Diseases--Atlases.
   2. Gastrointestinal system--Atlases. I. Taylor, Caroline, MD.
   II. Crawford, James M., 1954- III. Title. IV. Series.
     [DNLM: 1. Gastrointestinal Diseases--diagnosis--Atlases.
   2. Gastrointestinal Diseases--diagnosis--Case Report.
   3. Gastrointestinal Diseases--therapy--Atlases.
   4. Gastrointestinal Diseases--therapy--Case Report.
   WI 17 K17a 2002]
   RC801 .K34 2002
   616.3'3'00222--dc21
                                                    2002027084

British Library Cataloguing in Publication Data
Kapadia, Cyrus R.
   An atlas of gastroenterology - (The encyclopedia of visual
medicine series)
   1. Gastroenterology
   I. Title II. Taylor, Caroline III. Crawford, James M.
   616.3'3
   ISBN 1-85070-581-X

Published in the USA by
The Parthenon Publishing Group
345 Park Avenue South, 10th Floor
New York, NY 10010, USA

Published in the UK and Europe by
The Parthenon Publishing Group
23–25 Blades Court
Deodar Road
London SW15 2NU, UK

Copyright © 2003, The Parthenon Publishing Group

Composition by Siva Math Setters, Chennai, India.
Printed and bound by T. G. Hostench S. A., Spain

Contents

Preface

All too often in medical education the word atlas conjures up a mental image of a book containing pretty pictures. Gastroenterology lends itself readily to a compilation of neat endoscopic and radiological illustrations for the reader to behold and perhaps to use as an aid to the future recognition of the illustrated entities. That is not the purpose of the present atlas. The authors much prefer to assign the word a richer meaning, one perhaps not as celestial as the Homeric connotation, nevertheless one that implies more than a mere collection of colorful illustrations. The authors do not make pretensions to their work being any more scholarly or even more utilitarian than the conventional atlas of endoscopy or gastrointestinal radiology. Indeed, such atlases have a very important educational role and provide valuable learning experiences for gastroenterologists. All they wish to state is that this work is different. As the subtitle to this book states without apology, this is *A Guide to Diagnosis and Differential Diagnosis*.

The table of contents of this atlas is quite unlike that of other atlases in gastroenterology and, in fact, quite unlike that of a textbook on the subject. The reader will notice that it is patient-focused and deals with common gastrointestinal symptoms and symptom complexes seen by physicians, physicians assistants and nurse practitioners of all kinds, whether they be practitioners of internal or family medicine or subspecialists, such as gastroenterologists and even surgeons. In fact, the authors hope that several chapters will be of interest to their surgical colleagues as well. The authors have also had in mind the needs of house-officers, fellows and registrars in a variety of disciplines as they grapple to make sense out of what their patients tell them.

The information is presented largely using a series of case histories, with the reasoning used to arrive at the diagnosis, and the differential diagnoses considered on the way, clearly stated. The authors recognize that the explosion of technology in medicine, which has not escaped the practice of modern gastroenterology, has greatly enhanced the ability of the clinician to arrive at a diagnosis more rapidly than in years gone by. There can be no doubt that technology has been a great boon to patient and doctor alike. However, it has not come without cost. The cost is not only one that is measured in pounds sterling or dollars, but it has come at the great risk of the temptation to sacrifice one's clinical reasoning at the altar of technology. One of the main aims of the authors has been to encourage the prudent use of recent technology, but to stress the importance of the invaluable encounter at the bedside which ought to serve as the basis for ordering laboratory and imaging studies. The importance of pathology to the practice of medicine is recognized and presented in a way to meet the needs of the clinician. Above all, the authors are convinced that the practitioner who ignores developments in the basic sciences does so at his or her own peril and does not serve his or her patient well. Yet, textbooks of medicine and medical journals often assume a more sophisticated understanding of the ever-expanding knowledge in the basic sciences than can reasonably be expected from those engaged in the busy practice of medicine. The authors have tried to the best of their ability to present recent concepts in pathophysiology without complexity and as far as possible using illustrations. The only reward they seek is that their readers will have as much fun browsing through this atlas, as they have had putting it together.

Cyrus R. Kapadia, MD

CHAPTER 1

The patient with difficulty or pain during swallowing

The two major symptoms associated with swallowing recognized by patients are: difficulty swallowing (dysphagia) and painful swallowing (odynophagia). Of course, dysphagia and odynophagia may on occasion be present together.

DYSPHAGIA

Dysphagia may occur because of problems with the oral, pharyngeal or esophageal phases of deglutition.

ORAL PHASE

Problems with the oral phase of deglutition are shown in Table 1.1.

Clinical characteristics

The patient is unable to prepare a suitable bolus in order to swallow, resulting in difficulty in the passage of the bolus into the pharynx. Aspiration may occur.

Diagnosis   This is established clinically by history and physical examination.

PHARYNGEAL PHASE

Problems with the pharyngeal phase of deglutition occur because of either mechanical or neuromuscular impediments.

Mechanical

Mechanical problems with the pharyngeal phase of deglutition can result from severe pharyngitis or a retropharyngeal abscess.

Table 1.1 Problems with the oral phase of deglutition

Poor dentition
Lesions of mouth or tongue
Little or no saliva
medications with anticholinergic properties
Sjögren's syndrome

Table 1.2 Causes of neuromuscular or transfer dysphagia

Strokes – cortical, subcortical, brainstem
Tumor – brainstem
Progressive bulbar palsy
Degenerative – e.g. multiple sclerosis
Extrapyramidal lesions – e.g. Parkinsonism
Cranial neuropathies
Myasthenia gravis
Bulbar poliomyelitis
Dermatomyositis, polymyositis
Myotonia dystrophica
Occulopharyngeal dysphagia – ptosis and dysphagia

Clinical characteristics

The patient complains of a severe sore throat with or without systemic symptoms and pharyngitis, or a retropharyngeal abscess is obvious on clinical examination.

Diagnosis   This is established by examination of the mouth and pharynx for pharyngitis or a retropharyngeal abscess.

Neuromuscular or transfer dysphagia

This can result from various causes (Table 1.2).

Clinical characteristics of transfer dysphagia

Transfer dysphagia is the inability to transfer the bolus from the mouth or pharynx into the esophagus. Difficulty is greater with liquids than with solids. There can be nasal regurgitation. As a consequence, patients are likely to aspirate liquids, and perhaps solids as well, into the lungs and develop pneumonia and a lung abscess.

Diagnosis of aspiration   This is established by: history, as above – often a history of repeated episodes of aspiration pneumonia; videoesophagogram or pharyngeal intubation study (Figure 1.1).

ESOPHAGEAL PHASE

Problems with the esophageal phase of deglutition occur as a result of mechanical or motility disorders.

Clinical characteristics of esophageal causes of dysphagia depend upon whether the cause is secondary to a mechanical disorder or a motility disorder. In the case of mechanical disorders, solid food dysphagia always antecedes dysphagia due to liquids. When the dysphagia is secondary to a peptic stricture or esophageal squamous or adenocarcinoma, the solid food dysphagia is progressive, present with most meals unless the food is pureed and eventually leads to liquid dysphagia. The dysphagia due to a lower esophageal ring is intermittent and frequently follows the rapid ingestion of a bolus of meat or even bread. In contrast, symptoms in motility disorders arise as often with liquids as with solids, although the patient may perceive more problems with one or the other.

Mechanical disorders

Mechanical disorders causing problems with the esophageal phase of deglutition are shown in Table 1.3.

Diagnosis

A barium swallow will most often identify the cause. Early carcinomas can be missed if a barium marshmallow or barium soaked in bread is not administered to determine whether there is a hold-up in the passage of the bolus. A barium swallow is not generally indicated prior to the removal of a foreign body, although a chest X-ray is.

Endoscopy is almost always performed, even when the diagnosis is clear on a barium study. The two provide complementary information; when a tumor or stricture is present, endoscopic biopsies and cytology are obtained.

Table 1.3   Mechanical disorders involving the esophageal phase of deglutition

Upper third of the esophagus
Zenker's diverticulum
Webs (when in association with koilonychia and iron deficiency anemia, this is called the Plummer–Vinson or the Kelley–Patterson syndrome)
Cervical spine osteophyte (spur)
Thyromegaly
Dysphagia lusoria – aberrant right subclavian artery
Dysphagia aortica – aortic enlargement or aneurysm
Squamous cell carcinoma – post-cricoid carcinoma
Foreign body

Middle third of the esophagus
Right-sided aorta
Diverticula
Barrett's esophagus
Squamous cell carcinoma
Foreign body

Lower third of the esophagus
Diverticula – epiphrenic
Peptic stricture – from gastroesophageal reflux disease or scleroderma
Benign ulcer – frequently in Barrett's epithelium
Squamous cell cancer
Adenoma carcinoma arising from Barrett's epithelium
Adenoma carcinoma of the gastric cardia
Foreign body

Diffuse
Lesions described under Odynophagia

Case history 1

A 60-year-old Caucasian man presents with a history of dysphagia for the past 8 months. He first noticed difficulty with eating an apple, then with foods such as roast beef, over the past month with scrambled eggs and mashed potatoes, and now even has to swallow liquids slowly and feels them 'hold up' before they go down. He has not had chest pain. He has had moderate heartburn over the years, usually taken care of by antacid tablets taken when necessary, although he has off-and-on taken H_2 receptor antagonists. Barium swallow revealed an irregular, ulcerated circumferential mass in the lower third of the esophagus causing dilatation proximally. Endoscopy revealed narrowing of the lumen of the distal third of the esophagus with ulceration. Biopsy revealed an adenocarcinoma (Figures 1.2, 1.3 and 1.4).

Case history 2

A 66-year-old Caucasian man has a history of dysphagia over the past year, rather similar in terms of its progression to that in Case history 1. This patient, however, had a history of heavy smoking and alcohol consumption. The barium swallow revealed a long irregular stricture in the mid-esophagus with proximal esophageal dilatation. Biopsy upon endoscopy revealed an esophageal stricture (Figures 1.5 and 1.6).

Esophageal carcinoma   For years squamous cell cancer was more common than adenocarcinoma. Taken worldwide, that statement is still true. However, in Western countries over the past 10 years, adenocarcinoma, probably arising from Barrett's epithelium, is increasing in prevalence among middle-aged Caucasian males. It therefore appears to be related to chronic gastroesophageal reflux. Squamous cell cancer, in contrast, has been associated with heavy smoking and alcohol consumption, frequently both, as well as with tobacco chewing. Cancers of the esophagus tend to arise in the upper, middle or lower third of the esophagus. The hallmarks of the disease are:

(1)   Progressive solid food dysphagia. Ultimately difficulty with liquids also arises and patients may not even be able to swallow their own saliva.

(2)   Dysphagia that is not intermittent. Each time food of a certain size and consistency is eaten, the patient experiences dysphagia. For example, someone who has difficulty with apples or roast beef has trouble with apples and roast beef each time they eat it. If at the next meal they eat softer and more pureed food, they might not experience difficulty.

Case history 3

A 42-year-old man underwent a barium swallow for a complaint of solid food occasionally sticking in the region just below his sternal notch, at times causing him to choke. The symptoms occurred intermittently, were not progressive and had been present for some years. The barium swallow (Figure 1.7) shows an upper esophageal web. The patient's problems were no longer present after he underwent esophageal bougienage.

Esophageal webs   Most often a web is seen in the upper part of the esophagus, anteriorly, as an isolated finding of unknown etiology. A web may give rise to solid food dysphagia that is either not progressive or very slowly progressive. A rare syndrome, (the Kelley–Patterson syndrome, also termed Plummer–Vinson syndrome), is the presence of a web together with iron deficiency anemia and associated koilonychia (i.e. spoon-shaped nails that are seen with severe chronic iron deficiency

anemia of any etiology). The cause of the iron deficiency is not well understood. The Kelley–Patterson syndrome is seen in northern latitudes (Scotland, Sweden, Nova Scotia, Minnesota), and occurs more commonly in women. The patient reports the food being stuck just below the throat, at the site of the ring.

Case history 4

An 80-year-old man presented with dyspeptic symptoms and refused an endoscopy. A barium swallow was ordered and, in addition to gastroesophageal reflux, an incidental finding was a Zenker's diverticulum (Figure 1.8).

Esophageal diverticulum   Esophageal diverticula are of three types:

(1)   Upper esophageal – Zenker's diverticulum.

(2)   Mid-esophageal – at the level of the hilum of the lung. These are rare. They were thought in the past to be 'traction' diverticula, pulled by inflammation in the mediastinum, as in tracheobronchial tuberculosis.

(3)   Lower esophageal – epiphrenic diverticulum (see Case history 9) (Figure 1.9).

In Zenker's diverticulum, an area of weakness is normally present in the posterior part of the pharynx between the oblique fibers of the inferior constrictor and the horizontal fibers of the cricopharyngeus muscle. This area of weakness is called Killian's dehiscence. During swallowing, normally the cricopharyngeus opens easily. However, if for some reason it is tight or does not relax physiologically, pressure is transmitted in all directions. On account of Killian's dehiscence a small portion of the esophageal wall protrudes like a hernia and forms a diverticulum. This is the proposed mechanism.

A Zenker's diverticulum may be asymptomatic, as in the patient described here. In this patient the diverticulum was discovered when a barium study was ordered for the investigation of dyspeptic symptoms. On the other hand, many patients are very symptomatic (Figure 1.10).

Case history 5

A 40-year-old man presents to the emergency department of the hospital with acute dysphagia. He was at a buffet dinner party, had been drinking moderately and 'having fun with the boys'. He thinks he took a rather

Table 1.4 Food impaction of the esophagus may occur in the following situations

Behind a stricture
    benign – peptic or sequela of corrosive ingestion
    malignant – squamous or adenocarcinoma
Schatzki ring
Motor disorder of the esophagus
    diffuse esophageal spasm
    achalasia
No structural or functional abnormality discernible – bolus presumably too large for the lumen

Table 1.5 Disorders of esophageal motility

Achalasia
    primary
    secondary to:
        cancer of lower esophagus or gastric cardia
        Chagas' disease
Diffuse esophageal spasm
Nutcracker esophagus

generous bite of his steak and immediately noted it became 'stuck behind the lower part of my chest bone'. He pointed to the xiphisternum as the site of the obstruction. He has a history of episodic dysphagia to solid foods going back around 3 years. Normally he has no problem eating, but at variable intervals ranging from a week to several months apart, he suddenly chokes on solid food while eating a meal. Usually the food eaten is a piece of meat, but he has choked on bread as well. Most often he drinks a glass or two of water and feels the food entering his stomach. Thereafter, he is able to continue his meal. On a few occasions he has had to 'vomit up' the food stuck in his esophagus. This is the first time that his efforts have not succeeded and the food has remained impacted.

What is the most likely diagnosis? This is a typical history of a 'foreign body' obstruction of the esophagus behind a Schatzki ring. Food impaction can occur in several situations (Table 1.4). What strongly suggests a Schatzki ring in this case is the history of episodic dysphagia to solid food. The same sort of food may be eaten on other occasions without a problem, then suddenly, for one reason or another, it becomes impacted. Steak (hence the name 'steakhouse syndrome') is typical, but almost any type of solid food, including a piece of bread, can become impacted.

What was done for this patient? A chest X-ray was initially obtained to look for mediastinal or subdiaphragmatic air, to rule out an esophageal perforation. A chest radiograph also provides information as to whether bone is present in the meat that is stuck. It alerts the endoscopist to the fact that the impaction needs to be removed rather than being pushed into the stomach. Chicken bones, being cartilagenous, are frequently radiolucent.

An intravenous injection of glucagon, 1 mg, was then administered with the hope that the smooth muscle of

the esophagus would relax and allow the impacted meat to pass into the stomach. That did not happen. The patient then underwent an esophagogastroduodenoscopy (EGD) to remove the impaction. A Schatzki ring was seen after removal of the impaction.

A week later the Schatzki ring was ruptured using a large, 50 French bougie (Figures 1.11 and 1.12).

Esophageal rings Esophageal rings characteristically occur in the lower third of the esophagus. Two kinds are generally described:

(1) Type A (muscular ring): located in the lower 2 cm of the esophagus. It results from muscular hypertrophy. It is frequently seen in children if for some reason they require a barium swallow. It is seldom the cause of dysphagia.

(2) Type B (mucosal ring or Schatzki ring). Located at the squamocolumnar junction. The upper part of the ring has squamous mucosa and the lower part columnar mucosa. It may give rise to episodic solid food dysphagia. It is detected by both barium swallow examination and endoscopy.

Motor disorders (disorders of esophageal motility)

These can be divided into achalasia, diffuse esophageal spasm and nutcracker esophagus (Table 1.5).

Case history 6

A 45-year-old man complains of difficulty in swallowing. At this point his complaints are present with every meal, and he has problems almost equally with liquids and solids. A detailed history reveals that his problems began around 6 or 7 years ago when he intermittently experienced a feeling of fullness in his lower chest during eating. Over the years this developed into a feeling of obstruction, occasionally accompanied by a sharp spasm of pain in his chest. For quite some time he found relief by drinking a glass of water during the meal, and felt that this led to 'the food going down'.

As the years progressed and his complaints became worse, not only did he need to drink a glass of water to allow the food to pass down into his stomach, but he often needed to stand up and shrug his shoulders. Over the past year he has noticed that when he awakens in the morning he often sees a pool of 'spit' on his pillow. More recently, over the past month, some of the meal previously eaten is frequently, without warning, spontaneously regurgitated out of his mouth an hour or so after its consumption. This complaint is the one that has finally led this stoic to seek medical help. He admits to heartburn for the past 3 years or so, that has now become worse. Upon the advice of his friends he has tried over-the-counter H_2 blockers, but without relief. He has been eating less on account of the problems he now has with each meal, and has lost around 15 lb.

Based on the clinical features, a diagnosis of achalasia would be the first contender.

Achalasia What are the clinical features of this patient's dysphagia?

(1) It has been *gradually* progressive after the dysphagia first began. In dysphagia due to tumors, once the symptom is first noticed, progression is relatively rapid.

(2) It is about equal for solids and for liquids, unlike that from a benign or malignant stricture.

(3) He was able to help 'the food go down' initially with a glass of water, and later by a maneuver that involved standing up and shrugging his shoulders. This is typical in patients with achalasia. Various individualized maneuvers, in some cases elevation of the arms above the head, in others a Valsalva-like maneuver, often help the food go down.

(4) The puddle of saliva on the pillow upon awakening from sleep may be seen in patients with strictures as well.

(5) The weight loss that develops late in the course of the disease is quite typical.

(6) Chest pain with meals is not unusual.

(7) Heartburn is not uncommon. It is not due to reflux of gastric contents into the stomach, but rather the result of the food held up in the esophagus fermenting and producing organic acids. Hence the heartburn is not relieved by H_2 receptor antagonists or proton pump inhibitors.

Table 1.6 Features of achalasia seen on esophageal manometry

Upper esophageal sphincter
   pressure: normal
   reflex relaxation to air in the esophagus may be impaired, leading to difficulty with belching and chest pain
Upper third of body (skeletal muscle): normal manometry
Lower two-thirds of body (smooth muscle)
   low amplitude – often 20 mmHg or less (normal ~50–150 mmHg)
   non-peristaltic contractions
Lower esophageal sphincter
   pressure: normal or high
   relaxation: impaired on swallowing – *sine qua non* for the diagnosis of achalasia

Table 1.7 Types of achalasia

Primary achalasia
Secondary achalasia (pseudoachalasia)
   malignancy
      adenocarcinoma of the stomach infiltrating the esophageal wall
      paraneoplastic syndrome
   Chagas' disease (*Trypanosoma cruzi*)

A chest radiograph showed absence of the stomach bubble and an abnormal contour of the azygo-esophageal recess suggesting esophageal dilatation (Figure 1.13a). The barium swallow showed a dilated esophagus with a beak-like narrowing at the gastroesophageal junction and an air–fluid level in the upper esophagus. Ill-defined filling defects seen within the barium contrast represent retained esophageal contents (Figure 1.13b).

The pathology and pathophysiology of achalasia are shown in Figure 1.14. The features of achalasia on esophageal manometry are listed in Table 1.6 and shown in Figure 1.15. Types of achalasia are listed in Table 1.7.

Investigations to order when achalasia is suspected are shown in Table 1.8. Motor disorders that can mimic achalasia are shown in Table 1.9.

Case history 7

A young man, 23 years old, has a 4-year history of experiencing food impaction. On several occasions he has experienced food sticking behind his 'chest bone'. He generally points to the mid-sternal level as the site of hold-up of food. The nature of the food eaten appears to be irrelevant. He has had problems with meat, but has also had trouble on occasion with scrambled eggs and even with liquid beverages. Most of the time he has to wait for some time and the 'obstructed' bolus then seems to go down into his stomach. He has,

Table 1.8 Investigations for suspected achalasia

Chest X-ray
   absent stomach bubble (stricture or achalasia)
   look for sequela of repeated aspiration
Barium swallow: as described in the two cases above
Manometry
Endoscopy to rule out secondary achalasia as a cause

Table 1.9 Conditions that can mimic achalasia

Nutcracker esophagus
Amyloidosis
Eosinophilic esophagitis
Sarcoidosis
Neurofibromatosis
Juvenile Sjögren's syndrome

however, had to regurgitate food or drink a few times. Of late, during times of impaction, he has experienced sharp chest pain that has lasted a few minutes and has promptly disappeared upon regurgitation of the food that was causing the impaction. He has no history of heartburn or odynophagia. He has not lost weight. He has had two barium swallow examinations that have shown an esophagus of normal caliber. A few tertiary contractions were noted on the most recent barium swallow, a month ago. There was no evidence of a hiatus hernia and no reflux of barium was demonstrated despite maneuvers to try to induce it. An endoscopy had been performed 2 years earlier and was described as being normal. He had no Schatzki ring or stricture demonstrated. Finally, esophageal manometry was ordered. The patient found the procedure difficult to tolerate and the study was suboptimal. Some low-amplitude contractions were noted, but they were peristaltic for the most part. The lower esophageal sphincter appeared to relax in response to swallowing. The limited manometric evaluation was not consistent with either achalasia or diffuse esophageal spasm. The patient was not anemic. His hemoglobin was 14.3 g/dl, white blood cell count $7.8 \times 10^3/mm^3$) and platelet count 230 000/mm³. Serum electrolytes, blood urea nitrogen, serum creatinine, serum albumin and globulin and liver function tests were all normal. For an unknown reason a white blood cell differential count had been ordered and the patient had 14% eosinophils (absolute eosinophil count of 1092/mm³). At this point he underwent another EGD, and mucosal biopsies were taken at multiple vertical levels of normal-appearing esophagus, at the fundus, body and antrum of the stomach, and the third portion of the duodenum. The mucosal biopsies obtained from the upper, middle and lower thirds of the esophagus revealed some squamous cell hyperplasia, but the most prominent feature was an infiltration with many eosinophils. Several of these eosinophils were either located just below the surface epithelium, or actually infiltrating the surface epithelium, the so-called intraepithelial eosinophils (IEE). Biopsies from the stomach and duodenum were normal. The patient was treated for 10 weeks with proton pump inhibitors and an EGD was repeated with multiple biopsies from the esophagus. His symptoms had not improved. The biopsies were similar to those obtained 10 weeks earlier. A diagnosis of eosinophilic esophagitis was made. The patient was begun on oral prednisone. After a week on treatment he was greatly improved and after 2 weeks did not have further symptoms. After a prolonged course, the dose was gradually tapered. Symptoms returned when he reached a low dose of 5 g/day. He had to be restarted on corticosteroids. Later, he was administered fluticasone, a corticosteroid used in nebulizer form for the treatment of asthma. The patient was encouraged to swallow the medication after removal of the spacer on the nebulizer. With this treatment, he required very low doses of systemic steroids and remained asymptomatic.

Take home message: eosinophilic esophagitis needs to be excluded in patients who have complaints of dysphagia, have a normal esophagus when examined by barium swallow and EGD, and in whom a classic motility disorder is not diagnosed on manometry. A differential white cell count must be performed in all such patients, but if peripheral eosinophilia is absent, the patient must undergo an EGD and mucosal biopsies must be obtained at multiple levels of the esophagus and also from the stomach and duodenum. Eosinophilic infiltrate, including some IEEs, may also be seen in patients with severe reflux esophagitis. Differences in the mucosal biopsy in patients with gastroesophageal reflux disease and eosinophilic esophagitis are outlined in Table 1.10.

Gastroenteritis Symptoms of eosinophilic esophagitis include:

(1) Dysphagia to solids or liquids, leading to regurgitation, causing nutritional problems and weight loss in severe cases.

(2) Chest pain.

(3) Allergic symptoms – respiratory or food allergies in some patients.

Table 1.10 Differences between eosinophilic esophagitis and gastroesophageal reflux disease (GERD)

	Eosinophilic esophagitis	GERD
Histology	> 15 eosinophils/HPF	< 15 eosinophils/HPF
	abundant IEEs	few IEEs
	eosinophil aggregates commonly seen below surface	aggregates of eosinophils rare
	upper and middle third of the esophagus involved	eosinophilia mostly confined to lower third
24-h pH monitoring study	normal usually, unless two conditions present simultaneously	abnormal
Esophageal manometry	mild abnormalities may be seen; not typical of achalasia or DES	usually normal; rarely DES-like tracing
After 2 months of treatment with proton pump inhibitors	histology same	number of eosinophils diminished
Gastric or intestinal disease	the eosinophilic esophagitis may be part of a generalized eosinophilic gastroenteritis	eosinophilic involvement of other GI tissue absent

HPF, high power field; IEEs, intraepithelial eosinophils; DES, diffuse esophageal spasm; GI, gastrointestinal

(4) Other symptoms, depending on whether or not other areas of the gastrointestinal tract are involved.

Symptoms of eosinophilic gastroenteritis are shown in Figure 1.16. Peripheral eosinophilia is present in around 80% of eosinophilic gastroenteritis and perhaps in a lesser number in those with isolated eosinophilic esophagitis.

Case history 8

A 55-year-old woman seeks help for a complaint that began a few years ago for which she has seen several physicians before. Her main symptoms are intermittent episodes of either chest pain or dysphagia, or on occasion both, when she swallows either solids or liquids. She believes that cold liquids in particular seem to trigger these episodes, but often drinking cold beverages causes no problems at all. These episodes may occur at any time, and intervals between them vary, from days to weeks, and during those intervals she experiences neither dysphagia nor chest pain during swallowing. The condition has not been progressive over the duration of the complaints. The chest pain is very severe, lasts for a few minutes and radiates to the back. The severity of the pain diminishes, but the pain continues at a lower degree of severity for a time before completely subsiding. On occasion she regurgitates the bolus swallowed. After the pain subsides, she can continue eating the rest of the meal without further problems.

The above case history is typical for diffuse esophageal spasm.

Table 1.11 Manometric findings in diffuse esophageal spasm

Findings confined to the smooth muscle portion of the esophagus
  simultaneous contractions (i.e. not peristaltic) in > 30% of wet swallows
  repetitive contractions at the time of non-peristaltic contractions
    of prolonged amplitude
    of prolonged duration (> 6 s)
    multi-peaked

Diffuse esophageal spasm

Symptoms of diffuse esophageal spasm may be episodic. There is dysphagia in approximately 50% of patients, with solids or liquids, frequently leading to regurgitation. There is chest pain in > 80% of patients, lasting for variable periods of time, and being very severe. Chest pain and dysphagia may occur together.

The classic appearance of 'corkscrew' esophagus is shown in Figure 1.17.

Manometric findings in diffuse esophageal spasm are shown in Table 1.11.

Diffuse esophageal spasm may be primary or secondary (secondary to gastroesophageal reflux disease. These may become normal if the reflux is treated adequately).

Case history 9

A 64-year-old man presented with an 11-month history of progressive dysphagia to solids and liquids, with a

Table 1.12 Conditions associated with epiphrenic diverticula

Achalasia
Diffuse esophageal spasm
Hypertensive lower esophageal sphincter
Minor abnormalities noted on a motility study

Table 1.13 Manometric findings of nutcracker esophagus

Findings recorded in the distal esophagus
increased amplitude (> 180 mmHg) of peristaltic contractions
Increased duration (> 6 s) of peristaltic contractions

Table 1.14 Differential diagnosis of episodic dysphagia

Mechanical causes – dysphagia for solids only
esophageal web – solid foods only. Patient always points to just below the throat as the site of impaction
schatzki ring – solid foods only. Patient usually points to lower sternal region as the site of impaction
Motor disorders – dysphagia for solids or liquids
?nutcracker esophagus

Table 1.15 Causes of odynophagia

Infectious esophagitis
candida
herpes simplex
cytomegalovirus
Caustic injury to the esophagus
'Pill esophagitis'
aspirin
potassium chloride tablets
tetracycline, doxycycline
clindamycin
vitamin C
alendronate
(over 75 drugs reported)
Esophageal ulcers due to gastroesophageal reflux disease
in squamous epithelium
in Barrett's epithelium
Relapsing polychondritis

feeling of 'the food not getting into my stomach'. Endoscopy showed no stricture. The barium swallow revealed an epiphrenic diverticulum and tertiary contractions throughout (Figure 1.18).

Tertiary contractions are contractions of a short segment, irregular and non-propulsive, seen during fluoroscopy and captured on the radiograph (see Figure 1.18). The primary wave is the initial peristaltic wave seen normally during a swallow. A secondary wave is also normal and is triggered by local esophageal distension during normal deglutition.

What is an epiphrenic diverticulum? This is the name given to an esophageal diverticulum that occurs in the lower 5–10 cm of the esophagus, frequently at the lower-most portion of the esophagus.

What tests should the patient now undergo? Does the presence of the epiphrenic diverticulum explain the patient's symptoms? Seldom if ever does it cause symptoms because of food lodging in it. They are often entirely asymptomatic, being diagnosed incidentally on a barium swallow. However, when a patient has dysphagia with no other anatomic abnormality to account for it except the epiphrenic diverticulum, then one must search for a motility disorder of the smooth muscle of the esophagus (Table 1.12). It is essential to rule out a motor disorder of the esophagus in all symptomatic patients with an epiphrenic diverticulum. The patient described in Case history 9 had an underlying achalasia.

Nutcracker esophagus

Patients who have episodic dysphagia or episodic chest pain and have a normal barium swallow and EGD, and a normal cardiac work-up in the case of those with chest pain alone, are sometimes referred for esophageal manometry. On occasion they have manometric findings that are referred to as nutcracker esophagus (Table 1.13). It certainly appears that these abnormal findings are responsible for the patient's symptoms on occasion, but it is difficult to be certain (Table 1.14).

ODYNOPHAGIA

Pain during the act of swallowing occurs usually when the esophageal mucosa is inflamed. However, it is very seldom seen with gastroesophageal reflux disease, and when it is, it is in the setting of an esophageal ulcer. Inflammation of structures adjacent to the esophagus such as the thyroid, laryngeal or tracheal cartilage, as in relapsing polychondritis, may rarely be the cause of odynophagia (Table 1.15 and Figure 1.19).

Case history 10

A 55-year-old woman with known Crohn's disease has been on oral corticosteroids for some time. The symptoms of her Crohn's disease are better, but over the past fortnight she has noticed pain on swallowing and over the past week has developed dysphagia. She points to the mid-sternal region as the site of obstruction. The dysphagia was initially for solids only, but at the time the patient was seen she had difficulty swallowing liquids as well. A barium swallow was ordered. The swallow showed a cervical esophageal web and transient delay at the web during the swallowing of a barium tablet. In addition, she has submucosal pinpoint collections of barium and linear submucosal tracking of barium (Figure 1.20).

What is the cause of the patient's symptoms? The web is most unlikely to be the cause, despite the brief hold up of the barium tablet, as the condition has clearly been present for a long time and the patient's symptoms are acute. Furthermore, odynophagia would not occur with a web. The likely cause of the odynophagia and dysphagia is candidiasis. The patient underwent endoscopy and there was evidence of extensive esophageal candidiasis (Figure 1.21).

CHAPTER 2

The patient with heartburn

THE NORMAL ANTI-REFLUX BARRIER

Why is it that all of us do not have heartburn throughout the day? This is because we have an effective anti-reflux barrier. This barrier, which prevents regurgitation of gastric acid into the esophagus, is a zone of increased intraluminal pressure at the gastroesophageal junction. The increased pressure at the gastroesophageal junction is the result of two distinct mechanisms (Table 2.1).

The lower esophagus is anchored to the diaphragm's crural portion by the phrenecoesophageal ligament.

A part of the sphincter is within the esophageal hiatus and the other portion is intra-abdominal. When intragastric pressure increases in the proximal stomach, the oblique fibers of the gastric cardia form a flap around the lower esophagus, acting like a flap valve, further increasing the pressure of the lower esophageal sphincter (LES). In addition, contraction of the crural diaphragmatic muscle acts like a pinchcock, further enhancing the sphincteric mechanism and increasing the intraluminal pressure at the gastroesophageal junction area. During the act of swallowing the intraluminal pressure at the gastroesophageal junction falls as the 'sphincter' relaxes, allowing the solid or liquid bolus to enter the stomach.

Normally, from moment to moment, the intraluminal pressure at the gastroesophageal junction fluctuates slightly, on account of variable amplitudes of contraction of the LES (i.e. intrinsic mechanism). Also, with each inspiratory effort during normal breathing, neurons of the inspiratory center in the medulla send efferent messages to the phrenic nerve nucleus, which in turn stimulates the phrenic nerve to contract the crural

Table 2.1 The anti-reflux barrier

The anti-reflux barrier is a zone of increased intraluminal pressure at the gastroesophageal junction generated by two distinct mechanisms
  Intrinsic mechanism
    intrinsic muscles of the lower esophagus
    oblique muscle fibers of the gastric cardia
    together these constitute the lower esophageal sphincter
  Extrinsic mechanism
    the crural diaphragm wraps around the proximal 2 cm or so of the sphincter and forms a hiatus in the diaphragm through which the esophagus enters the abdominal cavity from the thorax

diaphragm. Thus, with each inspiration, the intraluminal pressure at the gastroesophageal junction rises slightly. In addition, in response to physiological and physical stresses, the intraluminal pressure at the gastroesophageal junction rises to protect against reflux of acid from the stomach into the esophagus. Such elevation of the intraluminal pressure may be secondary to:

(1) An elevation of the LES pressure (intrinsic mechanism). An example is the prevention of reflux during contractions of the stomach that normally occur in the fasting state.

(2) Contraction of the crural diaphragm at the esophageal hiatus (extrinsic mechanism). Reflux of gastric contents into the esophagus is prevented by contraction of the crural diaphragm during straight-leg raising, conditions that raise intra-abdominal pressure, coughing and the Valsalva maneuver.

Table 2.2 Theoretical causes of failure of the anti-reflux barrier

Failure of the intrinsic mechanism, i.e. a reduced resting lower esophageal sphincter pressure
Failure of the extrinsic mechanism, i.e. a failure of the crural diaphragm to contract normally
Failure of both the intrinsic and extrinsic mechanisms

Table 2.3 Mechanisms responsible for gastroesophageal reflux disease (GERD)

Mild–moderate reflux, non-erosive esophagitis
   normal resting lower esophageal sphincter (LES) pressure detected by esophageal manometry and normal pressure noted due to contraction of the crural diaphragm by diaphragmatic electromyography. Reflux due to transient relaxation of the LES and of the crural diaphragm transient relaxations last from 10s to 1 min
Severe reflux, erosive esophagitis
   low resting LES pressure and low-amplitude contractions of the esophagus, e.g. severe GERD, scleroderma

GASTROESOPHAGEAL REFLUX DISEASE

Mechanisms that induce reflux

Reflux of gastric contents occurs when the anti-reflux barrier fails (Table 2.2). It appears that patients with gastroesophageal reflux disease fall into two groups, based on the mechanisms responsible for reflux (Table 2.3).

Sliding hiatus hernia is a herniation of the proximal stomach into the chest through the diaphragmatic hiatus. It is present in most patients with moderate to severe gastroesophageal reflux disease. A hiatus hernia may play a role in the genesis of reflux (Table 2.4 and Figure 2.1).

Pathology

Gross appearance

Even a symptomatic patient with gastroesophageal reflux disease may have a normal-appearing esophagus on endoscopy. Like any other mucosa when inflamed, the esophagus too shows changes that vary from erythema to erosions to ulceration. The lesions may be patchy or diffuse. Clearly, the area most prone to injury, the lower esophagus, has the most lesions.

Histology

Histological criteria are listed in Table 2.5. Normal esophageal mucosa is shown in Figure 2.2, and reflux esophagitis in Figure 2.3.

Table 2.4 Role of a sliding hiatus hernia in the genesis of reflux

(1) Gastric acid is trapped in the hernial sac. During swallowing, the lower esophageal sphincter (LES) relaxes for 6–8s and the acid trapped in the hernial sac easily refluxes into the esophagus.
(2) The stomach in the chest becomes compartmentalized between the LES and the contracted crural diaphragm. Acid in the hernial sac refluxes through a weak sphincter or a sphincter rendered open by negative intrapleural pressure.
(3) A large sliding hiatus hernia enlarges the diaphragmatic hiatus and impairs the ability of the crural diaphragm to contract adequately, thus weakening the anti-reflux barrier.
(4) The herniation of a part of the stomach into the chest impairs an adequate functioning of the flap valve mechanism due to the oblique fibers of the gastric cardia.

Table 2.5 Histological criteria in gastroesophageal reflux disease

In order to make a diagnosis of esophagitis on an esophageal biopsy, at least two of the following three criteria need to be met:

(1) Hyperplasia of the basal cell layer > 15% of the mucosal height
(2) Increased papillary length > 66% of the mucosal height
(3) Infiltration by polymorphonuclear cells and/or eosinophils

Clinical features

Clinical features of gastroesophageal reflux disease are shown in Table 2.6. Figure 2.4 shows marked erythema and a benign stricture in a patient with GERD.

Complications

Stricture

Stricture in gastroesophageal reflux disease is described in Table 2.7 (Figure 2.5).

Regurgitation

Consequences of regurgitation are shown in Table 2.8.

Hemorrhage

This is uncommon. Causes are shown in Table 2.9.

Secondary diffuse esophageal spasm

Symptoms of chest pain while swallowing and/or episodic dysphagia and manometric changes identical to those of idiopathic or primary diffuse esophageal spasm (see Chapter 1) may develop as a consequence of gastroesophageal reflux disease. Symptoms frequently disappear after treatment.

Table 2.6 Symptoms of uncomplicated gastro-esophageal reflux disease

Heartburn
    acid reflux usually
    alkaline reflux on occasion, from reflux of biliary secretions
    reflux worse, depending on:
        position (supine, stooping, leaning forward)
        foods (orange and tomato juices, coffee, chocolate)
    reflux relieved somewhat by:
        sitting up and antacids
Regurgitation
    effortless regurgitation of sour fluid into pharynx or mouth
    often awakens patient from sleep
    differentiated from vomiting – no nausea, no retching, no effort
Waterbrash
    hypersalivation
    mouth fills up with watery saliva that is not regurgitated
        from the esophagus – it is a reflex initiated by acid in the
        lower esophagus
Chest pain
    may resemble unstable angina in character and radiation

Table 2.7 Characteristics of stricture

Site: usually of the lower third, rarely the middle third, of the
    esophagus
Mucosa: in squamous or in columnar metaplastic (Barrett's)
    epithelium
Symptom: progressive solid food dysphagia, progressing to liquids;
    frequently begins with difficulty with apples or roast meat

Sandifer's syndrome

Torsion spasms of the head, neck and shoulders can be experienced by little children with severe gastro-esophageal reflux disease. In early childhood these children vomit a great deal. As they spontaneously learn to posture in this fashion, for unclear reasons the vomiting ceases. Such children most often require surgical treatment (fundoplication).

Barrett's esophagus

As a consequence of chronic inflammation due to acid reflux, some patients develop columnar metaplasia of the lower third of the esophagus, occasionally extending to higher levels. For the columnar metaplasia to be termed Barrett's, goblet cells must be seen on biopsy. The metaplastic epithelium may be discontinuous, occurring as islands of pink columnar epithelium interspersed with the more pearly white squamous mucosa, or it may arise as a continuous cylinder or patch. The length of mucosa above the gastro-esophageal junction varies, extending to < 5 cm above the gastroesophageal junction (termed short-segment

Table 2.8 Consequences of regurgitation

Pulmonary
Aspiration pneumonia
Nocturnal wheezing, often simulating asthma

Pharyngeal
Edema, contact ulceration and granuloma formation of
    posterior vocal cords
Hyperplasia of basal layer
Symptoms: dysphonia, cough, globbus, soreness, throat clearing
Recovery upon treating reflux medically or surgically

Table 2.9 Origins of hemorrhage in gastroesophageal reflux disease

Severe erosive esophagitis
An esophageal ulcer in squamous or Barrett's epithelium
An ulcer or linear erosions in a large hiatus hernia

Table 2.10 Sequelae of Barrett's esophagus

Change in severity of heartburn
    On occasion, by no means always, the heartburn present
    initially may considerably diminish or even cease to occur
    once Barrett's epithelium develops. Rarely, the patient
    may never have experienced heartburn
Esophageal ulceration
Stricture
    The patient presents with progressive solid food dysphagia
Adenocarcinoma
    Clearly the most sinister complication. The patient presents
    with progressive solid food dysphagia

Table 2.11 Differential diagnosis of gastroesophageal reflux disease (GERD)

Differential diagnosis of heartburn
    dyspepsia: dyspepsia due to peptic ulcer is seldom confused
        with GERD, although non-ulcer dyspepsia frequently is
    bile reflux gastritis in patients with a previous partial
        gastrectomy (and a Billroth 1 or 2 anastomosis), or after
        vagotomy and pyloroplasty or gastrojejunostomy
    achalasia (see Chapter 1)

Differential diagnosis of chest pain
    angina pectoris or myocardial infarction
    diffuse esophageal spasm
    anxiety or depression

Differential diagnosis of the complications of GERD
    stricture – other causes of dysphagia (see Chapter 1)
    regurgitation – laryngitis, laryngeal neoplasm, asthma,
        pneumonia
    hemorrhage – other causes of upper gastrointestinal
        hemorrhage
    Barrett's – adenocarcinoma presenting with dysphagia

Barrett's), or to > 5 cm above the gastroesophageal junction (termed long-segment Barrett's). Figure 2.6 shows the endoscopic appearance in a patient with Barrett's esophagus. The histology of Barrett's epithelium is shown in Figure 2.7. The sequelae of Barrett's esophagus are shown in Table 2.10.

Diagnosis

A patient with uncomplicated gastroesophageal reflux disease with a typical history of heartburn does not require any investigation whatever prior to commencing treatment. Special diagnostic tests such as endoscopy, 24-h pH monitoring and esophageal manometry and motility are reserved for the following clinical situations:

(1) Symptoms are atypical or have changed, resulting in the need to exclude other upper gastrointestinal processes such as a peptic ulcer or cancer of the esophagus or stomach.

(2) A complication of gastroesophageal reflux disease is suspected.

(3) Prior to surgery (fundoplication) if medical management has failed.

(4) The work-up of atypical chest pain when the tests have excluded the heart as the cause of the pain.

Differential diagnosis

See Table 2.11.

CHAPTER 3

The dyspeptic patient

Dyspepsia is difficult to define. It is a term used to describe a variety of forms of chronic upper abdominal discomfort, pain or burning, which may or may not be accompanied by other symptoms such as bloating, nausea, a feeling of satiation and postprandial fullness, to mention a few.

Several ailments may give rise to dyspepsia, but the most common causes are the three mentioned below:

(1) Peptic ulcer;

(2) Gastroesophageal reflux disease;

(3) Non-ulcer (or functional) dyspepsia.

Less commonly, other conditions are responsible for dyspepsia as well (Table 3.1).

PEPTIC ULCER DISEASE

The integrity of the gastric and duodenal mucosa is a crucial balance between luminal aggressive factors that tend to damage the mucosa and mucosal defensive factors that are protective (Figure 3.1).

Peptic ulcers are those in whose genesis acid and pepsin play a role, even though excessive secretion of acid and pepsin may not necessarily be present. Ulcers develop when aggressive factors overwhelm defensive factors. Aggressive factors responsible for the genesis of peptic ulcers are:

(1) Acid hypersecretion;

(2) *Helicobacter pylori*;

(3) Aspirin or non-steroidal anti-inflammatory drugs (NSAIDs).

Table 3.1 Less common causes of dyspepsia

Foods and drinks
orange juice – by worsening symptoms of reflux
coffee
alcohol – usually greater than 40 proof
spices and peppers
Drugs – almost all drugs have been reported to cause dyspepsia
Aerophagia
Gastric neoplasms
Gastritides
eosinophilic gastritis
Crohn's disease of the stomach
Menétriér's disease
Conditions associated with flatulence
lactose intolerance
fructose/sorbitol intolerance
intestinal malabsorption – varied causes
irritable bowel syndrome
Disordered gastric motility
Parasites that inhabit the duodenum
giardiasis
strongyloidiasis

Acid hypersecretion

Acid is a crucial requirement for the genesis of all peptic ulcers, as opposed to ulcers due to conditions such as cancer or Crohn's disease. However, it is indeed a very small group of patients in whom acid hypersecretion is the only factor responsible for a peptic ulcer. Among these uncommon conditions the Zollinger–Ellison syndrome is by far the most prevalent (Table 3.2).

Helicobacter pylori

Helicobacter pylori is a Gram-negative, spiral shaped, flagellated organism (six to eight flagella) that resides on the surface epithelial cells of the gastric mucosa

Table 3.2 Acid hypersecretion as the primary cause of peptic ulceration

Due to excess gastrin
    Zollinger–Ellison syndrome
    antral G cell hyperplasia or hyperfunction
    antral exclusion: a retained rim of antrum at Billroth-type
       gastrectomy
Due to an excess of histamine
    mastocytosis
    basophilic leukemia

below the mucus coat. It is not invasive. It can be cultured under microaerophilic conditions (Figure 3.2).

How does H. pylori *survive in the acid gastric environment?*

H. pylori is a neutralophile (i.e. prefers a neutral environment) and not an acidophile. In ordinary circumstances *H. pylori* should die at the acidic pH in the gastric lumen. Likewise, when the pH of the stomach is completely neutralized by, say, a proton pump inhibitor, or in cases with atrophic gastritis of the corpus, the pH is too alkaline for the organism's liking and it does not multiply. It therefore needs to find a hospitable niche where the pH is between 6.5 and 7.0 to thrive and to multiply.

A hospitable niche   Such a niche is found at the surface of the surface epithelial cells of the stomach (Figures 3.3 and 3.4). These are the cells that secrete mucus and bicarbonate, and a mucus–bicarbonate gel lines the surface of the mucosa. The pH on the luminal side of this gel can be a foreboding 2.0, whereas at the surface of the cells the pH is around 6.5 and tends to provide a safe haven for *H. pylori*. As will be seen below, *H. pylori* through the urease mechanism contributes toward the generation of this safe milieu.

The flagella   As mentioned earlier, *H. pylori* is a flagellated organism. The flagella help it to move and find a welcoming place to survive in the stomach, adherent to the surface epithelial cells in the mucus–bicarbonate gel (Figure 3.3). Mutants of *Helicobacter felis*, a species similar to *H. pylori*, which colonize several mammalian stomachs and lack a flagellum, are apparently unable to colonize the mouse stomach. This is presumably because they cannot 'swim' to the safe haven adjacent to the cell surface.

Urease   There is considerably greater urease activity in *H. pylori* than in other Gram-negative organisms such as the *Proteus* species. Furthermore, the urease of *H. pylori* is a distinct molecule. Urease is absolutely essential for colonization to occur. It is ultimately

probably responsible for the creation of a cloud of ammonia around the organism that helps maintain an optimum pH to keep the organism viable (Figure 3.5).

The urease is composed of two subunits and contains nickel. There is both a surface urease and a cytoplasmic urease. The latter appears to be the important enzyme since the surface urease is inhibited at low pH. At pH > 6.2 the surface urease is probably active. At pH < 6.2 most of the NH_3 is probably generated by the cytoplasmic urease.

Recently, a new gene, the *ureI* gene, has been identified within the *H. pylori* urease gene cluster, which is not seen in the urease gene clusters of other microorganisms. UreI, the gene product of the *ureI* gene, functions as a pH-sensitive urea channel. When the pH falls in the stomach, this proton gated channel (UreI) opens and urea enters the organism from the outside into the *H. pylori* to reach the cytoplasmic urease. The urease produces ammonia, which then diffuses into the periplasmic space. Maintenance of the pH of the periplasmic space at physiological levels is key to the survival of the *H. pylori* (Figure 3.6).

How does H. pylori *cause mucosal damage?*

The cagA *gene and the* cagA *pathogenicity island*   The protein CagA is the product of the *cagA* gene (<u>c</u>ytotoxin <u>a</u>ssociated gene). CagA is a 128-kDa protein (antigen). The *cagA* gene is not present in all cases of *H. pylori* infection in the West. It is present in almost all *H. pylori* infection in the East (China and Korea). Does it confer pathogenicity toward peptic ulcer, atrophic gastritis and gastric carcinoma? It is impossible to tell in the East, as most *H. pylori* are CagA-positive. Epidemiological data vary in the West. A recent Eurogast study[1] showed no greater association between gastric cancer and CagA positivity than with prevalence of *H. pylori* alone. A possible mechanism by which CagA could be cytotoxic to gastric epithelial cells is shown in Figure 3.7. It is unclear whether such a mechanism is operative *in vivo* within the mammalian stomach.

The *cagA* gene is a marker for a larger region of DNA containing more than 40 genes, termed the *cag* pathogenicity island. Genes in this region of the *H. pylori* genome have homology to the so-called type IV secretion system. In fact, the translocation of the CagA protein seen in tissue culture (Figure 3.7) is under the influence of genes within the *cagA* pathogenicity island. The *cagE* gene is one of six genes located within the *cagA* pathogenicity island that can induce the infected host gastric epithelial cells to secrete interleukin 8. Interleukin 8 is a powerful neutrophil chemoattractant.

Vacuolating cytotoxin   Several strains of *H. pylori* produce vacuolation in the cytoplasm of cells in tissue culture, including gastric epithelial cells. Earlier studies suggested that strains of *H. pylori* isolated from patients with peptic ulcers were more prone to have the vacuolating cytotoxin VacA. This toxin binds to epithelial cells and is then internalized.

Lipopolysaccharide   Lipopolysaccharide is located on the outer leaflet of the outer membrane of the organism. *H. pylori* strains express type 2 blood group antigens, Lewis X (Le^x) and Lewis Y (Le^y). Various functions have been attributed to these blood group substances including immune evasion, colonization and adherence to the surface of the epithelial cell. The role of these blood group substances in initiation or perpetuation of disease is yet to be clarified.

Gastric epithelial cell apoptosis   *H. pylori* infection modulates the delicate balance between cell proliferation and programmed cell death or apoptosis (Figure 3.8). *H. pylori* also induces inducible nitric oxide synthase (iNOS) and cyclo-oxygenase-2 (COX-2). It is still unclear whether induction of iNOS and COX-2 promotes apoptosis or cell proliferation.

Ammonia   NH$_3$ generated by cytoplasmic urease (Figure 3.9) keeps the periplasmic pH of the organism at physiological levels, but some NH$_3$ diffuses out to the surface. This may be toxic to epithelial cells.

Increased gastrin release by G cells   Patients with *H. pylori* infection have higher levels of postprandial gastrin, which returns to normal levels upon eradication of the *H. pylori* infection. The increased circulating gastrin probably results in increased acid secretion, although this has been difficult to show in every case. The reason for the increased gastrin secretion by antral G cells is likely to be the result of diminished inhibition of gastrin release by somatostatin from adjacent D cells. The effect on the D cell is likely to be at the transcriptional level (Figure 3.10).

Does the hypergastrinemia cause an increase in acid and pepsin secretion? This has not been unequivocally substantiated, although it provides a convenient, though perhaps simplistic, explanation for ulcerogenesis.

Diminished bicarbonate secretion by mucosal cells of the duodenal bulb?   Surface epithelial cells in the duodenal bulb secrete bicarbonate (Figure 3.11) The amount of bicarbonate generated by the surface cells of the duodenal bulb goes a long way in neutralizing the acid that reaches the bulb. This is quite unlike the stomach, where the extent of acid generated overwhelms the quantity of bicarbonate secreted by the gastric mucosa. It has long been known that patients with a duodenal ulcer secrete less bicarbonate in the duodenal bulb than do control subjects. These studies were carried out by isolating the duodenal bulb proximally and distally between balloons and measuring the bicarbonate secreted, using titrimetric methods. After the discovery of *H. pylori*, these experiments were repeated before and after eradication of *H. pylori*. Bicarbonate secretion rose to control levels after eradication of *H. pylori*. Thus, *H. pylori* inhibits duodenal bulb bicarbonate secretion.

H. pylori *infection – the spectrum of lesions*

The acute phase – hypochlorhydria   Temporary hypochlorhydria occasionally develops after an acute infection following the ingestion of a large dose of *H. pylori*. Dyspepsia, nausea and some vomiting may accompany such an infection. This presentation has been noted in two separate experimental situations. In the first, subjects in a clinical study received the organisms presumably through contaminated equipment. In the second instance, the clinical syndrome was seen in volunteers who took *H. pylori* by mouth.

The chronic phase   For reasons that we yet do not understand clearly, chronic *H. pylori* infection gives rise to different types of lesions in different people (Figures 3.12 and 3.13). Whether host or environmental factors such as diet and lifestyle are the principal determinants that direct the process that leads to the development of a given type of mucosal lesion remains speculative (Figure 3.12). From Figure 3.12 it is evident that chronic infection with *H. pylori* appears to follow two distinct pathways. One segment of the population develops diffuse antral gastritis (DAG) and the other multifocal atrophic gastritis (MAG). DAG is a superficial chronic active gastritis that involves the antrum and for the most part spares the oxyntic mucosa. The word 'active' implies the presence of polymorphonuclear leukocytes in the lamina propria (Figure 3.14 a, b). Later in its course some atrophy and intestinal metaplasia may develop, but both are usually mild and sparse. Most patients who develop this type of lesion secrete more acid than those who develop MAG. Around 20% of those with DAG develop duodenal ulcers, the rest are asymptomatic. How such a lesion in the antrum may result in the development of duodenal ulcer is shown in Figure 3.13. MAG, in contrast to DAG, is a multifocal chronic atrophic gastritis involving both the corpus and the antrum and varies widely between individuals both in extent and degree of atrophy and intestinal metaplasia. The vast majority of those with this lesion remain asymptomatic. However, benign gastric ulcer, intestinal metaplasia, dysplasia and ultimately intestinal type gastric cancer probably develop from MAG in a few (Figure 3.12). It has recently been shown that the diffuse type of gastric cancer is also associated with *H. pylori,* although the type of lesion from which it develops is uncertain.

Figure 3.15a illustrates the normal histology of the body of the stomach, with its long glands containing parietal and chief cells, in sharp contrast to atrophic gastritis of the body of the stomach (Figure 3.15b). Such a lesion, while more typical for the autoimmune gastritis of pernicious anemia, may also be seen as the ultimate sequela of chronic atrophic gastritis of *H. pylori,* which probably begins as MAG. Intestinal metaplasia frequently develops in this type of lesion.

Intestinal metaplasia

Intestinal metaplasia may develop in the corpus or antrum of the stomach, resulting in gastric carcinoma (see Chapter 5 for a further discussion of this topic).

Lymphoid lesions associated with H. pylori

MALT (Mucosa Associated Lymphoid Tissue) lymphoma (MALToma) is by far the commonest type of gastric lymphoma. Mantle cell lymphoma, the second most common primary gastric lymphoma, is much less common and is not associated with *H. pylori* infection. Gastric MALTomas can be low grade or high grade.

Low-grade MALTomas When *H. pylori* colonizes the gastric mucosa and chronic active gastritis develops, reactive lymphoid follicles are frequently formed in the mucosa. Surrounding the follicles, in the parafollicular area, centrocyte-like (CCL) tumor cells develop and invade adjacent glandular elements ('lymphoepithelioid lesion', Figure 3.16). Eventually, the reactive lymphoid follicles become colonized by tumor cells: CCL cells, or CCL cells + blast-like large cells, or CCL cells transformed into plasma cells (Figure 3.17).

Table 3.3 Action of prostaglandins

Stimulate bicarbonate secretion from surface epithelial cells
Stimulate mucus secretion from surface epithelial cells
Protect the mucosal microcirculation and help mediate a reactive hyperemia in response to mucosal injury
Trophic action on gastric mucosa, possibly due to the direct stimulation of cell proliferation and prolongation of the life cycle of mucosal cells
Inhibit gastric acid secretion, but only at pharmacological doses

High-grade MALTomas Here no follicles are seen. Large clusters of confluent centroblastic cells are seen to comprise the tumor.

Aspirin and non-steroidal anti-inflammatory agents

The mechanism of ulcer formation by non-steroidal anti-inflammatory agents (NSAIDs) is as follows:

(1) They inhibit cyclo-oxygenase and thus the generation of gastric mucosal prostaglandins, which are protective;

(2) They promote neutrophil adherence to the endothelium of the small blood vessels that supply the gastric mucosa and mesentery.

Prostaglandins provide protection to the gastric mucosa against insult from the normally encountered aggressive factors (Table 3.3).

The location of peptic ulcers is shown in Figure 3.18. The symptoms of peptic ulcer are elaborated by the following case histories.

Case history 1

A 35-year-old man presents with a history of abdominal pain that comes on usually between meals, occasionally awakening him from sleep in the early hours of the morning. The patient points accurately to his epigastrium with one finger when asked to localize the site of his pain. When asked, he says it does not radiate anywhere. He describes the pain as a 'gnawing feeling that can be quite distressing'. Over-the-counter antacids relieve the pain within minutes of taking them, but when caught off guard without them, he is able to obtain relief with milk or a small snack. The pain is clearly brought on if, owing to pressure of work, he misses or is late for a meal. On further questioning he says that he has had this kind of pain lasting 6 weeks to 2 months each time for the past 5 years or so. The periods of remission between such episodes initially were around a year, but the episodes have become more frequent of late.

An analysis of the above history reveals the following important features about the patient's pain and the periodicity of the illness.

Pain The special features of this patient's pain are:

(1) Location: epigastric with no radiation. Note that, unlike some other types of upper abdominal pain such as those associated with non-ulcer dyspepsia and biliary colic, the pain of peptic ulcers is frequently accurately localized to a narrow area in the epigastrium, particularly when the patient is asked to point with one finger.

(2) Quality: 'Gnawing'. Patients may describe the pain differently, e.g. 'burning', 'aching', etc.

(3) Aggravating factor: acid acting on the ulcer on an empty stomach. Examples:

    (a) Occurs between meals ('hunger pains'), often starting an hour after meals when the products of protein digestion stimulate acid and pepsin secretion, but the food is no longer present in bulk to buffer the acid.

    (b) Nocturnal pain: nocturnal secretion of acid acts on the ulcer, awakening the patient.

(4) Relieving factor: food, milk or antacids neutralize acid. Once milk is digested, it may stimulate acid secretion via gastrin release and cause further pain later.

Periodicity The patient said these episodes of pain lasted 6 weeks to 2 months each time. This is about the time it takes for an ulcer to heal spontaneously. When large doses of antacids, H_2 receptor antagonists, proton pump inhibitors or sucralfate are used, the pain may be relieved sooner. When the cause of the ulcer is not eradicated (e.g. eradication of *H. pylori* or stopping of aspirin), then the ulcer usually recurs after a variable period of time.

Case history 2

A 75-year-old woman in otherwise good health was on a tablet of aspirin daily ever since she had her coronary artery bypass graft 5 years ago. Over the past month her family doctor had prescribed ibuprofen for her osteoarthritis. On most days she took from two to six tablets. She was admitted to hospital feeling weak and dizzy and having passed three black tarry stools. She gave no previous history of peptic ulcer disease, denied any pain or abdominal discomfort and had not retched or vomited. A perusal of her old medical records revealed that she had no history of liver disease. An esophagogastroduodenoscopy (EGD), performed after she was rendered hemodynamically stable after having received intravenous saline, revealed a 0.4-cm ulcer in the duodenal bulb that was not actively bleeding at the time but had an adherent clot on its base.

'Silent' (painless) ulcers What this patient had was a silent ulcer. While any patient may have a silent duodenal or gastric ulcer, it is especially common in the elderly who are on aspirin or NSAIDs. The initial presentation in such patients is a complication, most often hemorrhage, rarely perforation.

Nausea and vomiting These are less common in patients with peptic ulcer. Vomiting is seen when the pyloric–duodenal area is obstructed, either because of severe inflammatory edema as with a very active ulcer, or because of fibrotic stricturing from chronic ulcer disease. Particularly in the latter situation, the vomitus consists of food eaten at an earlier meal, often many hours earlier (see Complications of peptic ulcer, below).

Weight loss This is not usually seen with duodenal ulcer, but may be seen with benign gastric ulcers. In fact, benign gastric ulcers may give rise to as much weight loss on occasion as malignant ulcers. Radiographic, endoscopic and pathologic appearances of duodenal ulcers are shown in Figures 3.19–3.22.

Case hist ory 3

A 34-year-old man was seen by his family physician with a history of 2 weeks of severe abdominal pain radiating to his back, and vomiting. On closer questioning he mentioned that the abdominal pain had in fact been present for the past 3 months or so, but he had largely ignored it. The pain was not colicky, was located in the epigastrium and in the left upper quadrant. He described it as being a severe 'ache, like a tooth ache in my belly'. Initially it had been intermittent. For relief he had been taking a powder suggested by a friend, which, when dissolved in a glass of water, would effervesce. It was a preparation containing sodium bicarbonate and aspirin! Such preparations are unfortunately all too common in the 21st century and may be readily purchased over the counter. While this medication relieved his pain instantly, the pain would soon return.

The patient had a history of drinking fairly heavily. He had lost around 10 lb (4.5 kg) in weight since his pain had begun. He had lost his appetite and felt full at each meal after just a few morsels. Over the past week the pain had become more intense. It now radiated to the back, and the patient mentioned that he experienced some relief when he sat up and leaned forward. He had begun to vomit several times each day; the vomitus contained mucoid material and a little undigested food. He had been in good health until the onset of the pain. His history is significant for an appendectomy when he was 12 years old. He works as an automobile mechanic. On physical examination there was temporal wasting. While in some pain, he was not writhing in agony. He was able to move around in bed and walk without causing his pain to worsen. The abdomen was not distended and was soft on palpation, except on palpation of the upper abdomen, which caused the patient to tighten his abdominal muscles in voluntary guarding. There was tenderness to palpation of the upper abdomen, mostly in the epigastrium. The tenderness and tendency to guard his upper abdomen made it difficult to interpret an attempt to elucidate Murphy's sign. A succussion splash could not be elicited and no visible peristalsis was evident. Bowel sounds were heard normally. The rectal examination was also normal.

The differential diagnosis of this man's pain and vomiting would include:

(1) Peptic ulcer, perhaps with outlet obstruction. In such cases the obstruction may not be a permanent fibrotic obstruction, but rather one resulting from inflammatory edema of the distal antrum, pyloric channel or the first part of the duodenum, depending on the location of the ulcer. In such cases, a succussion splash may not be elicited and visible peristalsis would not be seen. The weight loss, anorexia and early satiety are causes for concern and without question require a broadening of the differential diagnosis.

(2) Gastric malignancy. Despite the patient's relatively young age, one would include it in the diagnosis on account of the history of weight loss, anorexia and early satiety. Unfortunately, all too often 'bad things' do happen to young people.

(3) An attack of acute pancreatitis. The radiation of the pain to the back is typical and vomiting could also be present. To explain the milder pain being present for the past 3 months, one would be

tempted to consider this an acute exacerbation of chronic alcoholic pancreatitis. If the patient were seen several days after the onset of the severe abdominal pain, the fact that the serum amylase and lipase were normal at the time they were obtained does not rule out acute pancreatitis.

(4) Alcoholic hepatitis. One should not forget alcoholic hepatitis. It certainly can present with upper abdominal pain. This patient's pain is not as typical for peptic ulcer as in the patient described in Case history 1. In particular, the association with meals is not as clear. The vomiting could be on account of an associated alcoholic gastropathy (so-called alcoholic gastritis). The liver function tests, if normal, would exclude the diagnosis, but if they are typical for alcoholic hepatitis it does not mean that the patient's symptoms are all explained by that diagnosis. This patient had serum levels of aspartate amino transferase (AST) and alanine amino transferase (ALT) obtained. The AST was 250 units/l and ALT 64 units/l. His prothrombin time was a little elevated too, with an international normalized ratio (INR) of 1.6. Could the tenderness on palpation of the upper abdomen be from tenderness over an enlarged liver? Therefore, do alcoholic hepatitis and gastropathy explain all of the patient's symptoms? This is a decision that the physician needs to make at the bedside after careful clinical evaluation. In this patient, the characteristics of the pain, the radiation to the back, a question of relief of the pain with antacids earlier, all caution against accepting alcoholic liver disease and gastropathy as the sole diagnoses.

In other situations, one would exclude:

(1) Alcoholic gastritis (gastropathy). The patient was drinking heavily, but the severity of the abdominal pain virtually excludes alcoholic gastritis as the sole diagnosis. Alcoholic gastropathy does not give rise to severe abdominal pain.

(2) Biliary colic could be excluded since the episodes of pain occurred several times a day each day, and antacids, at least in the early stages, relieved the pain. Furthermore, the quality of the pain was not characteristic for biliary colic (see Chapter 8).

(3) Intestinal obstruction. Vomiting and abdominal pain are characteristic features of intestinal obstruction. While clearly the patient could not

Table 3.4 Characteristics of sporadic vs MEN-1 gastrinomas in ZE syndrome

	Sporadic	MEN-1
Main sites	pancreas ~50% (head > body or tail)	duodenum 80%
	duodenum ~50% (bulb 70%, 2nd 20%, 3rd < 10%)	pancreas 20%
	almost never both	
Other sites	peripancreatic nodes, liver	
Numbers	single	multiple and multicentric
Metastatic potential	> 60%	> 60%
Metastatic sites	pancreatic → liver and lymph nodes	> 80% to regional nodes
	duodenal → regional nodes	< 20% to liver
Other metastatic sites	spleen, bone, mediastinum, peritoneum, skin	

have a complete obstruction that would go on for so long without a catastrophe, could he have a partial obstruction, for example from adhesions he might have developed following his appendectomy? However, the pain is not colicky nor is it periumbilical, as it usually is with small intestinal obstruction. The patient gives no symptoms of moving his bowels or not being able to pass flatus during times he has pain. The physical examination reveals no distension or altered bowel sounds at times the patient has pain. Furthermore, tenderness and guarding develop very late in the course of intestinal obstruction, all too often too late. Thus, one may fairly confidently rule out obstruction.

The patient's family physician asked for an upper gastrointestinal barium study (barium meal). It revealed a very large posterior penetrating gastric ulcer arising from the lesser curvature (Figures 3.23). Figure 3.24 reveals the gross (a) and microscopic (b) appearances from a different patient with a gastric ulcer. Figure 3.24(c) shows the endoscopic appearance of an antral ulcer in yet another patient.

Case history 4

A 22-year-old man was on H_2 receptor antagonists for epigastric pain of several months' duration. He returned with increased abdominal pain over the past month and presented with melena. He was offered an endoscopy, but he refused. He agreed to an upper gastrointestinal barium study, which revealed a duodenal ulcer and a post-bulbar deformity. Antral biopsy was negative for *H. pylori*. Despite this, *H. pylori* serology was ordered and was negative. He had not been taking aspirin or NSAIDs.

In the absence of a history of aspirin or NSAID use and with negative *H. pylori* serology and biopsy, it was felt that the patient may have Zollinger–Ellison syndrome. A fasting serum gastrin was obtained after the patient had been off H_2 receptor antagonists. The serum gastrin level was 2005 pg/ml, strongly suggesting a Zollinger ulcer (Figures 3.25 and 3.26).

Zollinger–Ellison syndrome

Zollinger-Ellison (ZE) syndrome was first described in a landmark paper in the *Annals of Surgery* in 1955 by Zollinger and Ellison[2]. It is now known to be caused by autonomous gastrin secreting tumors. There are two types of the syndromes: 80% sporadic and 20% with multiple endocrine neoplasia type 1 (MEN-1), although occasionally somatic mutations in the MEN-1 gene are seen in sporadic cases. Characteristics of sporadic versus MEN-1 gastrinomas are shown in Table 3.4.

Multiple endocrine neoplasia type 1 (MEN-1) or Wermer's syndrome

Features of MEN-1 include:

(1) Parathyroid hyperplasia → hyperparathyroidism (> 95%)

(2) Pituitary adenoma or carcinoma → (10–20%)

    (a) Prolactinomas

    (b) Growth hormone secreting tumors

    (c) Corticotropin secreting tumors

    (d) Non-functioning tumors

(3) Pancreatic or duodenal endocrine tumors (80–95%)

    (a) Non-functional or pancreatic polypeptide (Ppomas) in 80–100%

(b) Gastrinomas (~55%) – 80% duodenal (multiple) and 20% pancreatic

(c) Insulinomas (20%)

(d) Glucagonomas (~3%)

(e) VIPomas (1%)

(4) Other rare sites: adenomas of the adrenal or thyroid

Gastric carcinoids are seen in 15–30% of patients with MEN-1 who have gastrinomas, a prevalence 30 times greater than in those with sporadic gastrinomas. The mechanism for the development of these tumors is thought to be:

Hypergastrinemia → eneterochromaffin like (ECL) cell hyperplasia → gastric carcinoids.

The Genetic defect of ZE syndrome is loss of tumor suppressor gene on chromosome 11q12–13.

Figure 3.27 illustrates the *pathophysiology* of the ZE syndrome.

Clinical presentation in patients with gastrinomas

As shown in Figure 3.27, the three cardinal presentations of the ZE syndrome are peptic ulcer disease, gastroesophageal reflux disease (GERD) and diarrhea (often with steatorrhea). Cobalamin (Vitamin B_{12}) malabsorption also occurs.

Duodenal ulcer disease, often recalcitrant, is the commonest presentation. Peptic ulcers occur in over 90% of patients. Many patients with ZE syndrome also have severe symptoms of GERD with its complications of esophageal erosion, ulceration and Barrett's esophagus. Diarrhea is seen, frequently along with peptic ulcer disease, in one-third of patients, but may exist without peptic ulcer in a small number (5–10%). The diarrhea is frequently a secretory diarrhea with large amounts of watery diarrhea present.

Diagnosis

ZE syndrome should be suspected in patients with the following clinical presentations:

(1) Patients with peptic ulcers in whom at least two tests for *H. pylori* (usually serology plus either antral biopsy or a breath test) are negative and who have not been taking aspirin or NSAIDs.

(2) In patients with peptic ulcer associated with a large volume (secretory) diarrhea.

(3) In all patients with an unexplained secretory diarrhea.

(4) In patients with peptic ulcer disease associated with severe complicated GERD.

When the diagnosis is suspected for one of the reasons mentioned above and a fasting serum gastrin level is > 1000 pg/ml, the diagnosis of ZE syndrome is confirmed. When fasting serum gastrin levels are slightly above normal, or even within normal limits, and the diagnosis is clinically suspicious, a provocative test using pure porcine secretin intravenously (2 units/kg) is used. Serum samples are drawn for gastrin estimation at baseline and 1, 2, 5, 10, 15, 20, 25 and 30 minutes after the bolus dose of secretin is given. An increase by 200 pg/ml in any one sample (usually an early sample) clinches the diagnosis of the ZE syndrome.

Tests to locate the site of the gastrinoma

1. Somatostatin receptor scintigraphy: as for other neuroendocrine tumors, gastrinomas have an abundance of somatostatin receptors and are best identified by somatostatin receptor scintigraphy. Both the primary site and metastatic sites are identifiable.

2. Radiographic methods: CT scanning is not very sensitive. Nevertheless, larger tumors can be localized as can liver metastases. MRI has also been used and shows optimum results in the detection of liver metastases.

3. Ultrasonography: endoscopic ultrasonography is useful in the localization of both pancreatic and duodenal lesions provided they are of a reasonable size. Intraoperative ultrasonography is a very useful tool at laparotomy.

4. Angiography and selective venographic gastrin sampling should be reserved for cases where non-interventional methods have failed to identify tumor.

Prognosis

Large tumor size of the primary tumor, metastases, very high serum gastrin levels and onset at a young age are all bad prognostic features.

Complications of peptic ulcers

Complications of peptic ulcers are hemorrhage, penetration, perforation and obstruction.

Hemorrhage

Depending on the severity of the hemorrhage, the patient may present with 'coffee grounds' emesis or hematemesis and either bright red blood per rectum or the passage of black tarry stools (melena). In endoscopy for peptic ulcer hemorrhage the endoscopist may see:

(1) An actively bleeding ulcer.

(2) No active bleeding:

(a) An ulcer with a black spot at the base. The black spot represents old blood that has adhered to the ulcer base

(b) A 'visible vessel' present at the ulcer bed. A visible vessel is in fact a mini pseudo-aneurysm. The wall of the artery at the base of the ulcer is eaten away and is usually filled by a fibrin plug or clot. A visible vessel, once the clot or blood is washed away, appears as a translucent 'nipple' of tissue. Half to three-quarters of the patients with visible vessels rebleed during the same admission.

(c) Clot on ulcer bed. Ulcer frequently rebleeds.

Penetration

A duodenal ulcer may burrow very slowly through the duodenal wall resulting in free perforation and peritonitis. The ulcer bed will eventually lie on other structures, depending on the site of penetration of the duodenal wall. The commonest site of penetration is posteriorly into the pancreas, followed by the gastrohepatic omentum, the biliary tract leading to a choledochoduodenal fistula, greater omentum, mesocolon, hepatic flexure of colon, and finally the aorta or its branches which leads to spontaneous aorto-enteric fistula.

The pain pattern often changes when a duodenal ulcer penetrates. The periodicity is often lost, the pain being much more continuous. The pain radiates to the back being somewhat relieved by sitting up and leaning forward, much like pancreatic pain. Pain may radiate into the thorax. Nocturnal pain becomes more frequent.

Perforation

A gastric or duodenal ulcer may perforate through the wall of the stomach or duodenum (Figures 3.28 and 3.29). Chemical peritonitis resulting from the spillage of the acidic contents into the peritoneal cavity is the initial event. This is followed by a bacterial peritonitis if the patient is not operated on soon enough. The symptoms and signs of a perforated peptic ulcer are shown in Table 3.5.

Table 3.5 The symptoms and signs of peptic ulcer perforation

Early chemical peritonitis
    Dramatic onset of epigastric pain that soon becomes generalized
    Thready rapid pulse, hypotension, low temperature (~95°F, 35°C), cold sweat and an ashen appearance. These signs of probable catecholamine release subside after a couple of hours and the pulse and blood pressure return toward normal and the patient's ashen appearance improves for a while
    Shallow breathing
    Mild retching or vomiting
    Guarding develops immediately and rigidity within the first hour or two
    Liver dullness becomes obliterated on percussion
    Tenderness on gentle percussion of the abdomen or on shaking the bed
    Paralytic ileus sets in

Late bacterial peritonitis
    Abdomen becomes distended
    Paralytic ileus persists
    Vomiting becomes more persistent
    Labored breathing
    Shock sets in and persists

Obstruction

Case history 5

A 63-year-old patient presents with a history of 2 months of anorexia, and vomiting over the past 3 weeks. He vomits several hours after a meal, and at times in the early morning. The vomitus consists of undigested food eaten at the previous meal. He says his trousers have become too large for him and he has had to have more holes punched into his belt. The patient has had a history of duodenal ulcer disease in the past, treated initially with antacids but more recently with H$_2$ receptor antagonists. On examination the cardinal features are evidence of cachexia and a succussion splash. After he was given two glasses of water to drink, visible peristalsis, from left to right, was seen over the upper abdomen.

A plain X-ray of the abdomen revealed gastric outlet obstruction as shown in Figure 3.30. Endoscopy revealed a large pyloric channel ulcer (Figure 3.31).

Vomiting may occur as part of the symptom complex of a pyloric channel or duodenal ulcer when the ulcer is very active. The vomiting in this circumstance is the result of severe inflammatory edema of the pyloric–duodenal region. However, with chronicity, recurrent ulcers at the same location may give rise to fibrous stricturing of the pyloric–duodenal region, resulting in vomiting. The vomiting in such cases occurs several hours after eating, and consists of undigested food eaten at the previous meal. The vomitus is devoid of bile. Such patients require surgery, if an earlier trial of balloon dilatation of the pylorus fails.

GASTROESOPHAGEAL REFLUX DISEASE AS A CAUSE OF DYSPEPSIA

The symptoms of gastroesophageal reflux disease (GERD) are usually quite distinct (see Chapter 2). However, on occasion patients may present with burning or pain that tends to be more epigastric rather than substernal, and the presentation resembles one of dyspepsia.

FUNCTIONAL AND NON-ULCER DYSPEPSIA

Case history 6

A 30-year-old woman has had upper abdominal discomfort over the past 6 or 7 years. The complaint had not abated for periods of time in between, and occurred mostly every day or at least several days a week over these past few years. She describes the discomfort as a burning pain for the most part, although at other times it is a dull ache. The pain may come on at any time, sometimes while eating and at other times between meals. She may feel this discomfort at night if she does not fall asleep, but is seldom if ever awoken from sleep on account of pain. When asked whether antacids relieve the pain she initially said they did, but when asked in more detail mentioned that it often took about half an hour before she was able to appreciate relief. Furthermore, there were times when relief was not forthcoming. She often has a feeling of a little nausea, but vomiting is not a feature of her history. When asked to localize her pain on her abdomen, she uses the palm of her hand and outlines a rather broad area in the upper abdomen, mostly in the midline, but also a little to the left and right of it.

How do this patient's symptoms differ from those of the patient in Case history 1? The major differences are:

(1) The pain is not as accurately defined to a small area in the epigastrium. She had some trouble localizing it exactly with her index finger and preferred to use her palm to outline the general area.

(2) The pain was not clearly related to anything in particular. Hunger was not an aggravating factor, nor was food a relieving factor.

(3) Relief with antacids was not within a few minutes of taking them. Peptic ulcer patients experience relief with antacids, even if the pain does not completely abate, usually within a few minutes of taking them.

(4) There was no periodicity to the pain. It had occurred more or less every day for the past 6 or 7 years.

This patient has an ulcer-like variant of functional dyspepsia, or non-ulcer dyspepsia.

A large number of patients have chronic upper abdominal midline pain or discomfort, mostly without the characteristics of peptic ulcer disease described earlier and with no known organic cause detected when subjected to an endoscopic gastroduodenoscopy (EGD). The pattern and character of the pain is variable. The discomfort implies a 'negative' feeling not tantamount to pain and often accompanied by nausea, rarely vomiting, early satiety, upper abdominal fullness or bloating. Those patients with pain as the predominant complaint are sometimes referred to as having functional dyspepsia of the ulcer-like variant or 'ulcer-like dyspepsia'. Patients whose symptoms are more those of bloating, fullness, nausea and rarely vomiting are considered to have the 'dysmotility-like variant'. The differential diagnosis of the latter include other causes of gastroparesis, the most important among which is diabetic gastroparesis.

Gastroparesis

Case history 7

A journalist in his early fifties complains of 'feeling sick in my stomach most of the day'. The complaint was of insidious onset and has progressed slowly over the past 5 years. On further inquiry, he states that he feels most bloated after meals. Over the past 6 months or so he has not been able to complete a regular meal, and has been eating smaller portions more frequently. He feels nauseous for much of the time, especially when he awakens from sleep, jocularly describing that symptom as 'morning sickness'. He vomits only very rarely. He has had a diagnosis of type 2 diabetes mellitus for the past 15 years and has diabetic retinopathy and a fairly severe peripheral neuropathy. On physical examination no succussion splash or visible peristalsis are present.

The patient has the classic symptoms of diabetic gastroparesis. A succussion splash is usually not elicited because the emptying of liquids is generally normal. A radionuclide solid food emptying study may be done and would show delayed emptying, but with such a classic history this would not be necessary. Diabetic gastroparesis is the result of diabetic autonomic neuropathy. Other causes of gastroparesis are: amyloidosis; scleroderma; brainstem tumor or cerebrovascular accident; injury to the thoracic spine; Parkinsonism; multiple sclerosis; medications, e.g. opiates or anticholinergic agents; idiopathic. Non-ulcer dyspepsia must be considered in the differential diagnosis but symptoms are seldom as striking and clear cut as in true gastroparesis.

Aerophagia

Case history 8

A 30-year-old man complains of bloating and upper abdominal discomfort. The symptoms have been present for some years now. He also experiences heartburn and belches a great deal. He claims the belching helps relieve his symptoms a little. The physical examination was entirely normal, except that throughout the examination he was belching and the physician developed the impression of the patient being a very anxious person.

A plain X-ray of the abdomen revealed a large gastric bubble and some air in the upper small intestine but no dilatation of the intestinal loops. The diagnosis is aerophagia or the compulsive swallowing of air. This is frequently seen in very anxious people and even in those with mental retardation. Often making patients aware of the fact that they are swallowing air is enough to achieve relief of the very annoying symptom. More often, though, the physician prescribes a simethicone-containing antacid, under the illogical belief that it will take care of the air in the stomach. Worse still, the condition goes unrecognized and the physician takes the short cut of prescribing H_2 receptor antagonists or proton pump inhibitors.

REFERENCES

1. Webb PM, Crabtree JE, Forman D. Gastric cancer, cytotoxin-associated gene A-positive *Helicobacter pylori*, and serum pepsinogens: an international study. The Eurogast Study Group. *Gastroenterology* 1999:116:269–76
2. Zollinger RM, Ellison EH. Primary peptic ulceration of the jejunum associated with islet cell tumors of the pancreas. *Ann Surg* 1955;1423:709

CHAPTER 4

The patient with chronic diarrhea

Diarrhea is frequently defined as passing stools of larger weight (or volume) than experienced normally in the population. The normal for a Western population is 200–300 g (or ml in the case of liquid stool) per day. In developing countries where the diet contains much higher quantities of fiber, the normal daily stool weight may be much more. When does an acute diarrhea become chronic? The usual cut-off is 3 weeks.

APPROACH TO THE PATIENT WITH CHRONIC DIARRHEA

Key factors to determine

When approaching a patient with chronic diarrhea it is best to have a systematic approach to elucidate the cause (Table 4.1). This saves the patient needless inconvenience and a great deal of money and time.

Key question 1: Is it predominantly a colonic diarrhea?

The only way to be certain from the history alone is if blood is present in the stool along with the diarrhea. (NB Patients with non-bloody diarrhea may on occasion activate their hemorrhoids and the stool may be blood-tinged on that score.) The absence of blood in the stool does not rule out a colonic cause. However, the presence of a true bloody diarrhea does rule out the small bowel as the sole cause of the diarrhea. Ulcerative and Crohn's colitis would be the leading contenders with chronic ischemic colitis a possibility in the elderly. Radiation proctitis may also present with the passage of blood with bowel movements. Was the patient on antibiotics and could *Clostridium difficile* be the cause? *C. difficile* usually causes a non-bloody

Table 4.1 Key questions that need to be answered with each patient with chronic diarrhea

(1)	Is it predominantly a colonic diarrhea?
(2)	Is there an association with dietary factors?
(3)	Is there a history of taking medication?
(4)	Is it a parasitic diarrhea?
(5)	Is there a history of travel? Is there a history of residence in the tropics?
(6)	Is there reason to suspect a secretory diarrhea?
(7)	Is there an underlying endocrine disorder?
(8)	Could the patient have irritable bowel syndrome?
(9)	Could the patient have intestinal malabsorption?

diarrhea, but it may often be bloody as well. If a travel history is present, one most consider amebiasis.

Key question 2: Is there an association with dietary factors?

Foods to consider are:

(1) Milk and dairy products: lactose intolerance?

(2) Fructose- and sorbitol-containing foods and beverages: fructose/sorbitol intolerance?

(3) Alcohol: diarrhea may persist for several days after cessation of consumption.

Note: Patients with celiac sprue as a rule are unaware of intolerance to wheat, barley or oats until the diagnosis has been made. Thereafter, they may be able to associate exacerbations with dietary indiscretion.

Key question 3: Is there a history of taking medication?

A large number of drugs can cause diarrhea. Common examples are:

(1) *Antibiotics* Overgrowth with *C. difficile* is the best understood mechanism, but antibiotic-associated diarrheas may result from other as yet not well understood mechanisms.

(2) *Antacids* Magnesium-containing antacids may cause diarrhea.

(3) *Chemotherapeutic agents* Some of these cause diarrhea as a consequence of the side-effect of the drug, but on occasion *C. difficile* overgrowth may be the cause even in the absence of antibiotics.

(4) *Laxatives* These may be taken surreptitiously by patients.

Key question 4: Is it a parasitic diarrhea?

Is there a history of travel? The history of travel includes both travel abroad where a particular parasite is endemic, or travel within a developed country on camping trips or to rural areas. Of course, no history of travel is essential. On occasion both giardiasis and cryptosporidiosis may be acquired with no apparent travel history. The commonest parasite capable of causing diarrhea in the immunocompetent host is *Giardia lamblia*. *Cryptosporidium* and *Cyclospora* may also afflict immunocompetent hosts and persist for over 3 weeks, with the diarrhea thus becoming chronic. Amebiasis may give rise to a bloody or non-bloody diarrhea.

Is the patient immunocompromised? Patients with AIDS for instance may have diarrhea related to various protozoa such as *Cryptosporidium*, *Isospora belli* and *Microsporidium* or a helminth such a *Strongyloides stercoralis*.

Key question 5: Is there a history of travel to or of residence in the tropics?

The question is asked for two reasons. First, as mentioned above (under Question 4), one needs to consider parasites that can cause diarrhea or intestinal malabsorption. One of course does not have to go to the tropics to acquire giardiasis, but both giardiasis and amebiasis are certainly in the differential diagnosis for someone who might have developed a chronic diarrhea after returning from the tropics. Certainly, a history of travel is essential for someone with capillariasis.

Second, a more important reason to enquire about residence in the tropics is if one suspects a diagnosis of tropical sprue. Both in the UK and in the USA this becomes an important question. In the UK most of the cases reported have been in either civil service officers or

Table 4.2 Causes of chronic secretory diarrheas

Surreptitious laxative abuse
Ileal resection and disease
Contaminated bowel syndrome
    blind loop syndrome
    stagnant loop syndrome
Microscopic colitis
    collagenous colitis
    lymphocytic colitis
Tumors
    VIPoma (VIP, vasoactive intestinal polypeptide)
    Zollinger–Ellison syndrome (gastrin)
    malignant carcinoid syndrome (serotonin)
    medullary carcinoma of the thyroid (? prostaglandins)
    glucagonoma (glucagon)
    villous adenoma of the rectum (rare)
Giardiasis (very rare)

military personnel returning after spending a substantial time in the tropics, or in immigrants from South Asia. In the USA, most of the cases are from Puerto Rico, Honduras, Haiti, Guatemala or other central American countries.

Key question 6: Is there reason to suspect a secretory diarrhea?

While many acute bacterial diarrheas such as those due to toxigenic *Escherichia coli* and cholera are secretory, we are here considering only chronic secretory diarrheas.

A secretory diarrhea should be considered only when the daily stool volume is very large, of the order of at least 1–2 l of watery stools. The suspicion is confirmed by:

(1) The finding that if the patient fasts for 48 h it does not substantially reduce the stool volume.

(2) The serum osmolality being approximately equal to: stool $([Na^+] + [K^+]) \times 2$ (NB Do not measure stool osmolality, as bacterial metabolism of carbohydrate waste in stool will result in a false elevation of fecal osmolality).

Causes of chronic secretory diarrheas are shown in Table 4.2. Tumors that secrete humoral agents autonomously must be excluded. Surreptitious laxative abuse requires awareness on the part of the clinician. A secretory diarrhea is uncommon in giardiasis, but may occur. The diarrhea in conditions such as celiac and tropical sprue, contaminated bowel syndrome and ileal resection or disease, has a secretory component. However, in these conditions, on account of the accompanying malabsorption of foodstuffs, there will also be an osmotic component to the diarrhea.

Table 4.3 Endocrine causes of chronic diarrhea

Thyrotoxicosis
Addison's disease
Diabetes mellitus
Hypoparathyroidism (rare)

Microscopic colitis This entity affects patients of all ages, but especially the middle-aged and elderly. Patients present with a chronic, large-volume, non-bloody diarrhea. Frequently, but not always, the characteristics of a secretory diarrhea are present. Barium enema is completely normal and on colonoscopy the mucosa likewise appears normal in most instances, although some mucosal edema and vascular prominence may rarely be noted. However, biopsy of these normal areas shows an abundance of intraepithelial lymphocytes and infiltration of the lamina propria with plasma cells and occasionally also eosinophils. When such an appearance is seen, the condition is termed lymphocytic colitis. If, in addition to this cellular infiltration, a band of collagen (11–100 μm in thickness) is below the epithelial cell layer, then the condition is called collagenous colitis.

Key question 7: Is there an underlying endocrine disorder?

Endocrine causes are listed in Table 4.3.

Thyrotoxicosis Thyrotoxicosis is accompanied by mild to moderate diarrhea and perhaps mild steatorrhea. At other times there may be more hyperdefecation rather than diarrhea. Increased gut motility and perhaps stimulation of secretion by thyroxine-mediated increase in enterocyte or colonocyte cyclic AMP may be responsible for the diarrhea.

Addison's disease Corticosteroids are essential for the normal functioning of enterocytes.

Diabetic diarrhea Constipation is much more frequent in diabetics than is diarrhea. Diabetic autonomic neuropathy can give rise to diarrhea in those with severe diabetes mellitus, who often have peripheral neuropathy, retinopathy or nephropathy as well. While seen more often in type 1 diabetics, it is also prevalent in type 2 diabetics with severe disease. Other evidence of autonomic neuropathy such as postural hypotension and gastroparesis may also be present. Altered motility, poor sphincter function and perhaps poor colonic fluid and electrolyte absorption consequent to diminished α_2 adrenergic receptors may all be responsible. Bacterial overgrowth may be an occasional cause. Anywhere from

Table 4.4 Rome II criteria for the diagnosis of irritable bowel syndrome

Abdominal pain or discomfort must be present for at least 3 months, (*in toto* and not necessarily continuously), for at least the past 1 year, and be associated with at least two of the following three features

(1) Abdominal pain or discomfort is relieved by defecation
(2) Onset of the pain is associated with a change in the frequency of the stool
(3) Onset of the pain is associated with a change in the consistency of the stool

moderate to large volume diarrhea with considerable nocturnal diarrhea and incontinence is present.

Key question 8: Could the patient have irritable bowel syndrome?

Irritable bowel syndrome is a diagnosis of exclusion. However, the diagnosis must be thought of in the appropriate patient and made without needless investigations. The history and a high index of clinical suspicion are the key.

Definition Irritable bowel syndrome was defined at the Rome II (1999) multinational consensus conference as: 'A functional bowel disorder in which abdominal pain is associated with defecation or a change in bowel habit, with features of disordered defecation and distension' (Table 4.4).

Criteria used to diagnose irritable bowel syndrome The criteria enunciated by Manning in 1978 have been refined somewhat at the conference at Rome alluded to above. It is evident from the definition and the criteria that irritable bowel syndrome cannot be diagnosed if abdominal pain or discomfort is not a cardinal feature in the patient's history. Constipation or diarrhea without a primary cause would then have to be diagnosed as idiopathic constipation or idiopathic diarrhea, respectively, and not as irritable bowel syndrome.

Other clinical features that help in the diagnosis of irritable bowel syndrome Some of these (*) were mentioned by Manning in his criteria:

(1) *A perception on the part of the patient of bloating or abdominal distension;
(2) *A feeling of incomplete evacuation at the end of a bowel movement;
(3) *The patient reporting the passage of mucus in the stool. If patients do not spontaneously report the

Table 4.5 Beware of a diagnosis of irritable bowel syndrome when any of the following are present

Onset at an older age. Irritable bowel syndrome seldom begins after the age of 40 years
Weight loss
Occult or overt rectal bleeding
Anemia
Elevated erythrocyte sedimentation rate
Medications that can cause diarrhea
Diabetes, thyroid or adrenal disease
Nocturnal diarrhea is predominant

Table 4.6 Irritable bowel syndrome – disease patterns

Abdominal pain with diarrhea alternating with constipation
Abdominal pain with constipation (constipation predominant)
Abdominal pain with diarrhea (diarrhea predominant)
*Diarrhea alone with no abdominal pain (uncommon, beware of diagnosis)
*Constipation alone with no abdominal pain (uncommon, beware of diagnosis)

*Idiopathic diarrhea or constipation is now classified separately from irritable bowel syndrome

Table 4.7 Epidemiology of irritable bowel syndrome (IBS)

	Finding
Prevalence	survey data from questionnaires based on above criteria for IBS: 3–5%
Incidence	~ 1% per year; information inexact; < 25% of those with IBS (diagnosed in surveys) see a physician for their complaints
Race	no difference between races
Gender	female : male 1 : 1 in those diagnosed in surveys
	female : male 3 : 1 for those who see a physician
Time missed from work on account of IBS	approximates that for the common cold

passage of mucus, they will frequently admit to it when asked. This earned the condition the erroneous term, in days gone by, of 'mucus colitis'. There is no 'itis' of course in irritable bowel syndrome;

(4) Postprandial diarrhea with or without abdominal discomfort or pain (the so-called rapid gastrocolic reflex);

(5) The patient is generally not awoken from sleep to defecate.

Great caution needs to be exercised when diagnosing a patient as having irritable bowel syndrome if some of the symptoms mentioned in Table 4.5 are present. The disease may follow one of several different disease patterns in a given patient (Table 4.6). The epidemiology is shown in Table 4.7.

Pathophysiology Despite a great deal of research in recent times, we know less about the pathogenesis of irritable bowel syndrome then perhaps any other gastrointestinal disorder. For years psychological factors were considered to be the sole basis for irritable bowel syndrome. It is true that, among patients who regularly seek help from a physician for their symptoms, there is a marked increase in depression, anxiety, somatization and phobias. These patients also have higher hypochondriasis and neuroticism scores. However, as mentioned

earlier, those who regularly seek help for these symptoms are the tip of the iceberg. The majority of patients who could be identified as having irritable bowel syndrome based on questionnaires given on surveys never seek help. Most of these people deal with their problem themselves. Stress and day-to-day psychological pressures frequently result in mild gastrointestinal symptoms. It is more than likely that these psychological triggers cause more problems in those predisposed to irritable bowel syndrome. In fact, a vicious cycle may be perpetuated. Likewise, food allergies and intolerance to sugars (lactose, fructose and sorbitol) are also likely to cause more problems in such patients. There are recent studies that suggest in a small number of patients that irritable bowel syndrome begins after an acute attack of gastroenteritis. Did these patients, who were previously asymptomatic, have their symptoms brought on by an acute attack of gastroenteritis?

Overall, two major factors appear to distinguish patients with irritable bowel syndrome from people who do not have the syndrome, although these factors are by no means clear cut. These are: altered pain perception; and altered intestinal motility.

Altered pain perception The ways that pain perception may be altered are listed in Table 4.8. There is a role for serotonin or 5-hydroxytryptamine (5-HT) in altered

Table 4.8   Altered pain perception

Experimental evidence
Somatic sensory threshold same as, or even higher than, the normal population, e.g. response to painful stimuli like galvanic stimulation or appreciation of an extremely cold stimulus
Diminished threshold for the appreciation of visceral nociceptive stimuli, e.g. pain thresholds measured with dilatation of balloons in different areas of the gastrointestinal tract

Hypotheses
Peripheral visceral afferents
   ? more 'silent' nociceptors recruited
   ? either more dorsal column neurons excited, or dorsal column neurons excited at a lower threshold
Central processing of visceral sensory information altered

Table 4.9   Altered motility in irritable bowel syndrome

Constipation-predominant group
Delay in whole gut transit
Delay in emptying of ascending and transverse colon
Propagated colonic contractions decreased
Rectal tone and compliance normal
Altered vagal function

Diarrhea-predominant group
More rapid whole gut transit
More rapid emptying of ascending and transverse colon
Propagated colonic contractions increased
Postprandial contractions increased
Altered sympathetic function

pain perception. 5-HT$_3$ receptors are present on visceral afferents that travel with the vagus nerve to reach the nucleus of the tractus solitarius and also those that reach the neurons of the dorsal root ganglion. 5-HT$_3$ receptor antagonists, presumably by the competitive inhibition of 5-HT at these receptors, provide relief of pain in patients with irritable bowel syndrome. 5-HT is also released by enterochromaffin cells of the gastrointestinal mucosa and these probably act on 5-HT$_4$ receptors on mucosal neurons, which then may block the discharge of visceral afferent neuronal firing in response to painful stimuli.

Altered intestinal motility   Alterations in motility differ in the constipation-predominant group and the diarrhea-predominant group (Table 4.9). 5-HT released by enterochromaffin cells of the gut mucosa act immediately in their vicinity on 5-HT$_4$ receptors on neurons that release calcitonin gene-related peptide (CGRP) where they terminate on motor neurons in the myenteric plexus. These motor neurons may either be: excitatory (cholinergic), resulting in muscle contraction and the induction of peristalsis; or inhibitory (VIP-releasing or nitergic releasing nitric oxide), resulting in smooth muscle relaxation. Recent work using a 5-HT$_4$ partial agonist, tegaserod, suggests that contraction and stimulation of peristalsis is seen in the ascending colon and relaxation in the descending colon[1]. Such a situation would clearly benefit constipation-predominant irritable bowel syndrome.

'Designer' therapy for irritable bowel syndrome in the future   Based on what is currently known about gut innervation and the pathogenesis of irritable bowel syndrome, it may be possible to design specific treatment for abdominal pain, diarrhea and constipation for patients with different subtypes of the syndrome. Thus, 5-HT$_3$ antagonists may be useful for the relief of pain and diarrhea in patients with diarrhea-predominant irritable bowel syndrome, whereas 5-HT$_4$ agonists may be useful in the treatment of constipation-predominant irritable bowel syndrome. Newer anticholinergic agents that have fewer systemic effects may prove beneficial in providing relief from the spasmodic pains that are experienced by some patients with irritable bowel syndrome. Patients with a low threshold for pain experienced by rectal distension could benefit from a κ-opioid agonist such as fedotozine, which increases the threshold for the perception induced by rectal distension. Likewise, clonidine, an α_2-adrenergic agonist that diminishes smooth muscle tone as well as pain perception induced by balloon distension, may well prove useful in the management of some patients with pain. A working hypothesis of the pathogenesis of irritable bowel syndrome is shown in Figure 4.1.

Key question 9: Could the patient have intestinal malabsorption?

See the next section on Intestinal malabsorption.

INTESTINAL MALABSORBTION

Intestinal malabsorption is defined as the malabsorption of one or more components of the diet. How does one suspect intestinal malabsorption? The stereotypical patient with malabsorption shows:

(1)   Evidence of weight loss and/or malnutrition on the physical examination;

(2)   History of diarrhea with passage of large, bulky, greasy and malodorous stools;

Table 4.10 Why the diagnosis might be missed

It often takes a long time to develop weight loss as well as the overt effects of malnutrition such as glossitis, stomatitis, edema and skin and hair changes

Patients may be thin, having reached a low plateau with regard to weight years ago

Diarrhea may not be present, despite quite considerable steatorrhea

Nutritional anemia and hypoalbuminemia may take a while to develop

Isolated malabsorption of one component of the diet which may not result in diarrhea or the malabsorption of fat, carbohydrate or protein
Examples
isolated malabsorption of iron or calcium in celiac sprue, when the duodenum is severely involved, but much of the remaining small intestine is spared
isolated malabsorption of cobalamin (vitamin B_{12}), as in pernicious anemia
primary acquired lactose intolerance

Table 4.11 Suspicion of intestinal malabsorption

In the presence of chronic diarrhea, if one or more of the following are evident:
clinical evidence for weight loss or malnutrition
a grossly underweight patient who complains of fatigue
stools that are large, bulky, malodorous and difficult to flush
evidence of nutritional anemias or of hypoalbuminemia
intolerance to milk or dairy products
intolerance to fructose- or sorbitol-containing products
In the absence of diarrhea, if one or more of the following are present:
isolated weight loss
iron deficiency anemia with no cause clearly apparent
hypocalcemia or its sequelae with no cause clearly apparent
megaloblastic anemia – cobalamin or folate deficiency

(3) Evidence of nutritional anemia and hypoalbuminemia;

(4) Documentation of fat and D-xylose, and, on occasion, cobalamin malabsorption.

Based on this stereotype, many patients with intestinal malabsorption would be missed (Table 4.10).

Question Why do some patients with malabsorption, even those with marked steatorrhea, not have diarrhea?

Answer Under normal conditions, around 8 l of fluid passes through the small intestine in a day. It is able to reabsorb around 6.5 l of this, so that around 1.5 l enters the colon each day. The colon reabsorbs all but 100–200 ml of this fluid. Hence the daily fecal output on a normal Western diet is around 100–200 g/day. This property of the colon is termed colonic salvage (Figure 4.2).

The colon has the remarkable capability of being able to reabsorb several more liters of fluid and electrolytes than called upon to do so under normal conditions. In patients with intestinal malabsorption due to any cause, several liters may pass through the colon in a given day. Provided the colon is not diseased, colonic salvage can work so effectively that this entire additional load of fluid and electrolytes may be reabsorbed, and the patient does not experience diarrhea. A stool fat balance study may, however, show quite a considerable amount of steatorrhea. How then does one suspect that a patient has intestinal malabsorption? See Table 4.11.

Causes of intestinal malabsorption

Causes of intestinal malabsorption may be in the wall of the intestine; in the lumen of the intestine; outside the intestine; or due to small intestinal resection (Tables 4.12–4.15).

Jejunal resection

The effects of jejunal resection are due to the loss of absorptive surface, resulting in the malabsorption of fat, carbohydrate and protein. However, the ileum can take over much of the absorptive function of the jejunum and hence the severity of the malabsorption is minimized.

Ileal resection

Two of the functions of the ileum for which the jejunum cannot substitute are:

(1) Vitamin B_{12} absorption;
(2) The active absorption of conjugated bile salts.

In the discussion of the effects of ileal resection or disease, one could consider the disease involving the ileum, if substantial, to be similar to that of ileal resection.

Vitamin B_{12} malabsorption This is easily compensated for by periodic intramuscular injections of vitamin B_{12} for the rest of the patient's life.

Bile salt malabsorption In small ileal resections (< 100 cm), some bile salts are malabsorbed and enter the colon, inducing a colonic secretory diarrhea. The liver is able to compensate for the bile salt loss by synthesizing more conjugated bile salts. Thus, there are enough bile salts in the upper small intestine to form micelles and enable adequate fat absorption. With small ileal resections

Table 4.12 Causes of intestinal malabsorption in the wall of the intestine

Mucosal disease
'Structural'
  celiac sprue
  tropical sprue
  Whipple's disease
  idiopathic mucosal enteropathy
  systemic mastocytosis
  radiation enteropathy, chronic
  hypogammaglobulinemia
'Biochemical'
  abetalipoproteinemia
  amino acid malabsorption (e.g. Hartnup's disease, cystinuria)
  disaccharidase deficiency (e.g. lactase, sucrase–isomaltase)

Lymphatic abnormalities
Lymphoma
Lymphangiectasia

Wall of the intestine – deeper layers
Crohn's disease
Radiation injury
Ischemia, chronic
Scleroderma
Amyloidosis

Table 4.13 Causes of intestinal malabsorption in the lumen of the intestine

Hydrochloric acid – only extreme hyperchlorhydria as in
  Zollinger–Ellison syndrome
Lack of pancreatic enzymes and bicarbonate, as in chronic
  pancreatitis
Excessive bile acids in the colon, as after ileal resection
Excessive fatty acids in the colon, e.g. disorders associated
  with steatorrhea
Bacterial overgrowth
  blind loop syndrome – e.g. jejunal diverticulosis, Billroth II
    gastrectomy, surgical self-filling blind loop
  stagnant loop syndrome – scelroderma, amyloidosis, diabetes
    mellitus, etc.
  contaminated bowel syndrome
    fistula: gastro-jejunic-colic fistula secondary to peptic ulcer
      or cancer
    stricture: Crohn's disease, post-radiation, post-ischemia
Parasites
  giardiasis
  strongyloidiasis
  capillariasis
  Cryptosporidium
  Isospora belli

there is a watery diarrhea due to secretion induced in the colon, but no fat malabsorption. This condition would benefit by the oral administration of resins such as cholestyramine.

In large ileal resections (> 100 cm), the liver is unable to compensate adequately for the large loss of bile salts.

Table 4.14 Causes of intestinal malabsorption outside the intestine

Chronic pancreatitis (see Table 13)
Tumor-related diarrhea
  carcinoid syndrome
  Zollinger–Ellison syndrome
  VIPoma
  medullary carcinoma of the thyroid
Endocrinopathies
  thyrotoxicosis
Drugs

Table 4.15 Small intestinal resection as a cause of intestinal malabsorption

Jejunal resection
Ileal resection

The greater the extent of the resection, the greater the diarrhea/steatorrhea

Table 4.16 Summary of ileal resection or disease

Small resection* (< 100 cm)
Bile acid diarrhea. No steatorrhea

Large resection* (> 100 cm)
Fatty acid diarrhea. Steatorrhea

*'Resection' or equivalent amount of ileal disease, as with Crohn's disease

There is an inadequate amount of bile salts available to form micelles in the upper small intestine, resulting in fat malabsorption. The fatty acids entering the colon now cause a fatty acid diarrhea.

Ileal resection or disease is summarized in Table 4.16.

Diagnosis of the etiology of intestinal malabsorption

*The 'classical approach' to the diagnosis
of the etiology of malabsorption*

The economics of modern medicine no longer permit one to admit a patient who is ambulatory to a metabolic ward for the work-up of suspected intestinal malabsorption. There was a time when this was the practice and the classical two-step approach to the diagnosis of the etiology of malabsorption was used (Table 4.17).

*The 'modern approach' to the diagnosis
of the etiology of malabsorption*

Performing stool fat collections and urine collections for the D-xylose and Schilling tests in the out-patient

Table 4.17 The classical approach to the diagnosis of the etiology of malabsorption

(1) Perform tests to document malabsorption. Tests in general use were:

    (a) 72-h stool fat balance study – test of upper small intestinal function

    (b) D-xylose absorption – test of upper small intestinal function

    (c) Schilling test – test of ileal function

(2) Perform tests to determine the etiology of the malabsorption. Examples of such tests would be small intestinal biopsy, barium meal, provocative tests of pancreatic function, etc.

Table 4.18 The modern approach to the diagnosis of the etiology of malabsorption

(1) Based on the history, develop a strong suspicion that malabsorption may be present and also what might be causing it

(2) Perform tests directly to determine the etiology of the malabsorption based on an algorithm. Decisions in the algorithm are guided mainly from the patient's history and also to an extent by the physical examination

setting are inconvenient and often inaccurate. Therefore, a more prudent approach is called for (Table 4.18). Algorithms for elucidating the diagnosis are shown in Figures 4.3 and 4.4.

INFLAMMATORY BOWEL DISEASE

The spectrum of inflammatory bowel disease is shown in Figure 4.5. The differences between Crohn's disease and ulcerative colitis are shown in Table 4.19.

Clinical features of colonic involvement in ulcerative or Crohn's colitis

Clinical features of colonic involvement are:

(1) Diarrhea, most often with blood and mucus in the stool;

(2) Tenesmus in ulcerative colitis and in Crohn's colitis when the rectum is involved;

(3) Abdominal pain – generally colonic cramps. Steady pain with toxic megacolon;

(4) Fever – not uncommon during severe exacerbations (101–102 °F, 38–39 °C); higher fevers rare and might suggest perforation following a megacolon;

(5) Weight loss and anorexia – common with moderately severe disease.

Colonic complications of ulcerative or Crohn's colitis are:

(1) Fulminant colitis – the above symptoms unresponsive to medical treatment and requiring surgery;

(2) Toxic megacolon

Extraintestinal manifestations

Skin

Erythema nodosum is more commonly seen in children with Crohn's disease. Pyoderma gangrenosum is more commonly seen in ulcerative colitis. 'Metastatic' Crohn's disease – rare, nodular, necrotic, granulomatous skin lesions due to a vasculitis – is seen on the limbs and in women under the breasts or on the vulva. It is not seen in ulcerative colitis.

Buccal mucosa

Aphthous ulceration is more commonly seen in Crohn's disease but also seen in ulcerative colitis.

Eye

Anterior uveitis (5% with active colitis) is seen.

Joints

Seronegative polyarthritis usually involves larger joints asymmetrically. It responds when activity of disease diminishes or after colectomy. This manifestation is not associated with HLA-B27 preponderance.

Ankylosing spondylitis occurs in around 1% of cases of ulcerative colitis. There is an association with HLA-B27 in 80% of cases. Activity of spondylitis is not related to the activity of colitis and is not relieved after colectomy.

Sacroileitis occurs in 10–15% of cases of ulcerative colitis if evidence is sought for by using radiology. When symptomatic, this results in low back pain. Most patients with sacroilitis are HLA-B27 negative.

Muscle

This is a polymyositis-like syndrome.

Hepatic

Sclerosing cholangitis ocurs in about 3% of patients with ulcerative colitis. Of the patients with ulcerative

Table 4.19 Differences between ulcerative colitis and Crohn's disease

	Ulcerative colitis	Crohn's disease
Small intestine	not involved	often involved
Esophagus or stomach	never involved	rarely involved
Perianal disease abscess fistula fissure	infrequent	frequent – may be the initial presentation
Layers of bowel involved	predominantly a mucosal disease	all coats involved, disease often extending to serosa and to adjacent bowel loop
Granuloma	absent	present – often not seen on superficial biopsies
Strictures	very rare to have colonic stricture	small or large intestinal strictures frequent
Fistulae	absent	frequent enteroenteric enterocutaneous abdominal wall perinium enterovesicle enterouterine
Colonic disease	rectum always involved	rectum frequently spared
Colonic disease	involvement contiguous	skip areas of normal mucosa often seen between diseased areas

colitis who develop sclerozing cholangitis, 70% are HLA DR3 B8-positive. Cholangiocarcinoma is also seen.

Hypercoagulable state

Elevations in levels of factors V and VIII as well as fibrinogen, and lower levels of antithrombin III, have been described. Venous thromboses are more common than arterial. Examples are: deep vein thrombosis of the legs or pelvic veins, leading to pulmonary embolism; cerebral thrombosis in young patients without atherosclerosis, often cerebral venous thrombosis.

Secondary amyloidosis

This is more common with Crohn's disease than with ulcerative colitis. Nephrotic syndrome is the commonest presentation, but cardiac, gastrointestinal, liver and splenic involvement also occur.

Case studies

Case history 1

A 24-year-old man who has been thin all of his life has a history of diarrhea for the past several years. He usually passes from two to five fairly large, pale, mushy, malodorous stools every day. For some time now he has felt fatigued by some of his more strenuous daily activities. He denies recent weight loss, has an excellent appetite and claims he eats 'like a horse'. He is not on any medication. On physical examination there is no pallor. He is a little underweight for his height, but does not appear to be obviously cachectic. There is no ankle edema. The rest of the physical examination is unremarkable. He is mildly anemic with a hemoglobin level of 11.2 g/dl, a hematocrit of 33.1, a mean corpuscular volume of 84 fl. The blood smear shows a mixed population of cells. There are small hypochromic red blood cells, and other red cells appear larger and slightly oval in shape. His serum iron saturation is less than 10% and his serum ferritin is low. The serum folate is low, at 3.2 ng/ml. The serum vitamin B_{12} (cobalamin) level is normal. The serum electrolytes, blood urea nitrogen, creatinine and fasting blood glucose are all normal. Stools have tested negative for ova and parasites.

What is the likely diagnosis? To a seasoned clinician, this young man gives a history very suggestive of intestinal malabsorption. He is thin, he passes large pale and mushy stools and has both iron and folate deficiency. If one had a doubt, one could go through the process of asking oneself the nine questions mentioned above:

(1) Is it predominantly a colonic diarrhea?
Answer: no. There is no history of blood and mucus in the stool.

(2) Is there an association with dietary factors?
Answer: yes. Dairy products make him worse, but he is thin, he has iron and folate deficiency, and his stools are like those described in a malabsorption syndrome. He may have secondary lactase deficiency.

(3) Is there a history of taking medication?
Answer: no.

(4) Is it a parasitic diarrhea?
Answer: no. Stools have been tested negatively for ova and parasites. In any event, the chronicity makes this unlikely.

(5) Is there a history of travel to or residence in the tropics?
Answer: no.

(6) Is there reason to suspect a secretory diarrhea?
Answer: no.

(7) Is there an underlying endocrine disorder?
Answer: no. He is not diabetic and clinically has no evidence of an endocrinopathy.

(8) Could the patient have irritable bowel syndrome?
Answer: no. He is the correct age, but the character of the stool and the lack of abdominal pain make this unlikely. The iron and folate deficiencies rule it out.

(9) Could the patient have intestinal malabsorption?
Answer: very likely. Why? The patient has been thin all his life; he has a voracious appetite, yet is not gaining weight. He feels fatigued and he passes large, bulky, malodorous stools.

What tests should one order? Ideally one would like to demonstrate that the patient has intestinal malabsorption and then determine the etiology (Table 4.17). However, as mentioned earlier, the performance of tests such as a 72-h stool fat balance study, D-xylose excretion test and a Schilling test (for Schilling test, see Chapter 6) is difficult in out-patients. Therefore, one would use the approach outlined in Table 4.18.

Following the algorithm charted in Figure 4.3:

(1) Is there a history of abdominal pain?
Answer: no.

(2) Is there a history of previous abdominal surgery?
Answer: no.

(3) Is there a history of intermittent ileus or pseudo-obstruction?
Answer: no.

(4) Were parasites detected in the stool?
Answer: no.

The most likely diagnosis is a primary mucosal disease.

This now takes us to the algorithm for the elucidation of the diagnosis of a patient who is suspected of having a primary mucosal disease (Figure 4.4). A tissue transglutaminase antibody assay is obtained, and it is positive. This strongly suggests a diagnosis of celiac sprue. A duodenal biopsy is obtained. The findings are a characteristic flat mucosal biopsy. The diagnosis of sprue now appears fairly certain, but the diagnosis of celiac sprue is established only when improvement is seen on a gluten-free diet.

Who is affected by celiac sprue/non-tropical sprue/gluten enteropathy? In Caucasians, it was originally thought to be predominantly a northern European disease. Recent demographic studies have suggest a similar prevalence in more southern European countries as well. In Israel it is much more common in the Ashkenazi population. In Africans, it is uncommon. In Asians, it is uncommon overall, but variable. It is virtually non-existent in southern India, but cases have been reported from northern India. Strangely, immigrants to the UK from parts of northern and western India appear to be very prone.

Celiac sprue was originally believed to be a disease that began in infancy. However, the majority of cases now seen present between the end of the first decade and the beginning of the fifth.

Pathology The mucosal lesion in celiac disease occurs in three stages:

(1) *Stage I* Increase in the number of intraepithelial lymphocytes, many of which are γ/δ T cells. This is followed by an increase in lamina propria lymphocytes.

Table 4.20 Prolamines of cereals

	Amino acids
Wheat: gliadins ($\alpha,\beta,\gamma,\omega$)	glutamine > 35%; proline > 15%
Barley: hordeins	glutamine > 35%; proline > 15%
Rye: secalins	glutamine > 35%; proline > 15%
Oats: avenins	glutamine fairly high; proline low
Corn and rice:	glutamine low; proline very little or none

(2) *Stage II* Crypt hyperplasia.

(3) *Stage III* Villous atrophy.

Altered intestinal function is easily understood based on an examination of the pathology:

(1) Involvement: duodenum > jejunum > ileum.

(2) Ranges from partial villous atrophy to total villous atrophy ('flat intestinal biopsy') leading to loss of fluid-absorptive function and malabsorption of carbohydrates (mono- and disaccharides), dipeptides and fat, leading to osmotic diarrhea.

(3) Crypt hyperplasia with increased mitoses in crypt compartment, leading to enhanced secretion, since the major function of the crypt is secretion, giving rise to the secretory component of diarrhea.

(4) Damage to tight junctions, leading to increased mucosal permeability.

(5) Surface cells have lost their columnar nature and tend to look more cuboidal. Brush border is lost or attenuated, leading to impaired absorption.

(6) Decrease in Paneth cells.

Figure 4.6 shows the histology in celiac sprue.

Pathogenesis The consumption of wheat, barley or rye (and also oats in larger quantities in some patients) is related to the clinical activity of celiac disease. The protein fractions of these cereals are responsible for the 'toxic' mucosal lesion of celiac disease (Figure 4.7). While recent evidence suggests that glutenins may also be 'toxic', prolamines, the ethanol-soluble protein fractions, have been extensively studied and are the major culprits. The prolamines of most of the cereals that are 'toxic' in patients with celiac sprue are rich in the amino acids glutamine and proline. The prolamine of oats, not as 'toxic' as wheat, rye or barley, contains less of these amino acids, and the cereals that are not 'toxic' in celiac sprue patients contain even less (Table 4.20).

Inheritance and HLA association The disease is seen in first-degree relatives in approximately 15% of cases. The disease is seen among monozygotic twins in 70% of cases. It is associated with the HLA locus HLA-DQ2 in 95% of cases, and with HLA-DQ8 in about 5% of cases. Since HLA-DQ2 is present in around a quarter to a third of the people in populations where celiac disease is present, it is clear that non-HLA-linked genes must also play an important genetic role.

Autoimmunity Associated autoimmune diseases are dermatitis herpetiformis, thyroiditis, alopecia, type 1 diabetes mellitus, autoimmune hepatitis and systemic lupus erythematosus. Patients diagnosed in infancy and treated with a gluten-free diet have shown associated autoimmune diseases in approximately 5%. Patients diagnosed in their twenties (including silent cases) have shown associated autoimmune diseases in 35%. It is concluded that continued presence of celiac disease results in the development of autoimmune disease in other organs. A variety of autoantibodies have been detected in the serum of patients with celiac sprue:

(1) Antigliadin antibodies
IgG and IgA antibodies are commonly seen in celiac sprue.
IgA antigliadin antibodies are more specific than IgG antibodies.
It is unclear whether these play any role in the pathogenesis.

(2) Antiendomyceal antibodies
These are IgA and IgG antibodies directed against an epitope on the endomycium (smooth muscle connective tissue).
They are detected by an indirect immunofluorescence test using monkey esophagus or, now more commonly, human umbilical cord.
The specificity is 85%; the sensitivity is 95–98%.

(3) Anti-tissue transglutaminase (anti-tTG) antibodies
It is now known that tissue transglutaminase is the epitope against which the antiendomyceal antibody is directed.
The anti-tTG serum antibody (IgG or IgA) test, being an enzyme-linked immunosorbent assay, is cheaper than the antiendomyceal antibody test, which is a fluorescent antibody test.
The anti-tTG antibody test is at least as specific and sensitive as the antiendomyceal antibody test.

Tissue transglutaminase   There are two important functions of this enzyme. First, it cross-links proteins rich in glutamine (such as gliadin) to themselves or to other proteins. The enzyme forms isopeptidyl bonds between proteins by linking the γ-glutamyl (carboxyl) group of gliadin to the ε-amino group of lysine. In this way gliadin–gliadin links and even gliadin–tTG links are formed. Second, it deamidates gliadin, or gliadin–gliadin complexes or gliadin–tTG complexes. The deamidated molecules (complexes) often expose more potent antigenic epitopes, or bind gliadin peptides to HLA-DQ2. A likely mechanism responsible for mucosal damage and the generation of antibodies is shown in Figure 4.8. Tiny amounts of gliadin probably enter the lamina propria even in normal people. In people with the appropriate genetic make-up (i.e. HLA-DQ2 or HLA-DQ8 plus an appropriate non-HLA-linked gene) the following sequence occurs (see Figure 4.8):

(1)   Gliadin is acted on by tTG:

> Gliadin is deamidated. Neutral glutamine groups are converted to negatively charged glutamic acid residues. This results in a 'tight fit' of the gliadin into the αβ T-cell receptor, thus activating the receptor.
> Complexes are also formed between native or deamidated gliadin and other gliadin molecules or with tTG itself.

(2)   Dendritic cells and macrophages serve as antigen presenting cells, presenting processed antigen (gliadin, tTG and their complexes) along with HLA-DQ2 or HLA-DQ8 to CD4⁺ T cells (Th1 or Th2).

(3)   Tumor necrosis factor-α (TNFα) stimulates fibroblasts to produce metalloproteinases, causing matrix breakdown, mucosal remodeling, crypt hyperplasia, villous atrophy, stimulated lamina propria and increased mucosal permeability, allowing entry of more gliadin into the lamina propria.

(4)   Th2 cells stimulate B cells to form plasma cells secreting antibodies against gliadin and tTG. Interleukin (IL)-4 and interferon (IFN) γ produce enterocyte damage.

The clinical spectrum of celiac disease is shown in Table 4.21.

Diagnosis   See Figures 4.3 and 4.4.

Table 4.21   Clinical spectrum of celiac disease

Malabsorption of fat, carbohydrate and protein and malnutrition with diarrhea
Malabsorption and malnutrition without diarrhea
Isolated malabsorption of
    iron, leading to iron deficiency anemia
    calcium, leading to osteopenia
Skin findings of dermatitis herpetiformis in those with that disorder

Radiology   A barium meal with small intestinal follow through is not specific for celiac sprue. Similar radiographic findings may be observed in tropical sprue, Whipple's disease, malabsorption as a sequela of previous abdominal radiation, amyloidosis and a host of other conditions. It is not recommended, therefore, as part of the routine work-up. Figure 4.9 shows some of the typical findings that may be seen in celiac sprue.

Tropical sprue   This occurs after prolonged residence in the tropics. Natives and visitors may be affected. The etiology is unknown. There appear to be distinct differences between Western hemispheric tropical sprue and that described from Asia. The cardinal difference is that almost all patients who acquire their disease in the Western hemisphere (Puerto Rico, Guatemala, Honduras, Haiti, Salvador, the West Indies) have cobalamin malabsorption and universally respond to a long course of antibiotics (usually tetracycline). Asian tropical sprue does not always respond to tetracycline treatment, at least among the natives, although experience in Great Britain suggests that Europeans with the disease do tend to respond much better. Cobalamin malabsorption, though frequently seen in the Asian disease, is not nearly as frequently present. Gluten is not the cause of tropical sprue. The clinical manifestations are very similar to celiac sprue (Figure 4.10).

Whipple's disease   This is caused by *Tropheryma whippelii,* a Gram-negative actinomycete. Small intestinal biopsy shows, on, light microscopy, mucosal macrophages that stain magenta with periodic acid Schiff (PAS) stain; on electron microscopy, 2.0 × 0.3-μm rod-shaped, bacilliform bodies are seen in and around the macrophages. Symptoms in the gut are diarrhea and abdominal pain, malabsorption of fat and D-xylose, and protein losing enteropathy. Arthralgia and arthritis involve knees, ankles usually, but also hips, and large and small joints of the upper extremity. Presentation is acute, and migratory, and each episode lasts for a few days. It is seldom if ever chronic. Systemic symptoms are low-grade fever and wasting. Cardiac manifestations include endocarditis, cardiac failure and pericarditis. Cardiac symptoms when present usually accompany arthritis. Pleurisy usually accompanies a bout of arthritis. The central nervous system may be affected resulting in gradual memory loss, confusion, focal cranial nerve deficits, nystagmus and ophthalmoplegia. The eyes may show uveitis. In the skin there is often hyperpigmentation and subcutaneous nodules. Lymphadenopathy is occasionally seen. PAS-positive macrophages can be found in lymph nodes as well. Secondary amyloidosis may develop. Treatment is with long-term antibiotics (trimethoprim–sulfamethoxazole). See Figure 4.11.

Case history 2

A 42-year-old man presented with watery diarrhea of 6 months' duration. He would pass around six to eight fairly large bowel movements a day, on occasion having to awaken at night to pass a stool. Symptoms had been present constantly over this period. He did not experience abdominal pain. He had no major travel history, nobody in his family had diarrhea and he was not on any medications and even denied taking over-the-counter medications or herbal remedies. He had lost 12 lb (5.4 kg). He was not anemic. His serum albumin was 3.1 g/dl.

It appears that the cause of chronic diarrhea is organic and not functional, since it has been constant, and nocturnal diarrhea is present on occasion. Furthermore, the loss in weight suggests malabsorption. Following the algorithms in Figures 4.3 and 4.4, a sample of blood was sent for a test for serum tissue transglutaminase antibodies, and this was negative, thus making celiac disease highly unlikely. A barium small-bowel follow-through study was obtained. Several diverticula were noted in the duodenum and jejunum (Figure 4.12).

A diagnosis of multiple jejunal diverticulosis was suggested. A Schilling test was not performed in the patient in the interests of economy, but a Schilling test parts I and II would probably both have been abnormal. The cause of diarrhea in this condition is bacterial overgrowth resulting in deconjugation and dehydroxylation of bile acids (similar to blind loop syndrome). The bacteria also bind the intrinsic factor–cobalamin complex, making it unavailable for absorption in the ileum.

The symptoms disappeared after a course of tetracycline (an oral quinolone antibiotic plus metronidazole is also commonly used). A year later the symptoms recurred, and again responded to antibiotic treatment. On occasion these patients require cyclic antibiotics.

Case history 3

A 31-year-old addicted to cocaine developed intestinal ischemia due to a clot in one of the major branches of the superior mesenteric artery. He required resection of 120 cm of distal ileum. After a surprisingly uncomplicated and a relatively rapid postoperative recovery, he began to have diarrhea. He would have from six to 12 large liquid or mushy stools devoid of blood and mucus each day. Over the past year since the surgery, he has lost 15 lb (6.75 kg) and feels tired for most of the time. He had no history of chronic diarrhea. His hemoglobin is 11.2 g/dl. He was given a course of a bile acid-binding resin (cholestyramine), during which time his diarrhea worsened.

It is clear that this patient did not have diarrhea prior to the onset of his surgery. It is difficult to ignore the large ileal resection he underwent. Following the algorithm shown in Figure 4.3, one quickly establishes the etiology of this painless diarrhea to the patient's ileal resection. Since the resection was large (> 100 cm) it is not surprising that it was made worse with a bile acid-binding resin that was initially tried (Table 4.16). A typical case of short bowel syndrome is shown in Figure 4.13; in this case in a patient with Crohn's disease.

Case history 4

A young woman presented with a history of a 25-lb (11-kg) weight loss over the past 6 months associated with a non-bloody diarrhea. She would pass from three to ten bowel movements each day, that were pale colored, malodorous and would stick to the toilet bowl while flushing. For a year previously, she had noted a gradual onset of postprandial bloating, an increase in belching and gradually increasing constipation. For the past 2 or 3 years she had noticed that her fingers turned pale and numb when exposed to cold, and when warmed became very red and painful. On examination she had thickening of the skin over her hands. The characteristics of the diarrhea together with the weight loss suggested intestinal malabsorption. The Raynaud's phenomenon, the skin changes over her hands and a history suggestive of intestinal pseudo-obstruction (bloating, distension and constipation) prior to the onset of diarrhea suggested systemic sclerosis (scleroderma) as a possible cause of the patient's illness.

X-rays of the hands revealed acro-osteolysis. A small-bowel barium study was ordered (Figure 4.14).

Case history 5

A young man with duodenal ulcer disease, in the era before the role of *Helicobacter pylori* was elucidated, had several symptomatic recurrences of duodenal ulcers despite being on ulcer-prevention therapy with H_2 receptor antagonists (proton pump inhibitors were not available then). His serum gastrin levels had been measured several times and were always normal. A secretin provocation test was also performed and Zollinger–Ellison syndrome was ruled out. After his second episode of a large hemorrhage from a duodenal ulcer, it was decided to take him for elective surgery. He underwent a vagotomy and a Billroth II partial gastrectomy (Figure 4.15). He never developed an ulcer again, but several months after surgery developed a non-bloody diarrhea. For 2–3 years he and his physician wrestled with his alleged 'post-vagotomy diarrhea', the patient requiring opiates to control his frequent bowel movements. He then began losing weight and lost over 25 lb (11 kg). He developed ankle edema and his serum albumin was 2.2 g/dl. He was referred to a gastroenterologist for further investigation. It was apparent that the young man had intestinal malabsorption that had begun after gastric surgery. The gastroenterologist documented malabsorption of fat (steatorrhea) and of cobalamin (vitamin B_{12}). A 72-h fat balance study, with the patient eating a diet containing around 100 g of fat a day, revealed that the patient excreted 18 g of fat/24 h, indicating severe steatorrhea (normal < 5 g/24 h). Next, absorption of cobalamin was examined by performing both part I and part II Schilling tests on different days (the Schilling test is described in detail in Chapter 6). In the part I Schilling test the patient was administered free radiolabeled cobalamin and in part II radiolabeled cobalamin bound to intrinsic factor. Both part I and part II Schilling tests revealed very low excretions of radiolabeled cobalamin in the urine, less than 1% in 24 h (normal > 10% in 24 h). Following the algorithm outlined in Figure 4.3, it was apparent that this patient's malabsorption had begun after his surgery. When patients develop intestinal malabsorption after gastric surgery, two diagnoses need to be considered first:

(1)   Unmasking celiac sprue;
(2)   A blind loop syndrome with bacterial overgrowth if the surgery was a Billroth II (or Polya) anastomosis.

In this patient not only was there fat malabsorption and likely protein malabsorption (a very low serum albumin in the absence of known liver disease or a hypercatabolic state), but also malabsorption of cobalamin that was not corrected by the concomitant administration of intrinsic factor. Malabsorption of cobalamin is very uncommon in celiac sprue. It became apparent to the gastroenterologist that the cause of the malabsorption was bacterial overgrowth, with the blind end of the duodenum acting as a self-filling blind loop in which bacteria multiplied (Figure 4.15). He therefore placed a sterile tube into the upper jejunum, and obtained jejunal contents for aerobic and anaerobic cultures. An abundant growth of both aerobic Gram-negative bacteria and anaerobic bacteria was reported. The mechanisms of intestinal malabsorption of fat and cobalamin due to bacterial overgrowth are described in Chapter 6. For the present, it is sufficient to say that these bacteria, not normally present in the upper jejunum, which is normally almost sterile, result in the deconjugation and dehydroxylation of bile acids. As a consequence, micelle formation does not occur and steatorrhea is the result. Also, these bacteria avidly bind the intrinsic factor–cobalamin complex, thus making it unavailable for attachment to the special receptors present in the ileum. Hence, cobalamin malabsorption results. Despite the severe degree of cobalamin malabsorption, the patient's serum cobalamin (vitamin B_{12}) level was normal. This is because cobalamin stores in the liver take several years to be depleted.

Parasites as a cause of chronic diarrhea   Even in immunocompetent persons, parasitic disease may have a prolonged course. Examples are giardiasis (Figure 4.16), cryptosporidium (Figure 4.17) and amebiasis. Capillariasis may need to be excluded if there is a history of travel in rural South East Asia.

Case history 6

A young man, 26 years old, was known to have Crohn's disease. He was first diagnosed with ileocecal Crohn's disease 5 years previously when he presented with episodes of colicky abdominal pain and a non-bloody diarrhea of 6 month's duration. At the time an upper gastrointestinal barium study was performed and revealed considerable narrowing of the terminal ileum, a 'string sign' (Figure 4.18). This was consistent with the suspected diagnosis of Crohn's disease. A colonoscopy was normal, but it was not possible to enter the narrowed terminal ileum.

He responded to corticosteroids and did well over the ensuing 5 years. He completed his master's degree and worked for a bank. As a rule he was free of pain and passed one to two bowel movements each day. Occasionally he would experience some diarrhea accompanied by a little abdominal pain. He required short courses of oral corticosteroids on two occasions during the 5-year period. He was never hospitalized for any of these mild recurrences.

He now presents with bloating and colicky abdominal pain of 5 or 6 days' duration. A day prior to admission he began vomiting copious amounts of bilious material. Other than a few watery bowel movements passed 3 days ago, he has not had any bowel movement and has now become constipated. He denies passing flatus. Plain X-rays of the abdomen were obtained (Figure 4.19a and b). They showed evidence of lower small intestinal obstruction, almost certainly at the narrowed terminal ileum identified 5 years earlier (Figure 4.18). A barium small-bowel follow-through study was then carried out (Figure 4.19c) and the site of obstruction localized to the distal small intestine.

He was given a trial of nasogastric suction and intravenous corticosteroids for the next several days, but the obstructive symptoms did not improve and he underwent resection of the diseased segment.

Points to note from this case:

(1) This case illustrates a typical presentation of Crohn's disease. Despite the presence of a 'string sign' the patient was given a trial of medical therapy and in fact did well for 5 years. Several patients even with such severe narrowing of the small intestine are able to remain fairly asymptomatic, as did this patient, with occasional exacerbations responding to medical therapy. Therefore, one does not operate on the basis of X-rays in Crohn's disease, but on the basis of the patient's symptoms.

(2) For a similar obstruction due to any cause other than Crohn's disease, one would consider surgery immediately. In the case of Crohn's disease, it is often worth a trial of corticosteroids and nasogastric suction, as was briefly attempted in this patient.

Case history 7

A 35-year-old woman with long-standing Crohn's disease was being maintained relatively free of symptoms on 6-mercaptopurine and was leading a productive life. A barium study carried out 5 years previously showed extensive Crohn's disease involving the duodenum, jejunum and ileum. She now presents with colicky pain occurring after each meal of 2 months' duration. These symptoms were mild 2 months ago, but with time both the severity of the postprandial colic and its duration have increased. The patient was not markedly distended. A plain X-ray of the abdomen revealed a few dilated loops of small bowel. An upper gastrointestinal barium study was repeated and showed stricture of the proximal jejunum (Figure 4.20). The patient required surgery.

Points to note from this case:

(1) As emphasized in the previous case, despite widespread disease, one does not operate in patients with Crohn's disease unless one has to. Obstructive symptoms frequently resolve on intravenous steroids, while drugs such as 6-mercaptopurine and azathioprine, and occasionally 5-aminosalicylates, may prolong intervals between recurrences. In such cases obstructive symptoms are due to inflammation and edema of the bowel during acute attacks with or without some degree of fibrotic obstruction present. When, however, the fibrotic stricture compromises the lumen sufficiently, fixed obstruction results, requiring surgery. Surgery may involve resection of the strictured area or a stricturoplasty. One should not resect all diseased bowel.

(2) A small-bowel barium study frequently identifies the site of the obstruction much better than a CT scan. A CT scan is often a better choice if there are symptoms and signs of inflammation (high fever, elevated white cell count, a new palpable mass) or of a fistula (bladder or cutaneous). In this case it was clear the patient had a subacute intestinal obstruction. Prior to doing a small-bowel barium study, it is essential to rule out a large-bowel obstruction. This sometimes requires a colonoscopy. If, however, the presentation suggests a small-bowel obstruction, particularly a high small-bowel obstruction, barium may be safely administered.

Case history 8

This patient had been diagnosed with Crohn's disease 24 years ago (when he was 12-years-old); 18 years ago he underwent a small ileal resection for a stricture and 16 years ago he had surgery to drain an intra-abdominal abscess. Now aged 36, the patient is on 6-mercaptopurine, prednisone 5 mg daily and a 5-aminosalicylate preparation (Pentasa® 2 g/day). The patient now presents with fever, dysuria and pneumaturia. A CT scan was obtained (Figure 4.21).

Points to note from this case An enterovesicle fistula is a well-known complication of Crohn's disease. Either the small or the large bowel may form a fistula with the bladder. Communications between the bladder and the sigmoid colon may also arise during an attack of diverticulitis. Malignancy of either colon or bladder is a less common cause.

Case history 9

An 18-year-old woman presents with diarrhea with blood and mucus in the stool of 6 weeks' duration. She experiences only mild lower abdominal cramps prior to bowel movements, but this cramp is instantly relieved after she passes a stool. She has marked tenesmus. There is no history of recent travel. During the first week of her illness the patient's family physician had obtained a stool culture that had grown only normal colonic flora, and over the next few weeks had obtained two stool specimens for ova and parasites, and these had been negative. He then performed a rigid sigmoidoscopy in his office and noted inflamed rectal mucosa that was friable and covered with thick yellow exudate. He then ordered a barium enema (Figure 4.22), which showed active pancolitis with ulcerations.

Points to note from this case Ulcerative colitis or Crohn's colitis often presents for the first time with blood and mucus in the stool, and appropriately is initially felt to be an acute infective dysentery caused by an organism such as *Campylobacter jejuni*, *Salmonella* or *Shigella*. More rarely, particularly if there is a travel history, amebiasis may be considered. Acute bacterial dysentery, in immunocompetent subjects, seldom lasts longer than 2 weeks, frequently not much more than a few days. Amebiasis, on the other hand, can become much more chronic. Sigmoidoscopy does not always differentiate an acute dysentery from a first attack of colitis in inflammatory bowel disease. If the patient is very symptomatic, a barium enema is best withheld, as this may precipitate a complication such as toxic megacolon.

Case histories 10 and 11

Compare the barium enema from the previous case in a patient with active ulcerative colitis of recent onset with those in the following two patients. The first, Case history 10, is that of a patient with chronic and advanced ulcerative colitis (Figure 4.23). Here the colon is narrow, lacking in haustra. In addition, the terminal ileum is featureless and dilated, but with no ulcerations seen. This is the so-called 'backwash ileitis' described in chronic ulcerative colitis, and appears very different from the irregular, often narrow and ulcerated terminal ileum in Crohn's disease. It results from a diseased, fixed ileocecal valve.

Case history 11 is that of an unfortunate 11-year-old girl who has had remissions and exacerbations of ulcerative colitis for several years. Her barium enema, taken during a recent remission (Figure 4.24), reveals the typical features of chronic ulcerative colitis, that of a shortened colon without haustra. Often such an appearance on barium enema takes many more years to develop.

Crohn's colitis is shown in typical barium radiographs (Figures 4.25 and 4.26). Features that differentiate this from ulcerative colitis are the skip lesions (i.e. areas of normal intervening mucosa) and rectal sparing. Neither of these features are always seen in Crohn's colitis, but when present they serve to differentiate it from ulcerative colitis. Stricture is yet another feature that distinguishes Crohn's colitis from ulcerative colitis. Earlier descriptions of colonic strictures in ulcerative colitis were probably cases of Crohn's colitis.

Case history 12

A young woman, 25-years-old, with known ulcerative colitis who has had several exacerbations of her disease in the past, is admitted with a marked increase in bloody diarrhea over the past 2 days. At this time she is passing small amounts of blood and mucus with very little fecal matter around 20 to 30 times a day and through the night. She has intense tenesmus. She experiences lower abdominal pain, which is generally relieved by a bowel movement, although intervals between such movements are now becoming fewer and hence the bouts of pain are more frequent. On admission to the hospital she is maintained on intravenous fluids only, and intravenous corticosteroids are begun. After 2 days the frequency of her bowel movements declines rather dramatically, but the patient does not feel well. Her abdominal pain is no longer intermittent, but is present all of the time and is not relieved by the occasional bowel movement she has. She feels bloated. She develops a temperature of

100–100.5 °F (37.8–38.1 °C). On examination, her abdomen, which on admission had been soft and flat, is now clearly distended with marked hyper-resonance elicited on percussion. Her bowel sounds are now diminished, with a few high-pitched tinkles heard. A plain radiograph of the abdomen revealed an acute toxic megacolon (Figure 4.27).

Points to note from this case:

(1) Toxic megacolon may be a complication of chronic ulcerative or Crohn's colitis, or may rarely be the initial manifestation of these diseases. Toxic megacolon is not specific for inflammatory bowel disease, but may be a complication of any severe colitis and has been described with *Campylobacter jejuni*, *Salmonella*, *Shigella* and *Entameba histolytica* infections as well as with pseudomembranous colitis due to *Clostridium difficile*.

(2) When the muscle layer of the colonic wall becomes involved, the colon becomes atonic, distends and becomes aperistaltic. The patient was admitted with a severe exacerbation of her ulcerative colitis. The countless small bloody bowel movements such patients have is typical of a severe exacerbation. It is the tenesmus rather than an increased volume of stool that takes the patient to the toilet repeatedly through the day and night. At that time, her abdomen was flat.

(3) In our patient, the progression of severe colitis to toxic megacolon was quite typical:

    (a) The number of bowel movements declined dramatically due to the atonic colon

    (b) The intermittent crampy pain now became constant

    (c) The abdomen became distended and hyper-resonant on percussion

(4) The marked dilatation of the transverse colon as is usually the case, often quite out of proportion to other areas of the colon, does not imply that the transverse colon is more diseased. It is merely a physical phenomenon: air rising to occupy the highest area of the colon. In a person lying supine in bed, this happens to be the transverse colon. Moving the patient in bed from side to side and prone if possible, for periods of time, shifts the gas to other areas of the colon, and in fact takes the tension away from the wall of the transverse colon.

(5) These patients need to be watched very carefully and, if no relief is seen with medical management in 48 h, or if percussion tenderness develops sooner, they need to be taken to surgery.

(6) Medical therapy consists of rest to the bowel, nasogastric suction, turning the patient in bed periodically, intravenous fluids and corticosteroids and antibiotics. Some gastroenterologists recommend a trial with cyclosporin. In any event, if relief is not forthcoming in 24–48 h, surgery is recommended.

Pathology – inflammatory bowel disease

Endoscopic images and pathologic features of Crohn's disease are shown in Figures 4.28–4.32, and ulcerative colitis in Figures 4.33 and 4.34

Case history 13

An elderly man presents with watery diarrhea and crampy lower abdominal pain of 3 weeks' duration. The stools were watery, numerous and copious. They contained mucus and, while they did not appear bloody on inspection, they always tested positive for occult blood. He had had a prostatic biopsy done a few weeks earlier and had been given oral quinolones for not altogether clear reasons. The abdominal examination revealed no distension. There was, however, generalized tenderness all over the lower abdomen. Bowel sounds were normal. The peripheral white cell count was $22\,000/mm^2$. Stools contained a large number of white cells when examined microscopically. A sigmoidoscopy revealed some mucosal erythema but had the classic appearance of pseudomembranous colitis (Figure 4.35). The diagnosis thus established, no effort was made to advance the endoscope any further. The stools were sent for a *Clostridium difficile* toxin assay, which was positive at a high titer. Even prior to obtaining the results of the toxin assay, the patient was begun on metronidazole. However, his condition worsened in the next few hours and a CT scan was obtained (Figure 4.36).

The causes of a thickened colonic wall are:

(1) Acute infectious colitides;

(2) Ischemia;

(3) Inflammatory colitis;

(4) Lymphoma.

SPURIOUS OR OVERFLOW DIARRHEA

Case history 14

A 70-year-old woman complains of diarrhea. All her life her bowels have been well regulated. Normally she used to pass one well-formed stool a day. On a rare occasion, if she felt a little constipated, she would use an aperient with excellent relief. She did not need one more than once or twice a year. She certainly had no history of diarrhea until recently. She does mention when asked that over the previous 6 months to a year, she has had 'more difficulty with her bowels' and she needed to take her aperient a little more frequently, around once each month. Over the past month she says she has had 'diarrhea' frequently. Upon further enquiry she defines her diarrhea as passing small amounts of brown liquid stool several times each day. At nights she has noticed that she has soiled her underwear on several occasions and consequently of late she has been using a diaper. She was advised loperamide by a friend a few days ago. Taking the loperamide made her very constipated. After stopping it 2 days ago, her 'diarrhea' returned and was worse than earlier. Once again, careful questioning revealed that she did not appear to be passing large amounts of stool. Her abdominal examination revealed a soft abdomen that was not tender. Several mobile non-tender 'masses' were felt in the abdomen that almost certainly felt like stool. The rectal examination was normal. At the time, the rectal vault was empty, and so no stool was available to examine for occult blood. A plain X-ray of the abdomen revealed the right side and transverse colon full of stool.

How would you investigate the patient's diarrhea? Physicians define diarrhea as an increase in stool weight or volume over the patient's normal. Since most causes of diarrhea result in the stool becoming more liquid than normal, diarrhea is often defined as an increase in stool volume and a change in the consistency toward becoming more liquid. However, patients may not define diarrhea in that way, and instead may refer to a change in stool consistency without a change in volume as diarrhea. Perhaps the most important 'investigation' in this patient was the careful taking of a history, which revealed that the patient was passing frequent liquid but small stools. Such a history is typical of a phenomenon that is described differently by different people, but is usually referred to as either spurious diarrhea or overflow diarrhea. We prefer the former term, as it clearly conveys the fact that the patient does not have a

Table 4.22 Causes of spurious or overflow diarrhea

Fecal impaction in the left colon due to constipation from any cause
Stricture in the left colon from any cause

Table 4.23 Differential diagnosis of colonic stricture

In the young
Crohn's colitis
In the middle-aged
Crohn's colitis
cancer of the colon or rectum
In the elderly
cancer of the colon or rectum
ischemic stricture from a previous attack of ischemic colitis, often years previously
At all ages
post-surgical at an anastomotic site

real diarrhea as defined as an increase in stool weight or volume. In this particular case, the palpation of fecal 'masses' on abdominal examination added to the suspicion. Two conditions give rise to spurious (or overflow) diarrhea (Table 4.22). The first is severe constipation especially in older or debilitated patients, and the second is a left colon or even rectal stricture (Table 4.23).

The fact that no rectal impaction was found on rectal examination in this patient should not detract from the diagnosis. The obstruction or fecal impaction may be higher up, in the sigmoid or descending colon. A plain X-ray of the abdomen is often a very useful and cheap test to order. In the case of patients with severe constipation, the entire colon, including the rectum, will be seen to be full of stool. In our patient, the fecal matter was seen up to the upper sigmoid colon, with no stool beyond. This suggested a sigmoid colon stricture or fecal impaction. The next investigation was a limited colonoscopy. It is very important to remember, when a colonic stricture is suspected, not to use an oral large-volume polyethylene glycol based electrolyte cleansing solution to prepare the colon for the colonoscopy. Instead, an old-fashioned preparation consisting of a clear liquid diet and saline enemas, perhaps with small amounts of laxatives cautiously administered over several days, is recommended. In our patient, a sigmoid cancer was found, that was obstructing more than three-fourths of the lumen.

Points to note from this case:

(1) Patients may use words ('diarrhea' in this case) to describe their symptoms. It is essential to ask more

questions to elucidate what they mean. Physicians have often treated patients with overflow diarrhea secondary to a rectal fecal impaction with opioids!

(2) If fecal impaction is detected on rectal examination, a careful digital evacuation should be performed. A small-volume oil enema given before the digital impaction is often helpful.

(3) The stool may test positive for occult blood, or may be frankly bloody. The bleeding, occult or overt, may be due to a cancer, but is often from a stercoral ulcer of the rectum or sigmoid.

REFERENCE

1. Grider JR, Foxx-Orenstein AE, Jin JG. 5-Hydroxytryptamine 4 receptor agonists initiate the peristaltic reflex in human, rat, and guinea pig intestine. *Gastroenterology* 1998;115:370–80

CHAPTER 5

The patient with abdominal pain and weight loss

INTRODUCTION

Abdominal pain and weight loss is a common association of symptoms encountered by a physician. Pain due to functional causes such as in the irritable bowel syndrome (Chapter 4) and functional dyspepsia (Chapter 3) is almost never associated with weight loss. In the evaluation of patients with abdominal pain and weight loss, there is a tendency on the part of physicians to order an abdominal CT scan almost directly after they have shaken hands with such a patient. Frequently, it is a thoughtless kneejerk response. While it is often appropriate to order a CT scan as the first major investigation, the patient is likely to benefit the most if the physician has a rational basis for ordering the test. Intra-abdominal malignancy, while frequently the cause of abdominal pain and weight loss, is by no means the only cause. The physician must, in the appropriate context, think also of the four 'Is': inflammation, infection, ischemia and intestinal malabsorption.

AN INITIAL APPROACH TO THE EVALUATION

Is diarrhea present?

This should be the first question, since, if it is, then the causes of intestinal malabsorption that can occur with abdominal pain must be considered (see Chapter 4). Crohn's disease must be considered high in the diagnosis of patients in whom diarrhea accompanies abdominal pain and weight loss, even though overt intestinal malabsorption may not be evident. As mentioned earlier (Chapter 4), the absence of diarrhea does not rule out intestinal malabsorption.

When diarrhea is absent

Clearly the most important *inflammatory* disease in the Western hemisphere that causes abdominal pain and weight loss is Crohn's disease, particularly when the small intestine is involved, even when diarrhea is not present. The following history of one of the author's patients is illustrative.

Case history 1

A 28-year-old man presented with episodic abdominal pain and gradual weight loss amounting to 40 lb (18 kg) over the past 3 years. He was diagnosed with Crohn's disease 4 years previously and was on large doses of mesalamine, and received azathioprim 100 mg daily. He had no evidence of colonic involvement, but had documented ileal disease. He had never had diarrhea with any of his exacerbations of Crohn's disease that required corticosteroids frequently. During the current presentation he had epigastric pain and localized tenderness. There was a vague non-tender fullness present in the umbilical region that probably represented an old inflammatory mass. The CT scan revealed a large intra-abdominal fluid collection. He responded within 2 days to intravenous methylprednisolone. Interestingly, during none of these episodes did he have symptoms to suggest intestinal obstruction, such as vomiting, constipation or not passing flatus.

Even in the absence of diarrhea Crohn's disease should be considered when the abdominal pain occurs especially as distinct attacks or episodes. The pain may be steady and severe, and frequently accompanied by localized tenderness and fever, as in fistulous disease, or

Table 5.1 Abdominal tuberculosis – populations at risk

Residents in developing countries
AIDS patients
Women > men (peritonitis from tuberculous salpingitis)

colicky and frequently presenting as a subacute intestinal obstruction, as in the stricturing variety of disease.

Infection Tuberculosis is the classic example of a chronic infectious disease that can present with abdominal pain and weight loss. Fever frequently accompanies the illness, especially with tuberculous peritonitis. Diarrhea and malabsorption frequently accompany ulcerocaseating tuberculous enteritis (Figure 5.1).

Populations at risk are shown in Table 5.1. Tuberculous enteritis is generally caused by swallowing the tuberculosis bacillus in patients with lung disease. The hypertrophic ileocecal variety is seen in those highly resistant to the organism. The disease starts in the lymph follicles of the cecum, ascending colon and ileum and spreads to regional lymph nodes. Diarrhea, weight loss and abdominal pain follow, and later intestinal obstruction gradually develops. A mass is usually palpable in the right lower quadrant. The differential is Crohn's disease, but unlike Crohn's disease, fistula formation seldom occurs. In the ulcerocaseating type, longitudinal ulcers develop in the wall of the ileum. Tubercles can be seen on the serosal surface as well. Diarrhea and weight loss are the main symptoms.

Tuberculous peritonitis is often, but not always, associated with tuberculous salpingitis. Early on it presents with either painful or painless ascites, weight loss and often fever and night sweats. This can then go on to the dry peritonitis ('plastic' variety), where the abdomen has a doughy feel, and intra-abdominal masses may be palpated. Abdominal pain and weight loss are frequently present.

Case history 2

A 25-year-old man with a chronic cough and some mucoid expectoration developed abdominal pain and weight loss. He experienced abdominal distension, postprandial bloating and constipation. He had some dullness on percussion over the right supraclavicular and infraclavicular regions, with diminished vocal resonance, vesicular breath sounds and medium crackles. There was no egophony. The sputum was positive for acid-fast bacilli. The chest X-ray showed an apical infiltrate suggestive of apical tuberculosis (Figure 5.2a). Plain X-ray of the abdomen revealed air–fluid levels in the small bowel. A barium small-bowel study was performed which revealed abnormal loops of dilated small bowel, loss of mucosal pattern and angulation and focal dilatation, implying fibrosis and stricture formation (Figure 5.2b). The diagnosis of lung tuberculosis was confirmed when the sputum culture grew *Mycobacterium tuberculosis*. The patient underwent an intestinal resection and the diagnosis of intestinal tuberculosis was confirmed.

Ischemia

Case history 3

A 55-year-old man with ischemic cardiomyopathy and a left ventricular ejection fraction under 20%, peripheral vascular disease and hypercholesterolemia experiences severe periumbilical pain within half an hour of eating. The pain is severe, and lasts for an hour, before it slowly subsides over the following hour or two. It occurs with every meal, as a result of which the patient has been eating very little, largely because he is afraid to eat. He has lost over 40 lb (18 kg) over the past year.

The history is typical for chronic intestinal ischemia. Chronic intestinal ischemia presents classically as severe abdominal pain that has its onset shortly after eating. While these patients often show intestinal malabsorption if specifically tested for, the major reason they develop profound weight loss is because they have so much postprandial pain that they are afraid to eat. It was in the past considered to be a distinct but rare entity, often overdiagnosed. However, because of the demographic shift in the Western population toward the elderly, patients with atherosclerotic cardiovascular and peripheral vascular disease are living longer and are thus more prone to developing chronic intestinal ischemia in the superior mesenteric artery territory. The ostium of the superior mesenteric artery or one of its branches is occluded by an atheromatous plaque. Patients with severe left ventricular failure, with very poor forward flow, are more prone to developing symptoms.

An aortogram showed delayed filling with poor opacification, supporting the diagnosis of chronic intestinal ischemia (Figure 5.3a and b). The patient underwent surgery and received an end-to-side saphenous graft from the iliac artery to the superior mesenteric artery (Figure 5.3c). The patient's abdominal pain considerably improved and he was able to eat better.

Intestinal malabsorption Causes of intestinal malabsorption that are frequently accompanied by abdominal pain, and an approach to arriving at the diagnosis, are discussed in Chapter 4. It is important to emphasize how often these are overlooked.

Malignancy Malignancies most likely to present with abdominal pain and weight loss are:

(1) Pancreatic cancer;

(2) Gastric cancer;

(3) Lymphoma;

(4) Hepatocellular carcinoma;

(5) Any advanced intra-abdominal cancer;

(6) Any cancer with metastatic liver disease.

Malignancies in which weight loss is usually a *late* presentation are:

(1) Colorectal cancer;

(2) Small intestinal carcinomas;

(3) Cholangiocarcinoma;

(4) Ovarian cancer;

(5) Endometrial cancer;

(6) Stromal tumors and sarcomas;

(7) Carcinoid tumors;

(8) Other hormone-secreting tumors (gastrinoma, VIPoma, etc.).

Case history 4

A 45-year-old man with a long history of alcoholism presented with a month's history of abdominal pain, anorexia, bloating and a weight loss of 15 lb (6.75 kg). The pain was epigastric and was relieved somewhat while sitting up and leaning forward. Over the past week he had felt the pain radiating to the back. On examination he appeared thin. There was no lymph node enlargement evident. The abdomen was soft and non-tender, with no masses palpable and without organomegaly. His serum transaminases, alkaline phosphatase, bilirubin, amylase and lipase were normal.

Despite the fact that there was no jaundice, and the pancreatic enzymes were normal, as was the CA19-9, the highest clinical suspicion must be for pancreatic cancer. Painless jaundice is the presentation only in the case of those tumors in the head of the pancreas which are close enough to the common bile duct to obstruct it relatively early in the course of the tumor, before the lesion becomes painful. Tumors in other areas of the pancreas, including at times areas of the head away from the common bile duct, often present with abdominal pain long before jaundice develops. CA19-9 levels, though useful, are by no means uniformly elevated in pancreatic cancer. The quality of the pain (constant), with little variation with meals and somewhat relieved by sitting up and leaning forward, are typical of pancreatic pain, although by no means is the pain so typical every time. The differential diagnosis must include other intra-abdominal malignancies such as non-Hodgkin's lymphoma, stromal tumors, gynecological malignancies and gastric cancer. Gastric cancer is frequently painless to start with, but when pain develops, it has some of the characteristics of ulcer pain. The patient was referred for an abdominal CT scan. It revealed a mass in the tail of the pancreas with a metastatic lesion in the liver (Figure 5.4a).

A fine-needle biopsy of the pancreatic lesion revealed it to be a pancreatic anaplastic carcinoma (Figure 5.5).

Case history 5

A 48-year-old man who consumed four to six packs of beer every day complained of a continuous, dull mid-abdominal ache of recent onset. He was seen by his family physician who initially prescribed a proton pump inhibitor, which gave the patient no relief whatever. When seen approximately 2 months after the onset of his symptoms, he had lost 17 lb (8 kg). Other than for evidence of recent weight loss, the physical examination was normal. The patient was not jaundiced. The patient was mildly anemic (hemoglobin 13.0 g/dl, hematocrit 38.7, normochromic, normocytic). His serum electrolytes, liver function tests, amylase and lipase were all within normal limits. The symptoms, as discussed in Case history 4, here too suggested pancreatic cancer. The patient was referred for a CT scan that showed a 1.4 × 2.6-cm mass in the body of the pancreas (Figures 5.4b and c). The patient underwent an endoscopic ultrasound examination, rather than an endoscopic retrograde cholangiopancreatogram (Figure 5.4d).

PANCREATIC CARCINOMA

While most malignancies arising in abdominal viscera are painless in the early stages, eventually most become painful as the disease advances. Patients with intra-abdominal malignancies can on occasion present with weight loss and without pain. The most important malignancy to consider is pancreatic cancer (Table 5.2).

Table 5.2   Clinical presentation of pancreatic cancer

Painless jaundice – tumors of the head that compress the
  common bile duct early
Abdominal pain and weight loss
Jaundice, abdominal pain and weight loss
Pruritus from compression of the common bile duct, prior
  to jaundice developing
Acute pancreatitis – most consider cancer in the diagnosis
  in the middle-aged and elderly, when no cause is apparent
  for a first bout of acute pancreatitis
Vomiting with or without abdominal pain and weight loss –
  vomiting is secondary to either gastric outlet or duodenal
  or proximal jejunal obstruction
Thrombophlebitis
  deep vein thrombosis
  migrating superficial thrombophlebitis – Trousseau's sign
Depression may be an early symptom, usually when it is
  accompanied by one of the above

Pathology

See Figure 5.6.

Diagnosis

See Figure 5.7 for an approach to the diagnosis of pancreatic cancer.

Case history 6

A 77-year-old man presented with a 6-month history of fullness, bloating and early satiety. He had lost 12 lb (5.4 kg) in weight and his hematocrit was 33 (previously 49) and he had a mean corpuscular volume of 70 fl. Such a patient should receive endoscopy as the initial evaluation. However, his family physician ordered a barium meal, which revealed an antral lesion with a large ulcer (Figure 5.8a). Endoscopic biopsy subsequently revealed the 8-cm ulcerated mass on the lesser curvature to be a gastric adenocarcinoma. A CT scan was then ordered (Figures 5.8b and c).

The salient features in the history were fullness, bloating, weight loss, anorexia and early satiety, and iron deficiency anemia.

GASTRIC CARCINOMA

The tumors may appear as polypoid lesions or as ulcers. As a rule, malignant ulcers have rolled-out overhanging edges, unlike benign ulcers that appear more punched out. However, gross appearances can be deceptive. Adenocarcinoma is by far the commonest malignant gastric tumor. For the etiology and pathogenesis of gastric adenocarcinoma see Table 5.3

Table 5.3   Gastric adenocarcinoma – etiology

Chronic atrophic gastritis and intestinal metaplasia due to:
  Helicobacter pylori – antrum > body > fundus
  pernicious anemia – fundus and body (not antrum)
Adenomatous polyps
  isolated often in atrophic mucosa
  part of familial adenomatous polyposis coli
Hereditary non polyposis colorectal cancer syndrome (Lynch 2)
Previous (> 20 years) gastric surgery
  Billroth I or II partial gastrectomy
  Gastroenterostomy
Ménétrier's disease
Unknown

Table 5.4   Types of gastric carcinoma

Macroscopic
  polypoid – fungating
  ulcerating
  linitis plastica or leather bottle stomach
Microscopic (Lauren's classification)
  intestinal – glandular architecture
  diffuse – groups of malignant cells

and Figure 5.9. Intestinal metaplasia is shown in Figure 5.10.

Around two-thirds of gastric adenocarcinomas arise in the antrum of the stomach, around a quarter in the body and the rest in the fundus and cardia (Figures 5.9 and 5.10).

Gastric adenocarcinoma is on the decline in the West, the prevalence decreasing in the USA from 33/100 000 population prior to World War II to under 4/100 000 in the last decade of the 20th century. Even in Japan, where gastric adenocarcinoma is relatively very common, the incidence is on the decline. Of all the patients with pernicious anemia, only around 5–10% develop carcinoma. The increased prevalence of *H. pylori* gastritis in childhood in developing countries very probably contributes to the high prevalence of gastric cancer in these areas. However, the situation is more complex than that. A country such as India, where the *H. pylori* prevalence in childhood is high, as in other developing countries, does not have such a high prevalence of gastric cancer. Types of gastric carcinoma are listed in Table 5.4 (see Chapter 3 for more on *H. pylori* and gastric cancer).

In linitis plastica or the leather-bottle stomach, the mucosa may grossly appear normal. The gastric wall is very thickened and feels like leather, owing to extensive fibrous tissue proliferation in the submucosa. It may be generalized involving the entire stomach, or more

Table 5.5 Gastric cancer – clinical presentation

Symptoms
Iron deficiency anemia – symptoms associated with
   chronic anemia
Anorexia
Early satiety
Dyspepsia – peptic ulcer-like
Weight loss
Epigastric pain
Dysphagia
Gastric outlet obstruction – non-bilious vomiting of
   undigested food
Overt upper gastrointestinal hemorrhage – hematemesis,
   melena, etc.
Abdominal mass – late

Signs
Pallor
Cachexia
Epigasric mass – late
Jaundice – late
Enlarged liver – metastasis
Virchow's node (left supraclavicular) palpable – Troisier's sign
Left axillary node – Irish's node
Periumbilical skin lymph node palpable – Sister Mary
   Joseph node
Superficial thrombophlebitis of the leg veins – Trousseau's
   sign
Deep vein thrombosis of the leg veins – hypercoagulable
   state
Skin
   acanthosis nigricans
   seborrheic keratosis – (Leser–Trélat sign)
   dermatomyositis
Kidney – mild albuminuria or rarely nephrotic syndrome due
   to membranous glomerulonephritis
Microangiopathic hemolytic anemia

Table 5.6 Staging of gastric cancer

Tumor
T0: Carcinoma *in situ* or intraepithelial cancer
T1: Confined to mucosa or submucosa
T2: Involving the muscularis propria
T3: Penetrating the serosa
T4: Abutting an adjacent organ

Node
N0: No nodes involved
N1: Perigastric within a radius of 3 cm from primary tumor
N2: Perigastric and regional beyond 3 cm from primary
   tumor that will be removed at surgery
N3: Intra-abdominal nodes more distant, e.g. mesenteric,
   hepatoduodenal, peripancreatic
N4: Intra-abdominal distant, e.g. para-aortic, mid-colic, etc.

Metastases
M0: Absent
M1: Present

localized involving the antrum only. The appearance on barium meal is typical. On endoscopy, absence of peristalsis is striking and the lumen is difficult to keep open, despite attempts at inflation with air. The endoscopist may feel that there is a technical problem with the air inflation mechanism and of course none is found.

The clinical presentation of gastric cancer is shown in Table 5.5 and the pathology is shown in Figure 5.11.

Gastric cancer metastases may be:

(1) Lymphatic

   (a) local
   (b) distant intra-abdominal
   (c) superficial periumbilical – Sister Mary Joseph node
   (d) left supraclavicular – Virchow's node
   (e) left axillary node – Irish's node

(2) Peritoneal nodes leading to ascites

(3) Rectal shelf detected on digital examination – Blummer's shelf

(4) Peritoneal spread to ovaries – Krukenberg's tumor

(5) Invasion of transverse colon leading to gastrocolic fistula

(6) Distant – liver, lung, bone, brain.

The differential diagnosis of gastric carcinoma is:

(1) Benign peptic ulcer disease, especially giant ulcer of the antrum;

(2) Gastric lymphoma;

(3) Leiomyosarcoma;

(4) Pancreatic cancer;

(5) Duodenal and periampullary cancers.

For an approach to the diagnosis of gastric cancer, see Figure 5.12. The endoscopic findings for gastric carcinoma are: a friable exophytic mass or nodules (polyps) with or without ulceration of the surface, often on and surrounded by thickened folds; an ulcer with large rolled-out elevated edges; thickened folds of the fundus/body and/or antrum. The stomach, or part thereof, does not distend with air, initially suggesting to the endoscopist that there is a technical problem with the endoscope. This is the appearance of linitis gastrica. Anorexia and early satiety are almost always present.

Staging of gastric cancer

Final staging of gastric cancer is usually achieved at surgery. However, preoperative staging is best achieved by endoscopic ultrasonography and CT scanning using oral and intravenous contrast. The TNM classification is used (Table 5.6).

Early gastric cancer

These are gastric cancers confined to the mucosa or submucosa usually detected during screening endoscopic procedures in countries such as Japan where there is a high prevalence of gastric adenocarcinoma. Most of these patients are asymptomatic; a small minority have dyspeptic symptoms and rarely anorexia. They are detected on careful endoscopic observation of small elevations or depressions in the gastric mucosa. When detected at this stage, the prognosis is excellent, upward of a 90% 5-year survival rate.

Case history 7

A 43-year-old woman, who works as a salesperson at an elite clothing store for women, presented with a history of 'abdominal cramps' of 6 months' duration. The pain was mostly periumbilical. The episodes of pain would come on at any time, would last from a few minutes to an hour, were not particularly related to meals, and had a colicky quality to them for the most part. She would have several such episodes each day. More recently she had felt somewhat bloated. She had gradually lost her appetite and was eating less. She had not vomited earlier, but over the past fortnight she had felt nauseated and had vomited bilious material at least once or twice daily. The bloating in her abdomen subsided after she vomited. She did not notice any change in bowel habits. She was never one who had weighed herself regularly. However, she said it was clear that she had lost quite a considerable amount, as her clothes were now too loose for her. There were no other systemic symptoms such as fever, night sweats, joint pains or skin rashes. She did feel very tired. The main feature on physical examination was clear evidence of recent weight loss. The abdomen was soft and non-tender, no masses were palpable and there was no organomegaly. Bowel sounds at the time of the examination (the patient did not have pain at the time) were normal. The rectal and pelvic examinations were also normal, but occult blood was present in the stool. Apart from a hematocrit of 34% (normochromic, normocytic smear), the routine blood tests were normal. All of her liver function tests were normal as well. She had mild hypoalbuminemia with a serum albumin of 3.1 g/dl. Serum globulins were in the normal range.

Abdominal pain and weight loss, without diarrhea, are the major features of this woman's history. The pain is not of the peptic ulcer variety, hence it is unlikely to be due to a benign ulcer or gastric malignancy, nor is it the relentless severe pain seen typically with pancreatic cancer. The location of the pain, its colicky quality, duration and recurrence several times a day has none of the characteristics of biliary 'colic'. The pain pattern and the more recent history of vomiting both might suggest a low-grade small intestinal obstruction. If the rest of the history were appropriate, tuberculosis would certainly be a possibility. However, in an otherwise previously healthy Western woman with no travel history, intestinal lymphoma would loom large in the differential diagnosis. Whether to order a barium meal with a small-bowel follow-through or whether to go first to a CT scan are somewhat arbitrary. Both would eventually be required: the barium study to define the site of the lesion more precisely, and the CT scan to determine the extent of disease outside the luminal gastrointestinal tract. In most instances of primary small-bowel lymphoma, peripheral blood and bone marrow aspirate and biopsy are not helpful. A tissue diagnosis often requires a laparotomy.

INTESTINAL LYMPHOMA

Intestinal lymphoma may be classified as primary or secondary (Figure 5.13).

Secondary intestinal lymphoma

These patients have disease that began as a nodal lymphoma that has subsequently involved the gastrointestinal tract. Most often the diagnosis is established prior to intestinal involvement or, if not, the nodal involvement provides a clue to the diagnosis.

Primary intestinal lymphoma

These are extranodal lymphomas, which eventually may spread to surrounding lymph nodes and ultimately may disseminate further. The three major clinical subtypes are briefly discussed.

Immunoproliferative small-intestinal disease

Immunoproliferative small intestinal disease (IPSID) is also known as Mediterranean lymphoma or alpha heavy chain disease. It has recently been classified as a variant of mucosa-associated lymphoid tissue (MALT)-type

Table 5.7 Immunoproliferative small-intestinal disease (IPSID)

Population affected
Countries
  Sephardic Jews and Arabs from the Mediterranean littoral
  Iran
  Pakistan
  South Africa – among the Black population only
  Taiwan
Socioeconomic group
  Poor, living in unhygienic conditions

Site
Jejunum the most prominent site

Clinical presentation
Age: second and third decades
Symptoms
  abdominal pain
  diarrhea and malabsorption syndrome
  weight loss
  clubbing – frequently seen
  perforation, hemorrhage or obstruction are not features
    of IPSID
Laboratory abnormalities
  α heavy chain in serum or intestinal juice in 75% of patients
  serum IgG, IgM, IgA usually low

Treatment
Antibiotics: anthracycline-containing multi-drug
  chemotherapy (e.g. CHOP)

CHOP, cyclophosphamide, hydroxydaunomycin, Oncovin® and prednisone

Table 5.8 Classification of non-immunoproliferative small-intestinal disease, or 'Western' non-Hodgkin's lymphomas

Mucosa-associated lymphoid tissue (MALT) type
Mantle cell or lymphomatous polyposis
Burkitt's lymphoma
Burkitt-like lymphoma
Other (rare)

Table 5.9 Non-immunoproliferative small-intestinal disease, or 'Western' non-Hodgkin's lymphomas

Population affected
Developed nations

Site
Gastric > 50%
Small intestine (ileum > jejunum, ileocecal region) ~ 25%
Colon and rectum, 5–15%

Morphology
Masses
Ulcers (triangular duodenal ulcer is very suggestive
of lymphoma)

Clinical presentation
Symptoms
  abdominal pain
  weight loss – later
  diarrhea and malabsorption are infrequent
  perforation
  hemorrhage (occult or overt)
  obstruction and intussusception
Signs
  palpable abdominal mass in ~ 30% of patients
Laboratory abnormalities
  Anemia – chronic disease, iron deficiency, folate
  deficiency
  hypoalbuminemia
    malnutrition late in disease
    associated protein-losing enteropathy

lymphoma (Table 5.7). The mucosa of the diseased area of the intestine is diffusely involved with total or partial villous atrophy and lymphoplasmacytic infiltration of the lamina propria. Since a fair amount of the mucosal surface of the small intestine is involved, diarrhea and malabsorption are features of the clinical presentation of the intestine. The lesion involves mucosa and submucosa only.

Non-immunoproliferative small-intestinal lymphoma, 'Western' small-intestinal lymphoma

Most gastrointestinal lymphomas that occur in developed countries are of the non-IPSID variety.

Recent reclassification of 'Western'-type gastrointestinal lymphomas   These lymphomas were classified using the same classification schemes as used for nodal lymphomas, until the concept of MALT was described. Until then most small-intestinal 'Western' lymphomas were thought of as being diffuse large B-cell lymphomas. More recently, it has been recognized that the cells responsible for most low-grade B-cell lymphomas of the gastrointestinal tract are histologically similar to cells of MALT (Table 5.8).

The extent of mucosal involvement is not diffuse. Small areas are involved, forming masses, and skip lesions are present when more than one area of the small intestine is involved. The areas of the small intestine between lesions are normal. Since large contiguous areas of mucosa are not involved as they are in IPSID, diarrhea and malabsorption are seldom seen. Weight loss is a late presentation consequent on the patient not eating, on account of abdominal pain, the systemic effects of malignancy or the effects of chemotherapy. Since there can be transmural involvement, perforation,

Table 5.10 Causes of chronic pancreatitis

Alcohol
Hereditary
  Autosomal dominant (~80% penetrance)
    Mutations in the cationic trypsinogen gene (PRSS 1)
      mutation in codon 122 (R122H)** in exon 3
      mutation in codon 29 (N29I)** in exon 2
  Autosomal recessive (low penetrance) or disease modifier
    Mutations in the cationic trypsinogen gene (PRSS 1)
      mutation at codon 16 (A16V) in exon 2
      mutation at codon 22 (D22G) in exon 2
      mutation at codon 23 (K23R) in exon 2
    Mutation in SPINK1 (serine protease inhibitor kazal type 1)
      mutation at codon 34 (N34S) in exon 3
      mutation at codon 35 (P35S) in exon 3
    Mutations in cystic fibrosis transmembrane regulator (CFTR)
Idiopathic
Autoimmune
Tropical

**Represents amino acid substitution, e.g. R122H: arginine for histidine

hemorrhage and obstruction can occur, unlike in IPSID (Table 5.9).

Figure 5.14 shows radiographic studies from patients with primary non-IPSID lymphoma (a,b) and from a patient with secondary lymphoma (c,d).

Mantle cell or lymphomatous polyposis This is a rare type of primary intestinal lymphoma. Lesions may be purely submucosal nodules, or polyps, or polyps with a stalk. As the polyp enlarges, the surface may ulcerate. Mesenteric lymph adenopathy is frequent at presentation. These are fairly aggressive tumors, and spread by lymphatic spread and by hematogenous spread.

Figures 5.15 and 5.16 illustrate the pathology in cases of non-IPSID lymphoma.

Enteropathy-associated lymphoma

This type of lymphoma develops in a small number of patients with celiac sprue: 5–10% of celiac sprue patients in northern Europe. It is relatively rare in the North American continent. Enteropathy-associated lymphomas are T cell lymphomas – large, histiocyte-appearing cells, similar to intraepithelial lymphocytes seen in jejunal biopsies in celiac sprue. These lymphomas must be suspected in the patient with known celiac disease who no longer responds to a gluten-free diet, and develops abdominal pain.

Table 5.11 Cambridge classification of the severity of chronic pancreatitis – ERCP criteria

	Main duct	*Secondary branches*
Mild	normal	3 abnormal
Moderate	abnormal	3 abnormal
Severe	abnormal	> 3 abnormal

CHRONIC PANCREATITIS

Chronic pancreatitis must always be considered in the diagnosis of chronic abdominal pain and weight loss.

Definition

Chronic pancreatitis is a chronic inflammatory disease of varying etiology that is characterized by pancreatic fibrosis with destruction of the parenchyma and giving rise to permanent anatomic abnormalities (e.g. stricture or dilatation) in the peripheral ducts and/or in the main pancreatic duct.

The causes of chronic pancreatitis are shown in Table5. 10.

Clinical presentation

Chronic pancreatitis presents with abdominal pain and weight loss in 80% of cases. Cases of weight loss without pain are known as the 'wasting syndrome'. The abdominal pain is due to increase in intraductal pressure, and/or increased neural stimulation – more nerve fibres with impaired nerve sheaths. The weight loss is due to pancreatic exocrine malfunction resulting in intestinal malabsorption. Reluctance to eat owing to the severity of abdominal pain also contributes to weight loss.

Complications

(1) Pseudocyst formation can occur, pseudocysts are seen:

    (a) during an acute (recurrent) attack;
    (b) secondary to pancreatic ductal obstruction.

(2) Obstruction of the common bile duct as it traverses behind the pancreatic head;

(3) Venous thrombosis – splenic vein as a rule → prehepatic portal hypertension → gastric varices;

(4) Endocrine malfunction leading to pancreatic diabetes;

(5) Carcinoma – the prevailing view is that chronic pancreatitis does predispose to carcinoma.

Diagnosis

There are numerous methods of confirming a diagnosis of chronic pancreatitis. A plain X-ray of the abdomen (lateral view) will show pancreatic calcification. A CT scan can show calcification (very sensitive), ductal dilatation, parenchymal atrophy, acute changes in the pancreas and peripancreatic tissue following an acute (recurrent) attack, or any of the complications identified above (Figures 5.17 and 5.18).

Magnetic resonance imaging, or magnetic resonance cholangiopancreatography (MRCP) may also be used for the diagnosis. Endoscopic ultrasonography (EUS) is a useful technique often used in patients with chronic pancreatitis particularly when carcinoma is in the differential diagnosis (Figure 5.17b).

Endoscopic retrograde cholangio-pancreatography (ERCP)

Changes in the main pancreatic duct and its secondary branches are characteristic of chronic pancreatitis and vary with the severity of the disease (Table 5.11).

CHAPTER 6

Chronic anemia as a presentation of gastrointestinal disease

INTRODUCTION

All too often patients with low hemoglobin levels noted on a blood count, frequently obtained during a routine visit to a general practitioner, are referred to a gastroenterologist for work-up. If the patient is middle-aged or elderly, the referral is even more specific, the patient being referred for a colonoscopy. It is imperative on the part of both the practitioner and the gastroenterologist to inquire, prior to the initiation of any gastrointestinal work-up, whether the anemia is one that may be caused by a gastrointestinal disorder. For the most part, this amounts to making sure that the chronic anemia is due to iron, folate or cobalamin (vitamin B_{12}) deficiency. Of course, gastrointestinal disorders may be associated with the anemia of chronic disease, for example Crohn's disease, intestinal tuberculosis or the gastrointestinal complications of collagen vascular disease and the vasculitides. However, in the case of such patients the request for help from a gastroenterologist is usually directed to the elucidation of a specific problem rather than to the evaluation of the accompanying anemia.

Useful points to remember in the work-up of chronic anemias:

(1) A normal mean corpuscular volume (MCV) does not indicate that microcytosis or macrocytosis is absent. Both may be present. Check the red-cell distribution width (RDW) and blood smear.

(2) An elevated MCV does not necessarily indicate a megaloblastic anemia.

(3) Examine the blood smear for multilobed polymorphonuclear leukocytes. If they have six or more lobes, this suggests a megaloblastic anemia.

(4) If iron, folate or cobalamin deficiency anemias are suspected, send off a sample for testing of serum levels before transfusing the patient with packed red cells.

(5) Red blood cell folate is often more useful then serum folate in the detection of folate deficiency.

(6) Serum ferritin may be elevated with inflammatory or infectious states as an acute phase reactant, thus masking an associated iron deficiency anemia.

IRON DEFICIENCY ANEMIA

The commonest cause of anemia due to the lack of adequate availability of a nutritional factor to the bone marrow, both in developing countries and in developed countries, is iron deficiency.

Diagnosis

The complete blood count (CBC) usually suggests the diagnosis. On occasion, when a mixed population of red cells is present (both small and large cells) the MCV may be within the normal range, the RDW will be high, and it will be necessary to examine the peripheral blood smear. A low serum iron saturation and low serum ferritin will ultimately clinch the diagnosis (Table 6.1).

Table 6.1 Iron deficiency anemia – diagnosis

Investigation	Finding
Mean corpuscular volume (MCV)	low, unless associated with a macrocytic or normocytic anemia, when it may be normal
Blood smear	check smear if the MCV is not low for a population of microcytic and hypochromic cells
Iron saturation	< 16%
Serum ferritin	low (unless concomitant infection/inflammation)

NON-GASTROINTESTINAL CAUSES OF IRON DEFICIENCY

One should always think of the non-gastrointestinal causes of iron deficiency anemia. A carefully taken history of an excessive loss during menses, menorrhagia or dysfunctional uterine bleeding will often provide the clue to the diagnosis. With adequate antenatal care pregnancy or lactation are seldom the cause of iron deficiency anemia in the developed world, although they remain common etiologies of iron deficiency in developing countries. Dietary deficiency alone is seldom if ever the cause of iron deficiency in developed nations. In developing countries it certainly is a cause of iron deficiency, even when the total daily intake of iron appears to be adequate. This is because iron present in vegetables and grain is less available for absorption. Furthermore, marginal iron stores rapidly become depleted with the stress of pregnancy or lactation or a parasitic infestation.

GASTROINTESTINAL CAUSES OF IRON DEFICIENCY ANEMIA

These are illustrated in Figure 6.1.

Case history 1

A 51-year-old Japanese professor of chemistry on sabbatical at a North American University presents with a history of epigastric pain and a 10-lb (4.5-kg) weight loss. He says his problems began around a year earlier with a general feeling of malaise and a very gradual loss of appetite. Being busy with preparations for his forthcoming sabbatical, he did not see his physician. The abdominal pain is of more recent onset. He feels a gnawing upper abdominal pain most of the time, and over the past few weeks this has awoken him from sleep on a few nights. At the onset of the abdominal pain, on the advice of a colleague, he had tried over-the-counter ranitidine and had taken two tablets twice daily regularly for at least 6 weeks. His pain was completely relieved. It recurred after a month, however, and further treatment with ranitidine did not provide relief. There is no family history of a gastrointestinal cancer. On physical examination, other than a little pallor and temporal wasting, there were no other abnormalities noted. His hemoglobin was 8.8 g/dl, hematocrit 26.8, platelet count 550×10^9/l, and the blood smear showed microcytosis and hypochromia suggestive of iron deficiency anemia.

How should this patient be managed? Clearly this is not a conventional case of dyspepsia. There are an abundance of 'red flags': age over 40 years, anorexia, weight loss and iron deficiency anemia, and a failure of acid suppressive therapy. The presence of any one of these 'red flags' would signal the need for further investigation, as opposed to a trial of an H_2 receptor antagonist or proton pump inhibitor. In the West, the commonest cause of iron deficiency anemia is colon cancer. However, in this patient the pain is clearly epigastric, and was for a time relieved by a course of ranitidine, and there is a history of a loss of appetite. All of these point to an upper gastrointestinal source. Furthermore, the patient is from Japan, a country with a high prevalence of gastric cancer. Therefore, an esophagogastroduodenoscopy (EGD) should be the first investigation requested. On EGD a large gastric ulcer was present on the greater curvature. Biopsy of the edges of the ulcer revealed it to be an adenocarcinoma.

Points to note from this case:

(1) On H_2 receptor antagonists or proton pump inhibitors, dyspeptic symptoms are often relieved for a time, as the ulceration or inflammation surrounding a malignant tumor improves. Small malignant ulcers may on occasion completely heal. One of the authors has seen this happen not only with adenocarcinoma, but also with a gastric lymphoma presenting as an ulcer.

(?) Whenever any one of the following 'red flags' are present in a patient with dyspepsia, further work-up is called for and a therapeutic trial with acid-suppressive therapy should not be initiated:

(a) Age > 40 years
(b) Weight loss
(c) Anorexia or early satiety
(d) Iron deficiency anemia

(3) The nationality of the patient is very important. In countries such as Japan, China, Taiwan, Russia, Eastern Europe and South America, the prevalence of gastric carcinoma is still high.

Gastric carcinoma

The tumors may appear as polypoid lesions or as ulcers. As a rule malignant ulcers have rolled-out overhanging edges, unlike benign ulcers, which appear more punched out. However, gross appearances can be deceptive. Adenocarcinoma is by far the commonest malignant gastric tumor. (See Chapter 5 for details on gastric carcinoma).

Other gastric malignancies

Gastric lymphomas (see Chapter 5 for the classification of gastrointestinal lymphomas) and stromal tumors such as leiomyosarcomas may present much like gastric adenocarcinomas.

Benign peptic ulcers

Both gastric and duodenal ulcers may on occasion present with iron deficiency anemia resulting from the chronic oozing of blood from the ulcer surface. This is distinctly unusual, however. When benign peptic ulcers bleed, the bleeding usually results from the erosion of an arteriole in the ulcer bed and the patient presents acutely with a large hemorrhage. Therefore, in the work-up of iron deficiency anemia, if a small peptic ulcer is the only positive finding on investigation, the physician should be alert to the presence of another lesion, not yet identified, that might be responsible for the anemia.

Atrophic gastritis

Acid is required for the absorption of non-heme iron, especially that present in the ferric form. On occasion patients with achlorhydria due to atrophic gastritis will

Table 6.2 Mechanism of iron deficiency after gastric surgery

(1)	Slow oozing of blood from the erythematous gastric remnant
(2)	Food iron malabsorption

develop iron deficiency anemia. Cobalamin deficiency may be present concomitantly. Both adenomatous gastric polyps and gastric cancer may develop in areas of atrophic gastritis with intestinal metaplasia (see description of gastric cancer in Chapter 5 and Figure 6.2).

Gastrectomy

One long-term sequela of gastric surgery is iron deficiency anemia (Table 6.2). The incidence of developing iron deficiency anemia varies with the type of surgery performed: total gastrectomy > Billroth II > Billroth I or vagotomy + gastroenterostomy > vagotomy + pyloroplasty > parietal cell vagotomy. Since total gastrectomies are rare, the commonest operation as a consequence of which iron deficiency anemia develops is a Billroth II or Polya gastrectomy. There does not appear to be an increase after parietal cell vagotomy.

There are at least two specific pathways for the absorption of food iron:

(1) Iron in food bound to hemoglobin or myoglobin (heme iron);

(2) Ferrous iron, either in the elemental form or in a soluble chelated form.

Much of the iron in food is present as ferric iron, which needs to be reduced to the ferrous form in order to be absorbed. Ascorbate (vitamin C) in the diet is an excellent reducing agent. The acid pH of the stomach facilitates reduction to the ferrous state and its subsequent absorption in the duodenum. The most efficient site of iron absorption is the duodenum. The rate of absorption diminishes progressively down the small intestine. This simple understanding of the elements of iron absorption enables the mechanism to be understood of food iron malabsorption in humans after gastric surgery. Two factors play a major role:

(1) Elevated pH of the stomach, hindering the reduction of iron from the ferric state;

(2) Bypassing of the duodenum with gastroenterostomy and a Billroth II operation.

Benign gastric polyps

These may be hyperplastic, with no malignant potential (frequently resulting from foveolar hyperplasia), or adenomatous, with malignant potential. Adenomatous polyps often arise in atrophic gastric mucosa. Both hyperplastic and adenomatous polyps may occur as part of familial adenomatous polyposis syndrome (see below). In such patients adenomas of the colon usually precede gastric adenomas (Figures 6.3 and 6.4).

Other gastric malignancies

Gastric lymphomas (see Chapter 3 for details of MALT lymphomas and Chapter 5 for the classification of gastrointestinal lymphomas) and stromal tumors, such as leiomyosarcomas, may present much like gastric adenocarcinomas. Lymphomas of the stomach may appear as polypoid or ulcerated lisions or as large ulcerated masses (Figure 6.5). They may on occasion present as enlarged gastric folds of the body or antrum of the stomach.

Case history 2

A 56-year-old business executive, an American of Japanese ancestry (his grandparents having immigrated to the USA when they were young), was noted to be anemic during a routine medical checkup with his physician. He had neglected to see a physician in the past 3 years, since he had moved to New York City. Upon direct enquiry, he admitted to feeling tired with less than accustomed exertion. He had no history of weight loss, anorexia, early satiety, dysphagia, abdominal pain, or a recent history of a change in his bowel habits. His maternal grandfather had died of pancreatic cancer. The family history was otherwise not significant to the patient's current illness. His physical examination was normal and stool obtained during the rectal examination tested negative for occult blood. His hemoglobin was 10.3 g/dl. The work-up of the anemia revealed it to be due to iron deficiency.

How should this patient be managed? This middle-aged man with iron deficiency is almost asymptomatic, other than for minimal symptoms of fatigue, most likely to be related to his anemia. There is nothing in his history or physical examination to point to either an upper or a lower intestinal source for his iron deficiency anemia. However, there are two important factors to consider. The first is his age. He is 56 years old. The second is the fact that he was born and brought up, as were his parents, in the USA. The commonest cause of iron deficiency anemia in the USA, as in Western Europe, Australia and New Zealand, is colorectal cancer. Colon cancer is frequently asymptomatic, presenting with either the detection of occult blood in the stool upon routine examination or, later in the course of the disease, with iron deficiency anemia. The patient's Japanese ancestry is irrelevant in this context. Earlier studies carried out in Japanese immigrants to Hawaii have shown that the children and grandchildren of Japanese immigrants to the USA have the same predilection to developing colon cancer as do Americans of European ancestry, quite unlike first-generation immigrants. A similar study revealed that the children of Eastern European immigrants to Australia had a similar predilection for developing colon cancer to that of other Australians. The implication of the results of these studies is that factors related to the environment and/or life style are probably more important than genetic factors as far as sporadic colorectal cancer is concerned. The picture is of course different in families with a very high prevalence of colorectal cancer. Therefore, the investigation this patient needs is a colonoscopy. On colonoscopy, a cecal carcinoma was detected. The patient also had several other polyps in other areas of his colon that were removed using a snare. One of the polyps was a localized invasive carcinoma in the ascending colon and another was a small tubular adenoma in the sigmoid colon. Three other tiny polyps removed from the rectum during the colonoscopy were shown to be hyperplastic polyps. Liver function tests and a computerized tomography (CT) scan of the abdomen were normal. The patient underwent a right hemicolectomy.

Points to note from this case:

(1) In an asymptomatic person who has grown up in parts of the world where colorectal cancer is very prevalent, such as Western Europe, North America or the Australasian continent, colon cancer should be the first diagnosis to consider in a middle-aged person who presents with either iron deficiency anemia or occult blood in the stool. Colonoscopy is the investigation of choice. A barium enema should be reserved for people unable to undergo a colonoscopy for technical reasons.

(2) The patient described did not have occult blood noted on examination. This is not surprising at all,

since polyps and cancers bleed intermittently and the test is frequently negative. That is why annual screening for colorectal cancer for those over the age of 50 years using occult blood testing requires that three tests be done over the span of a few days. Also, factors such as taking large amounts of vitamin C may give rise to a false-negative test for occult blood.

(3) A patient's ancestry may be of great importance in the diagnosis of certain diseases, but for reasons explained above, in this case the fact that the patient had grown up in a part of the world with a high prevalence for colorectal cancer was more important than his ancestry.

(4) This patient had both a synchronous tubular adenoma and a synchronous invasive cancer, albeit within a polyp. Patients with colon cancer frequently have adenomatous polyps or a second cancer within their colon (i.e. synchronous adenoma or cancer). It is therefore necessary to evaluate the entire colon for a synchronous cancer prior to surgery. In the event that the colon is obstructed and it is not possible to evaluate the colon preoperatively, it is essential to do so as soon after surgery as is deemed safe.

(5) A preoperative CT scan should be obtained in every patient prior to surgery, to investigate the likelihood of liver and peritoneal metastases.

(6) The patient should continue to receive surveillance colonoscopies every 3 years, so that any adenomatous polyps that develop may be removed. This is because patients with colon cancer are prone to develop a metachronous cancer some time later. Many surgeons prefer the initial surveillance colonoscopy to be a year after surgery and, if that is negative, then one every 3 years.

Colorectal cancer

Adenocarcinoma of the colon is the commonest cause of iron deficiency anemia in developed nations, where the prevalence of this cancer is very high. By contrast, in developing nations the prevalence is low, and the commonest causes of iron deficiency in several developing nations are pregnancy and hookworm disease.

Dietary factors that may contribute to the causation

There is evidence from longitudinal cohort studies, case–control studies and cross-sectional studies that the following may contribute to colorectal cancer: red meat, high total caloric intake, saturated fat and cholesterol.

Dietary factors that may be preventive

There is evidence from longitudinal cohort studies, case–control studies and cross-sectional studies that the following dietary factors may prevent colorectal cancer: fish, poultry and fresh fruit.

Dietary factors with no evidence in support

There is no evidence from epidemiological studies as yet that fiber is protective.

Chemoprevention

There is experimental evidence as well as some based on epidemiological studies to suggest that chemoprevention may have a role in the future. There is considerable evidence in support of non-steroidal anti-inflammatory drugs (NSAIDs) and aspirin: ten out of 11 studies have shown a benefit of aspirin in reducing the risk for the development of colon cancer. Sulindac, an NSAID, has been used with limited benefit in familial polyposis coli. Work is underway to see whether selective cyclo-oxygenase-2 (COX-2) inhibitors will be effective.

The evidence for the following is less impressive, as to date various nutrition intervention trials and case–control studies have shown different results. The scientific rationale for many nutrients is good.

Vitamin E There is evidence from one case–control study.

Vitamin D Vitamin D has not conclusively been shown to be of benefit, despite excellent scientific data to suggest that it might well be useful. Vitamin D analogs inhibit growth and promote differentiation of colon cancer cell lines *in vitro*. The growth-inhibiting properties might be mediated by its effect on the vitamin D nuclear receptor.

Calcium Calcium has been shown to be of benefit in more studies than those in which it has not been shown to be of benefit.

The adenoma–carcinoma sequence and the genetics of sporadic colorectal cancer

The following statement may be accepted:

'Every colorectal carcinoma that develops in the absence of underlying inflammatory bowel disease arises in an adenomatous polyp.'

In that a polyp is defined as a lesion that is raised above the plane of the mucosal surface of the gastrointestinal tract, and the fact that an adenoma is a polyp whose mucosa is dysplastic, one could redefine the adenoma–carcinoma sequence in terms of dysplasia (Figure 6.6). The definition would then read as follows:

'Every colorectal carcinoma arises from dysplastic epithelium, irrespective of whether the dysplasia is present in a raised lesion, as in an adenomatous polyp, or in a flat lesion, as in inflammatory bowel disease.'

There is now evidence that suggests that the progression from normal mucosa through a hyperproliferative epithelium, early intermediate and late adenomas and ultimately to carcinoma takes place in stages. At each stage mutations or deletions in either oncogenes or tumor suppressor genes arise. It is important to recognize that, as a rule, the aggregate of such mutations or deletions would be acquired more in a carcinoma than, for instance, in an early adenoma. However, every carcinoma does not have the same genetic profile and may often lack genetic alterations that may be present in some other adenomas. It is important to stress that one is speaking here of somatic mutations and deletions and not of germline alterations, as would be seen, for example, in the familial adenomatous polyposis or adenomatous polyposis coli syndrome (Figure 6.7).

A somatic mutation or deletion (i.e. one in the involved tissue and not in the germ cell) in the adenomatous polyposis coli (*APC*) gene on the long arm of chromosome 5, is an early event along the pathway that leads to a cancer. *APC* is a tumor suppressor gene. Increased expression of the inducible cyclo-oxygenase enzyme (COX-2) also occurs very early in the dysplasia–carcinoma sequence. Another early event is a mutation in the K-*ras* gene. By contrast, a deletion on the long arm of chromosome 18 is a later event. This was thought to occur in the so-called *DCC* (*Deleted in Colon Cancer*) gene. It appears that another tumor suppressor gene at an adjacent locus on the long arm of chromosome 18, *DPC4/Smad* might be the culprit. At the stage where a highly dysplastic adenoma becomes a carcinoma, two other events have been recognized. The first is a deletion in the *p53* gene on the short arm of chromosome 17. More recently, mutations within the gene for the type II transforming growth factor (TGF)-β receptor (TGF-βRII) have also been described. In addition, the role of genomic instability in the development of some sporadic colon cancers has recently been explored. Alterations in target genes that possess microsatellite repeat sequences in their coding region results in microsatellite instability that would alter the mechanisms that regulate DNA fidelity. Thus, there are colon cancers in which microsatellite instability appears to play a major role in the development of the cancer (microsatellite mutator phenotype). Such cancers are diploid. On the other hand, in some cancers chromosomal instability appears to play a central role in tumorigenesis. Such tumors are aneuploid.

Table 6.3 Clinical presentation of colorectal cancer

Asymptomatic detection at screening sigmoidoscopy or colonoscopy
Occult blood in stool
    proximal cancers, even when large
    left-sided cancers, usually smaller
Iron deficiency anemia as the sole manifestation
    proximal cancers more frequently
Bright red blood per rectum
    more common with left-sided colon cancers and rectal cancers
Change in bowel habits
    more common with left-sided cancers
Tenesmus
    low rectal cancers
Obstruction (early symptoms include straining at stool)
    more frequent with the napkin ring-like left-sided cancers
Perforation
    uncommon presentation
Appendicitis-like syndrome
    cecal cancer obstructing the orifice of the appendix
    cecal perforation

Clinical presentation of colorectal cancer

Table 6.3 outlines the common presentations of colorectal cancer. Although none of the symptoms are specific for a cancer in any location, perhaps with the exception of tenesmus, which occurs only with low rectal cancers, some symptoms tend to occur more frequently with cancers of the left colon, whereas others are more frequent with more proximal cancers.

Diagnosis of colorectal cancer

(1) Rectal examination – most rectal cancers should be detected on rectal examination.

(2) Colonoscopy in most instances is the way in which cancers are detected (Figure 6.8).

(3) Barium enema is now generally reserved for those patients in whom colonoscopy was incomplete for technical reasons.

The role of the barium enema

Once the prime modality for the diagnosis of colon cancer, this is now reserved mainly for patients in whom, for technical reasons, it is not possible to complete a colonoscopy (Figures 6.9–6.11).

Staging colorectal cancers

Endoscopic ultrasonography may be used for staging rectal cancers in addition to CT scanning.

Case history 3

A 66-year-old man who had received a renal transplantation 6 years earlier of presented with a history of intermittent rectal bleeding and tenesmus. A firm mass was palpated on digital examination. Sigmoidoscopy revealed an ulcerated rectal adenocarcinoma. An endoscopic ultrasound examination was performed to stage the cancer (Figure 6.12). Transrectal ultrasonography is the best tool to stage rectal cancers for local extension.

CT scan   The CT scan is used to stage colon cancers and may show local, peritoneal spread and also spread to distant viscera such as the liver or lung.

Case history 4

A 65-year-old man, who had never had previous screening for colon cancer, presented with bloating and diffuse abdominal pain. He had not moved his bowels for several days. He felt nauseated and had a very small amount of emesis the morning he came to see his physician. The abdominal and rectal examinations were normal. Plain X-rays of the abdomen showed fluid-filled small bowel with dilated large bowel, air–fluid levels within the large bowel and no air in the recto-sigmoid region (Figure 6.13). These findings were consistent with a distal large bowel obstruction. The patient underwent a CT scan (Figure 6.14). Intravenous contrast could not be used as the patient had mild renal failure.

Case history 5

A 72-year-old woman complained of passing bright red blood in her stools. She attributed her symptom to an increased activity of her hemorrhoids. She had not noted any change in her bowel habits. At times she noticed rectal bleeding. The blood was seen to coat solid stool. Her abdominal and rectal examinations were normal. Occult blood was present at the time

Table 6.4   Types of colorectal polyp

Epithelial polyp
  Hyperplastic polyp – hyperplastic or dysmature epithelium
  Adenomatous polyp – dysplastic epithelium
    tubular adenoma – long, often branched, glands
    villous adenoma – papillary or finger-like processes
    tubulovillous – tubular with few papillary processes
    carcinoma within an adenoma
  Carcinoid tumor – gut endocrine cell
  Hamartomas
    juvenile polyp
    Peutz–Jeghers polyp
    Cowden's syndrome
    Cronkhite–Canada syndrome
Inflammatory tissue
  'Pseudopolyp' in inflammatory bowel disease
Non-epithelial polyp
  From lymphoid, smooth muscle, neural or fatty tissue

of rectal examination. Her blood count revealed a hemoglobin of 10.8 g/dl, a MCV of 70 fl with microcytosis and hypochromia on her blood smear. A work-up of her anemia revealed that she was severely iron deficient. She had never been screened for colon cancer. When her family physician suggested a colonoscopy, she initially opposed it, not wanting to make a fuss over her 'piles'. She ultimately yielded, and the colonoscopy revealed a 3-cm polyp with a short stalk, in the lower sigmoid colon. It was very friable and bled easily even on gentle contact with the colonoscope. It was safely removed at colonoscopy. The pathology report revealed the polyp to be a tubular adenoma with some villous elements. There was no evidence of malignancy.

Points to note from this case:

(1)   On occasion a large adenomatous polyp can bleed slowly and after a time can give rise to iron deficiency anemia, just as a cancer can.

(2)   If the polyp is located in the proximal part of the colon, bright red blood per rectum may never be seen, the bleeding always being occult.

(3)   Even though a patient might be convinced the bleeding is from hemorrhoids, one must always consider the possibility of colonic polyps or cancer.

Colonic polyps

Definition   A lesion that is raised above the plane of the mucosal surface of the gastrointestinal tract, irrespective of its histology, is termed a polyp.

Types of colorectal polyp are listed in Table 6.4.

Hyperplastic polyps   These polyps are generally very small, usually < 0.5 cm. They never undergo malignant transformation. They may occur anywhere in the colon, but are seen more frequently in the rectum (Figure 6.15a,b).

Adenomatous polyps   These occur in almost 30% of middle-aged and elderly people in Western countries. The prevalence in developing countries is very low. The condition is increasing in Japan. Polyps may be stalked or sessile, and vary in size from a millimeter or two to several centimeters. The usual clinical presentation is occult blood loss. Polyps in the descending colon or rectum may on occasion present with spotting of bright red blood per rectum much like hemorrhoidal bleeding. Bleeding from large polyps may eventually result in iron deficiency anemia. Large low rectal polyps (or cancers) may cause tenesmus. Very rarely, rectal villous adenomas may be the source of a secretory diarrhea that results in hypokalemia. The major concern of harboring adenomas is that they may develop into carcinomas (Figure 6.15c–f and 6.16). Facts to remember about adenomatous polyps are:

(1) Less than 1% of adenomas overall develop into carcinomas;

(2) The larger the size, the greater the malignant potential;

(3) Malignant potential of adenomas: villous > tubulovillous > tubular.

Case history 6

A 5-year-old boy is brought in by his mother who has noted her son has been passing bright red blood in his stools off and on for the past week. The boy was born at full term and has been in robust health. The blood appears to be mixed in with the stool, so she is unable to say how much blood is being lost each time. Stool consistency is normal. She has now noticed this on three separate occasions. The child has no abdominal pain and has not had rectal discomfort at the time of defecation. His appetite has been excellent and he has been eating as well as he usually does. His physical examination is normal. On asking him to strain, no prolapsed rectum is noted.

What is the source of the bleeding?   The history is clearly suggestive of lower gastrointestinal bleeding, since the child would have needed urgent care for hemodynamic

instability had an upper gastrointestinal source caused the bright red blood per rectum. For similar reasons a Meckel's diverticulum would not be the source of the hemorrhage. Also, the bleeding occurred only at the time of defecation. The history was not compatible with dysentery or an early onset of inflammatory bowel disease, since the patient had neither diarrhea nor abdominal discomfort. The absence of pain ruled out intermittent intussusception. The most likely cause was bleeding from a colonic polyp. The patient underwent a colonoscopy and a 1.5-cm globular-looking polyp was seen in the descending colon that was removed. The histology revealed it to be a juvenile polyp.

Colonic polyps in children   Rectal bleeding in young children, frequently in the 3–4-year age group, is due to the presence of juvenile polyps. In childhood, these are more common than adenomas. Juvenile polyps are seldom diagnosed after the second decade is over. They appear as small rounded masses at endoscopy. The cut surface of these polyps shows cystic spaces. Histologically these cystic spaces are cystic glands made up mostly of goblet cells that are located below an eroded surface epithelium. There is abundant stroma filled with granulation tissue and dilated lymphatics. By definition, if the juvenile polyp is a hamartoma, it ought not to become malignant. The fact that rarely juvenile polyps do become malignant suggests that on occasion there are adenomatous foci present within such polyps. Bright red blood per rectum is the commonest clinical presentation. Occasionally mild diarrhea with mucus in the stool or an intussusception with the polyp at the leading edge may be seen.

Other hamartomas   The Peutz–Jegher syndrome is another example of a condition where hamartomatous polyps are seen in association with a characteristic brownish pigmentation of the skin. There may be just an isolated polyp of the stomach, small intestine or colon, or more often the disease presents as a polyposis syndrome (i.e. when several dozen colonic polyps are present with or without small intestinal or gastric polyps). While it is uncommon for a Peutz–Jegher polyp to undergo malignant transformation, it may. Thus, a person with the Peutz–Jegher syndrome, whose iron deficiency anemia cannot be otherwise explained, should be suspected of harboring a cancer of the gastrointestinal tract. Several extraintestinal manifestations are also present (Table 6.5). The polyps grossly resemble adenomatous polyps, but

Table 6.5 Extraintestinal manifestations of the Peutz–Jegher syndrome

Dark brown, blue or black freckle-like pigmentation around the mouth, eyes or nostrils or over the bridge of the nose. Similar macular pigmentation of the hands and feet, especially over the fingers and toes may be seen.

Increased prevalence of extraintestinal tumors
    pancreas
    gallbladder and biliary tract
    breast
    Sertoli cell testicular tumor
    sex cord tumors of the ovaries (benign)

histologically they are true hamartomas. Hence polyps of the stomach are seen to contain mucus, parietal and chief cells. Small intestinal Peutz–Jegher polyps are made up of villous or crypt-like cells. Those in the colon are made up of goblet cells (see Figure 6.15g, h). The Peutz–Jegher gene has been mapped to chromosome 19p. However, at least one other locus appears likely.

The Cowden's syndrome is a rare autosomal dominant condition. Multiple hamartomas derived from ectodermal, endodermal and mesodermal elements are present mostly, but not confined to the distal colon and rectum. Polyps in the stomach are mostly hyperplastic. Other associations that can be present in Cowden's syndrome include fibrocystic disease of the breast, hypertrophic gums and hyperkeratotic papillomata of the lips, non-toxic goiter and thyroid cancer.

Cronkhite–Canada syndrome is a polyposis syndrome involving the stomach, small intestine and colon, with skin pigmentation involving the body creases, hands, alopecia and dystrophic nails. The polyps are similar to juvenile polyps. Patients are middle-aged or elderly and develop diarrhea, malabsorption and severe protein-losing enteropathy.

Case history 7

A 60-year-old man with a history of a myocardial infarction 5 years earlier presents with fatigue, moderate dyspnea on exertion and two episodes of exertional chest pain that subsided on rest. His father had died of colon cancer when he was only 45 years old. The patient had his colon removed over 20 years ago and is left with an ileostomy. He was told at the time that he had two small cancers and hundreds of polyps in his resected colon. On examination he appears very pale, has a mid-systolic murmur in the aortic area and along the left sternal border which is of moderate intensity. The abdominal examination is normal except for the ileostomy. The ileostomy effluent readily tests positive for occult blood. His hemoglobin is 8.5 g/dl and the work-up of the anemia reveals it to be due to iron deficiency.

What are the likely causes of iron deficiency anemia in this patient? A strong family history of colon cancer occurring in members of his family when they were young, and with the knowledge that the patient's colon contained 'hundreds' of polyps, makes the diagnosis of familial adenomatous polyposis or adenomatous polyposis coli almost certain. By definition, a polyposis syndrome is one in which the colon contains over a hundred polyps, although in most patients with familial adenomatous polyposis the colon contains from hundreds to thousands of small adenomas. These patients may develop adenomas, which could then go on to become carcinomas, in other regions of the gastrointestinal tract as well. Since the duodenum and ileum are the most common extracolonic sites, endoscopy should be the initial investigation. An esophagogastroduodenoscopy (EGD) usually identifies duodenal tumors, although on occasion a side-viewing endoscope is necessary to identify a carcinoma of the ampulla of Vater. Ampullary tumors may present with obstructive jaundice and/or iron deficiency anemia or even overt upper gastrointestinal hemorrhage. If the upper endoscopy is normal, the ileum may be inspected using a colonoscope through the ileostomy stoma or through an ileoanal pouch, should that be the operation performed at the time of the colectomy. A barium study of the small intestine should also be performed to be certain a cancer of the jejunum is not present. This patient had a 1.5-cm sessile polypoid tumor in the descending part of the duodenum, 1cm distal to the ampulla. It was a carcinoma.

Familial adenomatous polyposis or adenomatous polyposis coli

This is an autosomal dominant polyposis syndrome in which the colon is generally carpeted by hundreds to thousands of small adenomatous polyps by the time the person is in the second or third decade. Some of these polyps undergo malignant transformation, and those afflicted present with cancer at a young age (Figures 6.17 and 6.18). It is therefore necessary to perform a total colectomy once polyps are detected. The disease is the result of a germline mutation in the *APC* gene located on the long arm of chromosome 5 (5q21). *APC* is a tumor suppressor gene. Some patients with familial

Table 6.6   Familial adenomatous polyposis

Extragastrointestinal manifestations
Gardner's syndrome
  Skin
    epidermoid cysts
  Subcutaneous tissue
    fibromas
  Teeth
    supernumerary teeth
    multiple dental caries
  Bone
    osteomas of the skull and mandible, or generalized
  Desmoid 'tumors' – mesentery fibrosis leading to intestinal obstruction
Turcot's syndrome
  Malignant brain tumors
Retina
  Congenital hypertrophy of the pigment layer
Liver
  Hepatocellular carcinoma and hepatoblastoma
Thyroid
  Papillary carcinoma

Extracolonic gastrointestinal manifestations
Stomach
  Polyps due to cystic dilatation of gastric glands
  Adenomas
Duodenum
  Adenoma and carcinoma of ampulla of Vater
  Adenoma and carcinoma of duodenum
Jejunum
  Adenoma and carcinoma (ileum more common)
Ileum
  Adenoma and carcinoma
Gallbladder, bile duct, pancreatic duct
  Dysplasia leading to carcinoma

adenomatous polyposis have extraintestinal manifestations that constitute what is termed Gardner's syndrome. Gardner's syndrome is not a separate entity. In families with familial adenomatous polyposis, some members may present with extraintestinal features of Gardner's syndrome in addition to their polyposis (Table 6.6), whereas others may not.

Case history 8

A healthy 39-year-old woman is referred for a colonoscopy because of a striking family history. Her father had died of colon cancer at 44 years of age, her father's sister had colon cancer when she was 52 years and endometrial cancer at 58 years of age. The patient's older brother had been diagnosed with colon cancer 3 years previously at the age of 50 years and just a month ago a work-up for iron deficiency anemia revealed he had a duodenal cancer. Her colonoscopy revealed a cecal cancer and two adenomatous polyps in the ascending colon.

What diagnosis must be suspected?   The patient's history meets the clinical criteria used to diagnose hereditary non-polyposis colorectal cancer syndrome (HNPCC), also known as the Lynch syndrome (see below). In addition, one family member had endometrial cancer and another had duodenal cancer. These are relevant items of history, as discussed below.

Hereditary non-polyposis colorectal cancer or the Lynch syndrome

Clinical criteria required for diagnosis of HNPCC are:

(1)   Colon cancer must be present in at least three close relatives, at least one of whom is a first-degree relative of the other two;

(2)   Colon cancer must be present in at least two generations – i.e. evidence for vertical transmission;

(3)   At least one person in the family must be diagnosed with colon cancer at or before the age of 50 years.

Distribution and numbers of polyps and cancers in HNPCC:

(1)   Polyps tend to occur much more in the right side of the colon than in either sporadic colon cancer or in familial adenomatous polyposis;

(2)   Usually these are more polyps per colon than in sporadic colon cancer;

(3)   There are never close to as many as a 100 polyps per colon.

Other associated cancers

Families in which only colon cancer is inherited are termed to be suffering from Lynch I syndrome. Families in which other cancers are also inherited, such as endometrial, ovarian, duodenal, biliary and pancreatic cancers, are said to have the Lynch II syndrome.

The genetics of hereditary non-polyposis colorectal cancer

The genetic defect in HNPCC is a mutation occurring in one of several different DNA mismatch repair genes. DNA mismatch repair genes are responsible under normal conditions for repairing errors that occur in DNA that has been freshly copied. The polyps and cancers in HNPCC patients show evidence of genomic instability for short repeated sequences, a phenomenon called microsatellite instability. Germline mutations at four different gene loci have been described: MSH2, MLH1, PMS1 and PMS2. Of these, the first two are the most common and make up two-thirds or more of patients with HNPCC.

Screening for colorectal cancer

The United States Public Health Task Force recommends flexible sigmoidoscopy every 3 years and fecal occult blood testing annually for those aged 50 years and above. This conservative strategy recommends that screening colonoscopy be reserved for the following situations:

(1) Patients previously diagnosed with colorectal cancer;

(2) Patients with ulcerative colitis or Crohn's colitis with disease for 7 years or longer;

(3) Patients with a family history of HNPCC or familial polyposis coli;

(4) Patients with a first-degree relative with colon cancer;

(5) Patients with a first-degree relative diagnosed with colorectal cancer or an adenomatous polyp prior to the age of 60 years.

In the USA, Medicare and several private insurers will now pay for a screening colonoscopy in everyone over the age of 50 years. Several authorities believe that such screening every 10 years might suffice, although there are few data currently available to support the time interval.

Virtual colonoscopy or CT colography is presently an investigational tool. The preparation for the procedure involves colonic cleansing identical to that required for a colonoscopy. The colon is distended with air administered through a small rubber catheter inserted into the rectum. The patient then undergoes a helical or multi-slice CT scan in both supine and prone positions. Images are then reformatted for further three-dimensional image processing. The reformatted source images are viewed in axial, coronal and sagittal projections. One can then 'drive' through the colon obtaining a virtual endoscopist's view in three dimensions (see Figure 6.19).

Figure 6.20 illustrates gross and microscopic appearances of colonic cancer.

Case history 9

A 76-year-old woman presents with iron deficiency anemia. She is otherwise asymptomatic and her physical examination throws no light on the likely cause for her iron deficiency, other than the presence of occult blood in the stool on all three times it was tested for. She is unaware of whether any of her first-degree relatives ever had polyps. She is certain none of them had colon cancer. Nevertheless, because of her age it was mandatory to rule out colon cancer, so she underwent a colonoscopy, which was normal. She was then subjected to EGD, which was also completely normal. A carefully done barium study with a committed small-bowel follow-through was obtained, and was likewise normal.

What is the likely diagnosis and how should the patient be managed? The most likely diagnosis in an elderly patient is angiodysplasia, otherwise termed vascular ectasia. These vascular lesions can frequently be missed at endoscopy. The patient was begun on oral iron, and serial blood counts were obtained on an out-patient basis. For the next few months the patient did relatively well. The hemoglobin rose from 8.5 g/dl to 10.2 g/dl, but did not rise further. She continued to have occult blood in her stool. After about 6 months her hemoglobin started to drop and she became more anemic. She had to be restarted on oral iron. She became short of breath and required to be transfused on two separate occasions. The colonoscopy was repeated. The second time, angiodysplasia was seen in the cecum and also the ascending colon. The largest was seen to be oozing a little blood and was subjected to cauterization using a bipolar electrode.

Vascular lesions

The commonest of these are angiodysplasia or vascular ectasia. These lesions are most likely to be changes secondary to the degeneration of the venules in the wall of the gut that accompanies the process of aging.

Arterioles that supply the mucosa terminate in submucosal capillaries. These capillaries in turn form venules, which penetrate the circular muscle of the gut wall. The pressure resulting from the contraction and relaxation of the circular muscle of the gut in the course of normal peristalsis causes these ectatic venules to bulge and over time to become tortuous. This pressure is presumably transmitted to the capillaries, which dilate, giving rise to the characteristic mucosal tufts seen on angiography. Ultimately, the increased pressure results in the malfunctioning of the precapillary sphincters. At this stage in its natural history the vascular lesion behaves hemodynamically like an arteriovenous malformation.

Vascular ectasia or angiodysplasia is most commonly seen in the right side of the colon, but may occur elsewhere in the colon and in the stomach and small intestine. On occasion they may be the source of profuse acute hemorrhage, but more often they give rise to occult blood loss presenting as iron deficiency anemia. Gastric angiodysplasia, in particular, is more commonly encountered in patients with chronic renal failure often on hemodialysis, although such patients may have angiodysplasia in other areas of the gastrointestinal tract as well. There has also been an association of angiodysplasia with von Willebrand's disease. The diagnosis is usually made on endoscopy (EGD or colonoscopy) when the characteristic red lesions with a 'fern leaf' or a 'red ball of yarn' appearance are encountered. At times only cherry red spots may be noted and then the diagnosis may not be as definitive. Lesions are often missed on endoscopy. Documented chronic occult gastrointestinal blood loss, especially in an elderly patient or in a person on hemodialysis without a cause, even after EGD and colonoscopy, usually means that angiodysplasia has as yet not been identified. The lesions are more often missed on angiography too, but when present the following signs are indicative of angiodysplasia:

(1) A tortuous opacified vein seen in the late venous phase that does not empty – the so-called 'late emptying vein';

(2) A vascular tuft, with probably dilated capillaries, seen in the arterial phase of the angiogram;

(3) An early filling vein seen 4–5 s after contrast injection;

(4) Extravasation of contrast from a briskly bleeding lesion.

Endoscopy (colonoscopy or EGD), is the most sensitive way of identifying angiodysplastic lesions. They vary is shape and size. As a rule they have an appearance rather similar to spider naevi seen on the skin of patients with cirrhosis, or like telangiectasia on the buccal mucosa or lips of patients with hereditaty hemorrhagic telangiectasia (Figure 6.21a). Similar lesions when larger may have the appearance of a 'ball of yarn' or a 'fern leaf'. At other times they may resemble 'cherry red spots' (Figure 6.21b). Telangiectasias may also be seen in patients with scleroderma (Figure 6.21c).

In the 'watermelon stomach', bands of ectatic vessels are seen emerging from the pylorus and fanning out into the antrum like the stripes of a watermelon. Angiodysplasia-like lesions and cherry red spots may also be seen within the area of the lesion. These vessels bleed easily, resulting in either large or small hemorrhages or occult blood loss. The etiology is undetermined. The lesion is frequently seen in the middle-aged, more commonly in women. Achlorhydria often accompanies the lesion. A similar lesion is seen in patients with portal hypertension, and in such patients this may be a variant of portal gastropathy.

The lesions of hereditary hemorrhagic telangiectasia (HHT) or the Osler–Weber–Rendu disease appear very similar on endoscopy. This is an autosomal dominant condition and telangiectasia in the skin and mucous membranes is frequent. Nosebleeds, hemoptysis from pulmonary lesions and high-output failure from lesions in the liver, giving rise to shunting, are other features of the disease.

Case history 10

A 45-year-old man sees his physician because of a gradual increase in fatigue for over a year. His exercise tolerance has deteriorated quite markedly. His physical examination is normal other than for pallor. He has a hemoglobin of 9.5 g/dl and his anemia is shown to be due to iron deficiency. Stools tested three times for occult blood were negative each time. He denies any other symptom. He has experienced neither diarrhea nor constipation recently. Other than a business trip to the UK, he has not travelled. He has no family history of colon cancer, but his older brother, 10 years older than he is, had a colonic polyp detected on a screening sigmoidoscopy. He has no family history of HHT. He denies that any member of his family has a complaint of recurrent nosebleeds. Recurrent nosebleeds occur commonly in HHT. The patient underwent a colonoscopy that was completely normal. He next underwent an EGD, which revealed no ulcers, erosions, tumors or vascular lesions. Upon entry into the second part of the duodenum, the mucosa appeared somewhat atrophic, with the underlying vascular architecture appearing prominent. The valvular conniventes appeared scalloped and the mucosa had a slight cobblestone appearance. Five biopsies were obtained. All of the biopsies revealed a flat mucosa with cuboidal surface epithelial cells instead of the usual columnar cells. The nuclei of these cuboidal cells had lost their usual basal polarity.

What is the likely diagnosis? The likely diagnosis is celiac sprue. Serum tissue transglutaminase antibodies were positive, further supporting the diagnosis.

Celiac sprue – a cause of isolated iron malabsorption

The duodenum is the site for the most efficient absorption of iron. Iron is also absorbed in the rest of the small intestine, but not as efficiently. Therefore, any mucosal disease of the duodenum or jejunum has the potential to give rise to malabsorption of food iron. Therefore, iron deficiency anemia is frequently seen in conditions such as celiac and tropical sprue. However, when the anemia is part of the total presentation of a malabsorption syndrome with steatorrhea, malnutrition and weight loss, the anemia is a secondary manifestation. However, it is not uncommon for milder forms of celiac sprue, presumably affecting only the first few inches of the small intestine, to present with iron deficiency anemia as the sole manifestation, the patient not having any steatorrhea or weight loss (see Chapter 4). Thus, especially in young adults, but in fact at any age, a work-up for iron deficiency anemia is not complete until the possibility of celiac sprue has been excluded (Figure 6.22).

Hookworm disease

This is the commonest cause of iron deficiency anemia in large parts of the developing world. *Ancylostoma duodenale* is seen in Southern Europe, North Africa, especially Egypt, Northern India, Northern and Central China, the Pacific Islands and southern USA. *Necator americanus* is prevalent in Southern India, Sri Lanka, the Far East, Australia and Southern Africa. Hookworm disease largely affects the inhabitants of countries where farm work is carried out without protective footwear. The filariform larvae enter through the skin between the toes and enter a venule or lymphatic. At the site of entry there is occasionally a transient rash. The larvae migrate via the venous system, the right side of the heart and into the pulmonary capillaries. They break the lining of the pulmonary capillaries to enter the alveolar spaces. They travel up the bronchial tree, trachea and larynx, and curve around the epiglottis to enter the pharynx and thence into the gastrointestinal tract. The average time of migration is around 10 days and during this time eosinophilia may be present. The larvae settle in the duodenum and small intestine and develop into the adult worm, which burrows its teeth into the mucosa, giving rise to mucosal bleeding. In the case of *A. duodenale* the blood loss is of the order of 0.2 ml/worm per day and for *N. americanus* it is around 0.03 ml/worm per day. Hookworm infestation is a chronic disease, because the life span of an adult worm is around 3–4 years. The diagnosis is generally made by stool examination, often using a concentration method. The characteristic oval egg with four blastomeres is seen under the microscope. Eggs or the adult worm on occasion may be seen in fluid obtained from duodenal aspiration. The adult worms are a third to half an inch long (8–12 mm) and can therefore be visualized at endoscopy.

Crohn's disease

Patients with active Crohn's disease involving the small intestine frequently have anemia of chronic disease. However, on occasion occult blood loss resulting from mucosal ulceration may result in iron deficiency anemia as well. This is especially important, as the cause of the anemia is frequently not recognized.

Carcinoma of the ampulla of Vater

For the most part these tumors present with obstructive jaundice, mimicking a carcinoma of the head of the pancreas. On occasion they may bleed intermittently with episodes of melena. In time this may result in iron deficiency anemia.

Adenomas and carcinomas

Adenomas and carcinomas of the small intestine are relatively uncommon lesions. They are seen quite frequently, though, in patients with familial adenomatous polyposis, often many years after the colon has been resected. Many of these occur in the ileum (Case history 7).

MEGALOBLASTIC ANEMIAS

Whenever one encounters an elevated MCV, one needs to suspect a megaloblastic anemia due to folic acid or vitamin B_{12} (cobalamin) deficiency. However, it is crucial to remember that an elevated MCV does not in and of itself mean that the patient has either a folate or cobalamin deficiency anemia. In fact, small elevations in the MCV are more often due to other causes (Table 6.7).

Table 6.7 Causes of macrocytosis

Macrocytosis without megaloblastosis
Reticulocytosis
    hemolysis
    following blood loss, including from a gastrointestinal source
Increased red blood cell membrane surface ('thin macrocytosis')
    chronic liver disease
    cholestasis
    splenectomy
Alcoholism
    folate deficiency
    chronic liver disease
    likely direct effect of alcohol on marrow (commonest
        reason)
Myelodysplastic anemias
5q- / refractory anemia syndrome
Myelophthisic anemias
Hypothyroidism (usually a normocytic anemia)

Megaloblastic anemias
Folate deficiency
Cobalamin deficiency
Rare causes
    thiamine-responsive megaloblastic anemia
    deficiency of enzymes involved in folate metabolism
    orotic aciduria
    transcobalamin II deficiency
    congenital causes of methylmalonic aciduria
    congenital causes of homocystinuria
    Lesch–Nyhan syndrome
    drug induced – chemotherapeutic agents

Table 6.8 Causes of folate deficiency

Dietary
    In developing countries with diets rich in high-starch foods
        and relatively few green vegetables and fruit. Especially
        exacerbated by the requirements of pregnancy
        and lactation
    Alcoholism with or without cirrhosis
Intestinal malabsorption due to mucosal disease of the proximal
small intestine
    Celiac sprue
    Tropical sprue
    Whipple's disease
    Small intestinal resection – extensive
Drugs
    Sulfasalazine
    Phenytoin, primidone, phenobarbital

Megaloblastic anemia due to folate deficiency

A good history usually points to the cause (Table 6.8). The work-up of intestinal malabsorption is described in Chapter 4. When folate deficiency accompanies a cause of intestinal malabsorption such as celiac disease, either the anemia or the symptoms of malabsorption syndrome (diarrhea, steatorrhea, weight loss, etc.) may be the initial presentation. In the latter case the etiology of the malabsorption is established (Chapter 4) and the anemia is diagnosed and treated. When folate deficiency anemia is the initial presentation, it is important to determine the etiology and not just to treat the folate deficiency (Figure 6.23).

Prior to initiating folic acid replacement therapy, it is essential to rule out an accompanying cobalamin deficiency as well. If the cobalamin deficiency is not treated concomitantly, then a neuropsychiatric crisis may be precipitated.

Megaloblastic anemia due to cobalamin deficiency

Every cell in the body requires cobalamin, since cobalamin is essential for DNA synthesis. All cobalamin in nature is of microbial origin. All mammals derive their cobalamin either directly or indirectly from microbial sources.

Cobalamin in the food chain

See Figure 6.24.

Biological role of cobalamin in mammalian metabolism

Two coenzyme forms of cobalamin, 5′ deoxyadenosyl cobalamin and methyl cobalamin, play key roles in mammalian metabolism (Figure 6.25).

This reaction links cobalamin to amino acid and odd chain fatty acid metabolism via propionyl CoA, and to heme synthesis and gluconeogenesis. In cobalamin deficiency, because an inadequate amount of 5′ deoxyadenosyl cobalamin is available, the serum level of methyl malonyl CoA would be elevated and an excess of methyl malonyl CoA is excreted in the urine.

In the reaction shown in Figure 6.26, cobalamin metabolism is related to that of folate and through the latter to DNA synthesis. In cobalamin deficiency an inadequate amount of methyl cobalamin is available and therefore the serum level of homocysteine is elevated and an excessive amount of homocysteine is excreted in the urine.

Role of cobalamin in the nervous system

In cobalamin-deficient animals and humans, demyelination and later axonal damage occur. The exact mechanisms are not well understood. Since adult nerve cells do not divide, it is clear that the inhibition of DNA synthesis is not the cause. Methylation reactions are important in the brain and *S*-adenosylmethionine is the key methyl group (CH_3) donor in the nervous system.

S-adenosylmethionine donates methyl groups to proteins, including myelin basic protein, and to fatty acids, phospholipids, polysaccharides, nucleic acids, porphyrins and biogenic amines such as catecholamines. In cobalamin deficiency the conversion of homocysteine to methionine and therefore the synthesis of *S*-adenosylmethionine is reduced. There is a surplus homocysteine resulting in the synthesis of *S*-adenosylhomocysteine in place of *S*-adenosylmethionine. *S*-adenosylhomocysteine in turn inhibits several of the methylation reactions in which *S*-adenosylmethionine is normally the methyl donor. Thus, a diminished availability of *S*-adenosylmethionine appears to be an important explanation for the neuropathology seen in cobalamin deficiency. Other mechanisms may also be at play in the pathogenesis of neuropathy induced by cobalamin deficiency, such as homocysteine-related damage to the vascular endothelium and the inhibition of *N*-methyl D-aspartate (NMDA) receptors.

Cobalamin absorption

Cobalamin absorption may be considered to occur in several stages:

(1) Gastric phase

   (a) release of food-bound cobalamin
   (b) binding to R protein;

(2) Duodenal phase;

(3) Small intestinal luminal phase;

(4) Ileal enterocyte phase

   (a) events on the enterocyte surface
   (b) events within and exit from the enterocyte.

The gastric phase   The gastric phase of cobalamin absorption has two components (Figure 6.27):

(1) Release of food-bound cobalamin. Cobalamin in food is present tightly bound to proteins. In the stomach by the action of hydrochloric acid and pepsin on food, cobalamin is released from its bound form.

(2) R protein–cobalamin complex formation. In the lumen of the stomach this free cobalamin meets two different glycoproteins:

   (a) The first is a large sialic acid-containing glycoprotein that is called R protein. It was initially so called because it moved rapidly on electrophoresis. R protein is very similar to transcobalamin I (TCI) and transcobalamin III (TCIII) which are cobalamin-binding proteins present in serum. R protein is mostly of salivary origin.

   (b) The second is gastric intrinsic factor (IF), a 45-kDa glycoprotein. Its existence was first described by the classic experiments of William Castle. In humans it is synthesized and secreted by parietal cells, which are present in the fundus and body of the stomach.

At the pH of the stomach, free cobalamin preferentially associates with R protein, forming the R protein–cobalamin complex. Thus, the R protein–cobalamin complex and free IF enter the duodenum.

The duodenal phase   In the lumen of the duodenum, where the pH is around 6.5, the R protein is destroyed by pancreatic proteases, and free cobalamin is released and binds to IF (Figure 6.28). IF is a very sturdy glycoprotein that withstands pancreatic and brush border proteases.

The small intestinal luminal phase   The IF–cobalamin complex formed in the duodenal lumen travels in the lumen of the jejunum, since there are no receptors for this complex on the surface of the jejunal enterocyte. The complex is sturdy and withstands digestion.

The ileal enterocyte phase   This phase has two components:

(1) Events on the enterocyte surface. The IF–cobalamin complex binds specifically to receptors on the microvillous membrane on the brush border of ileal enterocytes.

(2) Events within and exiting from the enterocyte. The entire IF–cobalamin complex is then internalized by receptor-mediated endocytosis. Within a vesicular compartment in the enterocyte the cobalamin is released from IF. The free cobalamin is then bound to TCII within the enterocyte. The TCII–cobalamin complex is released from the basilateral side of the enterocyte into the portal circulation. Cobalamin thus makes its way to the liver, where it is stored. There is an enterohepatic circulation of cobalamin.

Cobalamin malabsorption

Cobalamin malabsorption is summarized in Table 6.9.

Table 6.9 Cobalamin malabsorption

The gastric phase of cobalamin absorption
Failure of release from food-bound cobalamin
   atrophic gastritis
   subtotal gastrectomy
Absence of intrinsic factor (IF)
   pernicious anemia
   congenital absence of IF
   congenitally defective IF
     biologically inert
     rapidly degraded

The duodenal phase of cobalamin absorption
Diminished pancreatic proteases and bicarbonate
   chronic pancreatitis
   total pancreatectomy
Low duodenal pH rendering pancreatic proteases ineffectual
   Zollinger–Ellison syndrome

The small intestinal luminal phase of cobalamin absorption
Binding of IF–cobalamin complex by:
   bacteria
     blind loop syndrome
     stagnant loop syndrome
   fish tape worm *(Diphyllobothrium latum)*
Low ileal pH ?
   Zollinger–Ellison syndrome

The ileal enterocyte phase of cobalamin absorption
Surface events
   ileal resection
   ileal mucosal disease
     tropical sprue
     celiac sprue (rare)
Events within the enterocyte
   congenital deficiency of transcobalamin II
   Immerslund–Gräsbeck syndrome
   drugs
     colchicine
     biguanides
     para-aminosalicylate

The detection of cobalamin malabsorption

The Schilling test This is named after Robert F. Schilling, who first described the test.

(1) *Part I Schilling test*

The test

(a) Radiolabeled free cobalamin is administered orally to a patient after an overnight fast (1 μCi in 0.5–1.0 μg).

(b) An hour later an injection of 1000 μg of non-radiolabeled cobalamin is administered intramuscularly. This saturates liver binding sites for cobalamin, so that the absorbed radiolabeled cobalamin is not held up in the liver and has the opportunity of being excreted by the kidneys.

(c) Urine is collected for 24 h after the administration of the radiolabelled cobalamin.

Interpretation

If less than 7–10% of the administered radiolabelled dose of cobalamin is excreted in the urine, it suggests cobalamin malabsorption. It does not discriminate between a gastric or a small intestinal cause for cobalamin malabsorption.

(2) *Part II Schilling test*

The test

Performed like the part I Schilling test except that, instead of administration of radiolabeled free cobalamin, the radiolabeled cobalamin bound to IF (usually hog IF is used) is administered orally.

Interpretation

If more than 7–10% of the administered dose of radiolabeled cobalamin is excreted in the urine, it would mean that the patient most probably has pernicious anemia. The congenitally defective IF is a very rare condition and would be seen in young children. If the results of the part II test are still low (i.e. < 7 to 10%) the cause of the cobalamin deficiency is not a lack of IF. In such cases the cause would be a disorder affecting either the duodenal, luminal small intestinal phase or the ileal enterocyte phase of cobalamin absorption. If, clinically, the cause is believed to be bacterial overgrowth, then the part II Schilling test should be repeated after treatment with antibiotics, at which time it should be normal.

Note: It is now possible to perform parts I and II of the Schilling test using two different isotopes of cobalamin, one to label the free cobalamin and the other to label the IF-bound cobalamin.

(3) False-positive Schilling test (falsely low urinary radiolabeled cobalamin excretion)

(a) If the patient has severe megaloblastic anemia due to either folate or cobalamin deficiency, the ileal enterocytes are not normal and a falsely low Schilling test result would be obtained. Therefore, Schilling tests should be

Table 6.10 Interpretation of the Schilling test

Disorder	Schilling test, part I	Schilling test, part II	Modified Schilling test (testing for food-bound cobalamin)
Failure to release food cobalamin	normal	normal	abnormal
Pernicious anemia	abnormal	normal	—
Chronic pancreatitis	abnormal	abnormal	—
Bacterial overgrowth	abnormal	abnormal	—
Bacterial overgrowth after a course of antibiotics	normal	normal	—
Ileal resection	abnormal	abnormal	
Ileal mucosal disease, e.g. tropical sprue	abnormal	abnormal	—

performed only after correcting the folate or cobalamin deficiency.

(b) If the patient has edema or ascites or has renal failure, then the absorbed radiolabeled cobalamin may not be adequately excreted. Therefore, a normal serum creatinine level and the absence of edema or ascites are prerequisites for the performance of a Schilling test.

(4) False-negative Schilling test (normal urinary radiolabeled cobalamin excretion in the face of cobalamin malabsorption)

This occurs in what is probably the commonest cause of cobalamin malabsorption, atrophic gastritis, and is generally seen in the elderly population. It may also be seen many years following a subtotal gastrectomy. In such patients, as mentioned earlier, the cobalamin is not released from its bound form in food, owing to achlorhydria, even though enough endogenous IF is present. Increasingly, a group of patients with food cobalamin malabsorption is being described in whom the cause of the non-release of cobalamin from its bound form in food is not a lack of acid and pepsin, but some yet unknown mechanism. *Helicobacter pylori* infection of the stomach may play some role in such patients. In any event, when a regular part I Schilling test is performed in these patients using crystalline free radiolabeled cobalamin, it is adequately absorbed, because endogenous IF is present in the stomach. There are ways of performing a modified Schilling test with the radiolabeled

cobalamin bound to meat or egg. If such a modified Schilling test were performed, then it would show an abnormally low excretion of cobalamin compared to that seen in a normal person.

The interpretation of the Schilling tests is summarized in Table 6.10.

Case history 11

A 76-year-old widower living by himself has been brought in by his daughter, who currently works in Europe. She had come to see her father after receiving a telephone call from a neighbor, who said that of late her father appeared to be considerably 'slower' than his normal self. Her father now did not always recognize his old neighbors and on occasion appeared confused, having been observed trying to enter the wrong apartment at least twice over the past 3 months. Formerly meticulous about his dressing, he now frequently appeared dishevelled. The daughter found that he did recognize her. On the whole, he remembered events from the past, but his recent memory was poor. It was difficult to hold his attention over a prolonged conversation. He tended to become irritable over small issues, which she felt was totally out of character with his usual pleasant disposition. He also appeared quite depressed. He had been in good physical health but for some osteoarthritis in both knees and mild systolic hypertension. He had had an appendectomy and cholecystectomy several years previously. He was never known to have abused alcohol and was not a smoker. It was unclear how much he had been eating, but he looked distinctly thinner. Physical examination revealed a thin-built elderly gentleman. The blood pressure was 175/85 mmHg.

Examinations of the heart, lungs and abdomen were normal. He was oriented to person and place but was not precise with time. His speech was normal and he was not confabulating. On a modified Folstein Mini-Mental Status Examination he scored 22 (< 24 suggests the possibility of dementia). His cranial nerve function, motor system examination, coordination, gait and deep tendon reflexes were normal. The Babinski test was negative and there were no involuntary movements. Tactile sensations were intact, he denied any 'pins and needles' or pricking sensations in his hands or feet, and vibration sense was lost in the toes but preserved in the fingers. Position sense was normal and the Romberg's test was negative. The hemoglobin was 11.4 g/dl, MCV 97 fl, and platelet and white cell counts were normal. The blood smear appeared normal. His serum electrolytes, blood urea nitrogen, creatinine and liver and thyroid function tests were all normal. A Venereal Disease Research Laboratories (VDRL) test was negative. A CT scan of the head revealed cerebral atrophy appropriate to the patient's age without marked hippocampal atrophy. A few old lacunar infarcts were evident. His red cell folic acid level was 155 ng/ml (> 150 ng/ml normal) and his serum vitamin B_{12} (cobalamin) level was low normal at 230 pg/ml (normal > 200 pg/ml).

What other tests should be ordered? The physician appropriately decided on a work-up for an etiology of dementia. Other than the assessment of higher mental functions, the physical examination was quite normal, except for a loss in vibration sense over the toes. The patient was mildly anemic, with an MCV that was at the upper limits of normal. Most endocrine and metabolic causes of dementia are excluded by the history, physical examination and the laboratory tests ordered. Likewise, multi-infarct dementia, Parkinson's disease and other neurological disorders that can cause dementia in the elderly are also excluded. The physician, perhaps guided by the failure of the patient to appreciate vibratory stimuli in his toes, had ordered a serum vitamin B_{12} level, which had returned in the low normal range. In any event the patient did not report paresthesias, nor was there evidence of ataxia, spasticity or a positive Romberg's test to sustain a diagnosis of subacute combined degeneration of the cord. Nevertheless, since a diagnosis of cobalamin deficiency had been entertained, it was mandatory to rule it out despite a normal MCV, the absence of macro-ovalocytes or multilobed polymorphonuclear leukocytes on the blood smear or evidence of a marked sensory neuropathy or posterior and lateral column disease of the spinal cord. Serum levels of methylmalonic acid and homocysteine were ordered, and were reported to be very high in both instances.

Cobalamin deficiency – serial progression A negative cobalamin balance can be present for years before a low serum level of cobalamin is detected. The earliest markers are perhaps measurements of red blood cell cobalamin and holotranscobalamin II (holo TCII). The latter is the sum of TCII-bound cobalamin and unbound TCII in serum. Both red cell cobalamin and holo-TCII are tests currently available only in research facilities. Serum levels of methylmalonic acid (MMA) and homocysteine, on the other hand, are now readily available and high levels are frequently present even before macrocytosis is evident (Figure 6.29).

Points to note from this case:

(1) Cobalamin deficiency must be suspected in elderly patients who present with irritability, agitation, apathy, somnolence, intellectual deterioration, confusion or symptoms suggestive of depression or dementia.

(2) Cobalamin deficiency should likewise be considered in patients with known dementia who present with a worsening of their symptoms.

(3) When anemia or macrocytosis is not present and when serum cobalamin levels are in the normal range, it is essential to take the next step and to order serum levels of MMA and homocysteine.

What is the likely cause of this patient's cobalamin deficiency state? From the history it appears that the patient does not have chronic pancreatitis or a disease involving the ileal mucosa such as tropical sprue. His age precludes a diagnosis of several of the congenital syndromes mentioned earlier. Either pernicious anemia or an inability to absorb food-bound cobalamin is the most likely etiology. A Schilling test would distinguish between the two.

Addisonian pernicious anemia

Pernicious anemia, initially described in 1849 by Thomas Addison, is an autoimmune disease. The hallmark lesion is an autoimmune atrophic gastritis that affects the fundus and body of the stomach (type A or type I atrophic gastritis).

On endoscopy, the normal gastric folds in the fundus and body of the stomach are found to be either absent or greatly diminished. Because of the mucosal atrophy, the underlying vascular architecture appears very prominent and easily visualized.

The microscopic appearance shows that parietal and chief cells are lost and replaced by mucus cells. The lamina propria is infiltrated with plasma cells, T lymphocytes and B lymphocytes. The mucosa of the antrum of the stomach is spared.

Physiological consequences of mucosal atrophy are parietal cell loss and chief cell loss. Parietal cell loss leads to achlorhydria. The normal feedback inhibition of gastrin secretion by acid is impaired, leading to hypergastrinemia. Absent IF secretion causes impaired cobalamin absorption, leading to megaloblastic anemia. Chief cell loss leads to low levels of serum pepsinogen I.

Pathogenesis – an autoimmune disease

Factors that favor autoimmunity as the pathogenesis of the disease:

(1) There are associated autoimmune diseases such as Hashimoto's thyroiditis, systemic lupus erythematosus, type I diabetes mellitus and Addison's disease.

(2) Treatment with immunosuppressive agents such as corticosteroids and azathioprine reverses the histological lesion. Thus, parietal and chief cells can regenerate from stem cells as long as the immune-mediated process is suppressed.

(3) Three types of serum antibodies to normal antigens are seen in patients with pernicious anemia:

(a) Parietal cell antibodies. These are autoantibodies against the proton pump. Briefly, it is a H^+/K^+ ATPase that constitutes most of the protein lining the secretory canaliculi of the parietal cell where acid is produced. Autoantibodies are made against both the α and the β subunits of H^+/K^+ ATPase. While these antibodies can be shown *in vitro* to lyse parietal cells by a complement-mediated mechanism, *in vivo* there is no way that circulating autoantibodies can have access to the secretory canaliculi. Therefore, they are unlikely to be responsible for the gastric lesion in pernicious anemia.

(b) Intrinsic factor type I or blocking antibodies. These are autoantibodies against the portion of the IF molecule to which cobalamin is bound. Thus, when these antibodies attach to IF, they block the binding of cobalamin to IF. They are seen in about 70% of patients with pernicious anemia.

(c) Intrinsic factor type 2 or binding antibodies. These are autoantibodies against the portion of the IF molecule that attaches to the receptor on the surface of ileal cells. They are identified in only 20–30% of patients with pernicious anemia using older methods of assay, although recently, using more sophisticated methods, they appear to be identifiable in a much larger number of patients.

(4) Several immune-mediated models of gastric atrophy can be generated in animals that resemble the lesion of pernicious anemia. One such example that throws considerable light on the pathogenesis of pernicious anemia is a gastritis model in BALB/c mice.

(a) Gastritis and serum antibodies against gastric H^+/K^+ ATPase develops when normal 2–4-day-old BALB/c mice undergo a thymectomy or are treated with cyclophosphamide.

(b) Gastritis and serum antibodies against gastric H^+/K^+ ATPase develop in normal adult thymectomized mice that are irradiated or immunized against gastric H^+/K^+ ATPase.

(c) Transfer of CD4 cells from these mice with gastritis produce gastritis and serum antibodies against gastric H^+/K^+ ATPase in recipient mice.

(d) A single injection of neutralizing anti-interferon-γ antibody prevents the development of gastritis, suggesting that Th1-type cytokines are related to the pathogenesis of the gastritis.

(e) When transgenic BALB/c mice that express the β subunit of H^+/K^+ ATPase in their thymus are similarly treated (i.e. 2–4-day-old mice with thymectomy alone or adult mice with thymectomy plus radiation or immunization with gastric H^+/K^+ ATPase), they do not develop gastritis.

Based on the above, it appears that immune gastritis in BALB/c mice and perhaps human pernicious anemia

Table 6.11 Neuropsychiatric manifestations of cobalamin deficiency

Brain (psychiatric)
Irritability, agitation, apathy, somnolence, depression-like symptoms, intellectual deterioration, confusion, dementia

Peripheral nerves
Paresthesias, loss of vibration sense, loss of position sense and loss of tactile sensations (uncommon)

Spinal cord
Posterior columns
   loss of vibration sense, loss of position sense (later)
Lateral columns
   ataxia, spasticity

Optic nerve
Rare. Begins with symmetrical centrocecal scotomata from atrophy in the papillomacular bundles

have the following pathogenesis: a complex of a major histocompatibility complex (MHC) class II molecule and the β subunit of the proton pump (H⁺/K⁺ ATPase) on antigen-presenting cells binds to the T-cell antigen receptors of CD4 Th1 cells. The latter are activated and release Th1-type cytokines. Among these, interferon-γ appears to be important in producing the gastric lesion (Figure 6.30).

Epidemiology

Pernicious anemia has been reported largely in Western countries in Caucasians over the age of 60 years. However, the condition has now been reported with some frequency in young Latino women in the USA.

Clinical presentation

Neuropsychiatric manifestations Many of the psychiatric features and even some neurological manifestations such as paresthesias may develop at a time of negative cobalamin balance and early cobalamin deficiency (Table 6.11). At this phase the serum cobalamin level is in the normal range, macrocytosis or multilobed polymorphonuclear cells are not yet evident on the peripheral blood smear and anemia is yet to develop (Figure 6.29). These clinical manifestations are those of cobalamin deficiency due to any cause, not just pernicious anemia.

Symptoms related to anemia Fatigue, shortness of breath and high-output cardiac failure.

Mucous membranes of the mouth Glossitis and stomatitis.

Skin Hyperpigmentation of the skin, especially of the palms, digits of hands and feet and flexure creases. This is due to increased deposition of melanin in the skin and may occur with a megaloblastic anemia due to folate or cobalamin deficiency. Interspersed patches of vitiligo are much more specific for pernicious anemia, both being autoimmune disorders.

Hair Premature graying of the hair has been mentioned since the earliest descriptions of the disease.

Gastrointestinal Manifestations may be a carcinoid tumor or adenocarcinoma.

(1) Carcinoid tumors arise from enterochromaffin-like cells. There was a 13-fold increase in gastric carcinoid tumors (fundus and body) in one Swedish study in pernicious anemia patients. Of pernicious anemia patients, 2% develop carcinoid tumors. Only 2% of carcinoid tumors overall arise in the stomach; 80% are asymptomatic. Most of them are submucosal, and hence may be missed at endoscopy. The sequence is: achlorhydria leads to feedback inhibition of antral gastrin release being abolished, causing hypergastrinemia, leading to enterochromaffin-like cell hyperplasia, and finally to carcinoid tumor.

(2) Adenocarcinoma. There was a three-fold increase in patients with pernicious anemia in one Swedish study. The prevalence of gastric cancer is low in Western countries, where pernicious anemia is common. Therefore, screening endoscopy is not recommended (Figure 6.31).

Diagnosis

Determine cobalamin deficiency There are tests available in most clinical services that would establish the diagnosis of cobalamin deficiency: lowered levels of serum cobalamin, elevated MCV and macrocytosis on blood smear; hypersegmented polymorphonuclear leukocytes and frank megaloblastosis on bone marrow.

Determine the etiology Very high levels of serum gastrin are very suggestive. The Schilling test part I is low, almost zero. The Schilling test part II corrects with concomitant administration of IF.

Failure to release food cobalamin

The most likely diagnosis for the patient described in Case history 7 is either pernicious anemia or the failure to release food cobalamin.

Epidemiology This is the commonest cause of cobalamin deficiency seen. It affects the elderly more commonly.

Pathogenesis The pathogenesis is as follows:

(1) *Atrophic gastritis. H. pylori* infection of the antrum causes chronic active superficial gastritis, leading to antral atrophic gastritis. *H. pylori* infection of the fundus/body causes fundus/body superficial gastritis, leading to fundus/body atrophic gastritis. Both can develop simultaneously. The degree of atrophic gastritis is less severe than in full-blown pernicious anemia. Patients have achlorhydria but do secrete enough IF to give a normal Schilling test (Table 6.10).

(2) *Partial gastrectomy.* These patients do not as a rule become cobalamin deficient for years after the partial gastrectomy. Very likely, the gastric remnant over time becomes atrophic.

(3) *Unknown etiology.* When gastric acid secretory tests are performed, some patients who are unable to release cobalamin from food are found not to be achlorhydric. It is unclear as to why they are unable to release cobalamin from food. A possible role for *H. pylori* by a mechanism little understood has been proposed as one cause.

Diagnosis This requires a high index of clinical suspicion. Older individuals with signs of new-onset dementia or worsening of old dementia should be considered (Table 6.11). Confirmatory tests are:

(1) Low serum cobalamin level. A normal level does not rule it out;

(2) Elevated levels of serum homocystine and methyl malonic acid;

(3) Achlorhydria often present (no need to check for it);

(4) Serum gastrin level may be high, seldom anywhere near the elevations seen in pernicious anemia;

(5) Normal Schilling test parts I and II;

(6) Abnormal modified Schilling test using food radiolabeled cobalamin.

CHAPTER 7

The patient with acute rectal bleeding

INTRODUCTION

Acute bleeding from the rectum does not always imply that the source is colonic: frequently the source may be a large hemorrhage proximal to the ligament of Trietz. Figure 7.1 outlines the questions that need to be asked when encountering a patient with acute bleeding from the rectum, and also the order in which they should be asked. The first two questions need to be asked simultaneously when encountering a patient with acute rectal hemorrhage:

(1) Does the bleeding arise from an upper (proximal to the ligament of Trietz) or a lower (distal to the ligament of Trietz, but mostly colonic) source?

(2) Is the blood being passed from the rectum due to a bloody diarrhea or is it due to hematochezia?

IS IT AN UPPER OR A LOWER SOURCE?

When hemorrhage from an upper source, such as from esophageal or gastric varices or a peptic ulcer, is large and brisk the patients may pass bright red blood rectally. When the bleeding is smaller and slower, the patient has melena (black tarry stool). It is therefore essential to exclude an upper source of gastrointestinal hemorrhage when one sees a patient with hematochezia (Figure 7.2).

The most efficient way to exclude an upper source when the patient's presentation leaves doubt is by an emergency esophagogastroduodenoscopy (EGD). The procedure is performed after the patient has been hemodynamically stabilized as far as possible. A nasogastric tube is a poor substitute, as it is more uncomfortable than an EGD and often does not provide the answer.

BLOODY DIARRHEA OR HEMATOCHEZIA?

When a lower (usually colonic) source is suspected, one needs to ask the question as to whether the rectal bleeding is due to hematochezia or to a bloody diarrhea.

Usually the differentiation between a bloody diarrhea and hematochezia is easy to make based on the presence or absence of the symptoms listed in Figure 7.3. However, on occasion the difference may not be readily apparent and a sigmoidoscopy or even colonoscopy may be needed. Patients with colitis due to enterohemorrhagic *E. coli* will often present with a bloody diarrhea that may be very difficult on history alone to differentiate from a diverticular hemorrhage, for example.

BLOODY DIARRHEA

The common causes of a bloody diarrhea, referred to as dysentery when infectious, are listed in Table 7.1.

Infection

All of the bacteria listed in Table 7.1 may cause only non-bloody diarrhea. When they do give rise to dysentery, (a term commonly reserved for an infectious diarrhea with blood and mucus in the stool), the bloody diarrhea often develops later (Figure 7.4). If the organism does not invade or does so only minimally, the diarrhea is not bloody.

Systemic symptoms most often accompany and may even antecede the diarrhea. Mild fever often accompanies an episode of dysentery. Abdominal pain, often quite severe and frequently colicky, together with vomiting is invariably present. Patients almost always

Table 7.1 Conditions that may give rise to a bloody diarrhea

Infection – acute infectious diarrheas
   Campylobacter jejuni
   Salmonella
   Shigella
   Enterohemorrhagic *Escherichia coli*
   Clostridium difficile
   Entamoeba histolytica
Inflammatory – non-infectious
   Ulcerative colitis – first presentation
   Crohn's colitis – first presentation
Ischemic colitis

Table 7.2 Causes of hematochezia

Upper GI sources
Peptic ulcer
Esophageal, gastric or duodenal varices
Mallory-Weiss tear
Dieulafoy's lesion
Previous abdominal aortic aneurysm repair
Tumor eroding into an artery (rare)
Hemobilia (rare)
Pseudoaneurysm rupture into GI tract (rare)
Gastric or duodenal angiodysplasia (rare)
Hereditary hemorrhagic telangiectasia (rare)

Lower GI sources
Diverticular hemorrhage
Colonic or small intestinal angiodysplasia
Hemorrhoids
Rectal varices in portal hypertension
Colonic carcinoma (uncommon)

complain of malaise and lassitude. A low-grade fever is frequently present with *Salmonella* and *Shigella* species. The fever may be high on occasion.

Inflammatory, non-infectious causes

Inflammatory bowel disease, either ulcerative colitis or Crohn's colitis may present for the first time as a bloody diarrhea. Again, systemic symptoms and abdominal pain of the type described for acute infectious diarrheas are usually present.

Ischemia

Ischemic colitis and not ischemia in the small bowel is part of the differential diagnosis of hematochezia. Iscemic colitis is discussed at length later in this chapter.

HEMATOCHEZIA

The common causes of hematochezia are listed in Table 7.2.

Case history 1

A 77-year-old man awoke in the morning feeling light-headed. Shortly after breakfast he felt an urgency to move his bowels. When he did, he noted passing some fecal matter at the start, but most of the bowel movement consisted of passing large amounts of bright red blood. He now felt very dizzy and was just able to reach his bed. His son called for the city's Emergency Services, but before the ambulance could come he had two more bowel movements, this time passing red to maroon "stool". The second of these bowel movements was described as a mix of blood and blood clots. He had no history of having eaten outside his home in the past week, nor of travel. He had been in his usual state of health, and had not noted any lethargy or malaise until the light-headedness in the morning. He felt no abdominal pain or discomfort and had not vomited, nor even felt nauseated. He had no fever. He suffered from ischemic cardiomyopathy, but his cardiac failure was well controlled on an angiotensin converting enzyme inhibitor, a diuretic and a low dose of a beta-blocker. He had not noted any recent change in his exercise tolerance. He appeared pale, had a systolic blood pressure of 85 mmHg, (his usual blood pressure being around 140/70 mmHg), a small volume rapid pulse that was irregularly irregular. His jugular venous pressure was not elevated and no third heart sound was noted on auscultation of the heart. Auscultation of his lungs revealed vesicular breath sounds of good intensity and a few crackles at the bases of both lungs. The abdominal and rectal examinations were completely normal except for red blood on the glove noted after the rectal examination. On admission his hematocrit was 40, hemoglobin 13.2 g/dl, white cell and platelet counts, prothrombin time and partial thromboplastin time were all within the normal range. Serum electrolytes and blood glucose were also normal, his blood urea nitrogen (BUN) was 45 mg/dl and serum creatinine 1.6 mg/dl.

Following the algorithm outlined in Figure 7.2, an upper GI source cannot be excluded since the patient is hemodynamically unstable with a supine systolic blood pressure of 85 mmHg. The fact that the patient is not vomiting blood nor has 'coffee grounds' emesis does not rule out an upper source. One could lavage the

Table 7.3 Once an upper GI source is excluded as the cause of hematochezia the following situations require an urgent evaluation of the cause of bleeding

Patients with obvious continuing hematochezia
Patients who remain hemodynamically unstable despite
    resuscitation and transfusion
Patients who may be stable but who continue to
    require blood transfusions beyond 5 units of packed cells
Patients whose bleeding recurs after having
    initially ceased

stomach using a nasogastric tube to try to distinguish between an upper and a lower GI source of bleeding. For reasons mentioned earlier this is not the intervention of choice. Once the patient is hemodynamically stabilized he would benefit most from an upper endoscopy. In this man the upper endoscopy is normal. Now what should one do?

When to do further investigation? The vast majority of lower GI hemorrhages stop on their own. Such patients may undergo elective colonoscopy after the colon has been cleaned out well. There is no urgency for immediate investigation.

When is investigation of the etiology of lower GI hemorrhage urgently required? Some situations requiring urgent investigation are listed in Table 7.3. There are two methods available to evaluate the source of lower GI hemorrhage when urgent evaluation is deemed essential: urgent colonoscopy, and radionuclide imaging followed by angiography.

Urgent colonoscopy

Until a decade ago or less, radionuclide imaging followed by angiography, if the former test suggested the site of hemorrhage, was the standard of practice. Whereas some clinicians still prefer this approach, an increasing number of gastroenterologists are moving towards urgent colonoscopy. Such patients need to have their colon well cleaned out using a large amount of orally administered polyethelene glycol based cleansing solution (or via a nasogastric tube). Frequently the volume required to clean the colon adequately is considerably more than for a routine colonoscopy, between 2 or 3 gallons. The patient described in Case history 1 underwent an urgent colonoscopy after an adequate colonic cleansing and a bleeding diverticulum was detected. The site of hemorrhage was injected

with 2 ml of 1:10 000 dilution of epinephrine and the bleeding stopped (Figure 7.5).

Radionuclide imaging

Two types of radionuclide imaging are available, each with their own advantages and disadvantages. The first is ^{99m}Tc sulfur colloid scintiscan: the radionuclide is directly injected intravenously and the patient scanned by a gamma camera. This technique has the advantages that it is easier to organize than a labeled red blood cell scan, and gives excellent results if the bleeding is occurring at the time the scan is done and at a rate of 0.1 ml/min or greater. The disadvantages are that the scan is negative if the bleeding has temporarily stopped or slowed down at the time the scan is done. However, lower GI bleeds are often intermittent, thus the window for obtaining a positive result is short. Also, since activity of the radionuclide is present in the liver and spleen, sources of hemorrhages at the colonic flexures may be difficult to appreciate. Likewise, activity in the bladder may interfere with bleeding form the ileum.

The second type is ^{99m}Tc pertechnetate labeled red cells, where the patient's red blood cells (RBC) are labeled *in vitro* and reinjected. The advantages in this case are that, since the isotope stays in the circulation for much longer, it is possible to inject the tagged RBCs into the patient and periodically observe the patient for evidence of bleeding. Also, there is no interference at the colonic flexures and no bladder activity. However, the technique is much more of an organizational problem than a sulfur colloid scintiscan. Furthermore, it calls for considerable manpower utilization. If bleeding is not seen at the time of injection of the isotope, then this technology has an advantage over the sulfur colloid scintiscan only if the patient is observed under the gamma camera at relatively short intervals. Otherwise, if bleeding occurs between scanning intervals, the source of the bleed will not be identified. As mentioned below, this patient received a colonoscopy. Figure 7.6 shows the result of a positive RBC scan done on another patient who had bleeding at the site of a polyp resected 7 days previously.

Angiography

This involves selective injection of the celiac, superior and inferior mesenteric arteries (Figure 7.7). The advantages of this method are that an accurate identification of the site of hemorrhage is made and even more

Table 7.4 Differentiation between diverticulitis and diverticular hemorrhage

	Diverticulitis	*Diverticular hemorrhage*
Site	Predominantly in the sigmoid colon	Right side of colon: 75% Left side of colon: 25%
Pathogenesis	A minute perforation of a single diverticulum that is usually confined and not free. May resolve gradually on antibiotic therapy or else an abscess could develop	The bleeding is not the result of inflammation or infection, but is from an ectatic arteriole coursing the dome or neck of a diverticulum that bleeds

precise localization is achieved by selective injection of smaller arterial branches. It is much more specific than a radionuclide scan and the false positive rate is very low. It may provide identification of angiodysplasia even when the lesions are not bleeding (see Chapter 6). In the event a lesion is seen bleeding, the hemorrhage can be arrested by angiographic embolization techniques. However, the disadvantage is that the method is useful only if the patient is bleeding at around 1 ml/min at the time the dye is injected. Since most lesions bleed intermittently, the bleeding site is often not visualized.

Diverticular hemorrhage

Diverticula in Western countries are much more frequent in the sigmoid and descending colon than in the right side of the colon. In Japan, where diverticular disease is much less common, but is an emerging disease, right-sided diverticula are more commonly seen. It is therefore not surprising that in Western countries most attacks of diverticulitis are most commonly seen in the sigmoid colon. This is not the case for diverticula that bleed. Diverticula located in the right side of the colon are more likely to bleed than those in the left side of the colon (Table 7.4).

Case history 2

A 73-year-old man was brought to the Emergency Department complaining of passing a large amount of bright red blood and clots per rectum. He had not had non-bloody diarrhea prior to passing red blood nor any similar episodes previously. No systemic symptoms were present. He had no abdominal pain, nausea or vomiting. He had no history of recent travel, family members with diarrhea or of eating out recently. There is no abdominal tenderness or distension. No masses are palpable. Bowel sounds are normal. He continued

to bleed and required urgent colonoscopy, like the patient in the previous case. A bleeding angiodysplastic lesion was seen (Figure 7.8). Bleeding ultimately stopped after injection of the lesion with epinephrine (1:10 000).

Angiodysplasia

Angiodysplasias (or vascular ectasia) have been discussed in Chapter 6 as sources of slow or occult bleeding giving rise to iron deficiency anemia. They may on occasion present with brisk hemorrhage, the patient presenting with a large amount of bright red blood and clots per rectum (Figure 7.9). For more details on angiodysplasia see Chapter 6.

Colonic adenomatous polyps and cancers

Colonic adenomas and cancers, when symptomatic, generally present with occult blood loss and iron deficiency anemia. More proximal lesions are more likely to present in this fashion. Larger left colon lesions, and occasionally large lesions more proximally too, may present with hematochezia. Usually though, the bleeding is not nearly as brisk as with diverticula and angiodysplasias (Figure 7.10).

Case history 3

An 86-year-old man with dementia and several comorbid medical conditions, who was generally constipated and required enemas and laxatives to move his bowels, was transferred from a nursing home after having passed large amounts of bright red blood and clots rectally. The bleeding did not stop in hospital and after several tap water enemas and a polyethylene glycol–saline clean-out administered through a nasogastric tube, the patient underwent a colonoscopy. Blood was seen filling the lumen of the left colon and transverse colon. The ascending colon and cecum contained much less blood and were adequately examined and found not to contain any lesion. Despite the rather heroic effort to clean the colon, due to the patient's constipation there was a fair amount of stool in the left colon and transverse colon. No site of bleeding was found while advancing the colonoscope. However, on the way out, a deep actively bleeding stercoral ulcer was noted in the rectum. The bleeding stopped after the injection of epinephrine, but recurred the next day. A sigmoidoscopy was done the second time and the bleeding stopped once again, only to recur several hours later. The patient had required several units of packed red cell transfusions. He was ultimately referred to surgery, where the bleeding site was localized and the vessel plicated. An endoscopic image of a stercoral ulcer is shown in Figure 7.11.

STERCORAL ULCERS

Stercoral ulcers occur in severely constipated people who have fecal impaction. As a direct consequence of the impacted stool, pressure necrosis of the mucosa and submucosa occurs. Deep ulcers result which can hemorrhage massively at times. These ulcers are frequently missed at colonoscopy on account of the stool. The rectum and sigmoid colon are the most common sites, although they may develop in other areas of the colon as well. Rarely these ulcers may perforate.

Case history 4

A 40-year-old patient with a history of quite considerable alcohol use and two previous attacks of alcoholic acute pancreatitis in the previous year was admitted for passing large amounts of blood per rectum and had thereafter become very lightheaded. On this occasion he did not have any abdominal pain, nausea or vomiting. He had stopped using alcohol since his last hospitalization for pancreatitis 4 months earlier. He was not taking aspirin or non-steroidal anti-inflammatory medications. He had no previous history of peptic ulcer disease or chronic heartburn. The patient was clammy, had a pulse rate of 120/min with a very small pulse pressure and a systolic blood pressure of 75 mmHg. There were no peripheral stigmata of liver disease such as icterus, palmar erythema, spider navei, Dupuytren's contractures, gynecomastia, parotid enlargement or testicular atrophy. Other than the tachycardia, the heart and lung examinations were normal. The abdomen was soft, non-tender, not distended, no masses were palpable and there was no evidence clinically for organomegaly. Bowel sounds were increased. The rectal examination was normal except for bright red blood on the glove. The patient's hemoglobin was 11.5 g/dl, hematocrit was 35, WBC $5.1 \times 10^9/l$, platelet count $210 \times 10^9/l$, prothrombin time and partial thromboplastin time were normal, serum electrolytes were normal, BUN 70 mg/dl, serum creatinine 1.7 mg/dl.

The cause for the massive hematochezia was not immediately evident, yet since he was hemodynamically unstable, an upper gastrointestinal source of hemorrhage (i.e. one proximal to the ligament of Trietz) had to be excluded, even though the patient had not vomited blood. The patient's young age made the likelihood of the two commonest causes of massive hematochezia, diverticular hemorrhage and angiodysplasia, extremely unlikely. The markedly elevated ratio of BUN to serum creatinine of 41 also suggested an upper gastrointestinal source.

A nasogastric tube could have been passed but instead it was appropriately decided to endoscope the patient as soon as he had been stabilized. The stomach was full of blood and clots. The endoscope was removed, and the stomach was lavaged with a large volume of water using a large-bore stomach tube before reinserting the endoscope. While much better visualization was obtained after the lavage, there were still large clots in the fundus of the stomach that made visualization of that region and the cardia very difficult. Nevertheless, esophageal varices, or an antral or duodenal ulcer could be excluded with confidence. The hemorrhage had stopped and no fresh oozing of blood was noted. The endoscopist could not exclude a Mallory-Weiss tear or a lesion under the fundic clots such as a Dieuafoy's lesion, angiodysplasia, a high gastric ulcer, tumor or gastric varices.

The patient was adequately stabilized overnight and endoscoped again 24 hours later. Good visualization was possible this time, there being no blood or clots in the stomach. Gastric varices, in particular one very large fundic varix, were seen on endoscopy. These had not been visualized at endoscopy the previous day as they had been hidden by clots in the fundus of the stomach. No esophageal varices were evident and no other lesions were seen. As the endoscopist was about to complete the procedure, he saw blood beginning to spurt from the large varix (Figure 7.12). Hemorrhage was stopped by injecting a sclerosant.

Points to note from this case:

(1) Even patients who present with massive hematochezia from an upper gastrointestinal source may on occasion not vomit blood.

(2) An upper gastrointestinal source must be excluded when a patient with hematochezia presents as hemodynamically unstable. It is unlikely that a patient presenting with bright red blood per rectum in large quantities will have an upper gastrointestinal source responsible for the hemorrhage and be hemodynamically stable.

(3) A markedly elevated BUN/creatinine ratio is very suggestive of an upper gastrointestinal hemorrhage. Here the elevated ratio is due not only to prerenal azotemia, but in addition is an expression of the rapid synthesis of urea by the liver in response to the products of protein digestion from blood in the stomach.

Gastric varices and splenic vein thrombosis

Why did the patient in Case history 4 with no previous history of liver disease and no esophageal varices have gastric varices?

When gastric varices are seen in the absence of esophageal varices, one most always suspects a splenic vein thrombosis as the cause. This patient could certainly have acquired a splenic vein thrombosis at the time of one of his rather severe attacks of acute pancreatitis. Acute pancreatitis and pancreatic cancer are well known causes of splenic vein thrombosis. A review of the computed tomography (CT) scan done during the patient's second episode of acute pancreatitis revealed that he did indeed have a splenic vein thrombosis (Figure 7.13).

How can a patient with splenic vein thrombosis have gastric but not esophageal varices?

When splenic vein thrombosis occurs in the absence of portal vein thrombosis as is the case in pancreatitis or pancreatic cancer, the left coronary vein remains in communication with the portal vein which is still patent. Thus collateral blood flow may occur via:

(1) Short gastric veins → the plexus in the gastric submucosa (gastric varices) → left coronary vein → portal vein ('sinistral' or left sided portal hypertension). (Thus patients with isolated splenic vein thrombosis often develop gastric varices without esophageal varices.)

(2) Gastric veins → esophageal submucosal veins (gastroesophageal varices) → blood thus shunted to portal vein or inferior vena cava.

(3) Gastroepiploic system → omental veins (omental varices).

Diagnosis of splenic vein thrombosis

While the gold standard is venous-phase angiography, it is not always necessary to order such an invasive procedure. Whenever a splenic vein thrombosis is suspected one could request a Doppler ultrasound to make the diagnosis. A contrast-enhanced CT including portal phase images is frequently required both to confirm the thrombosis and to shed light on the etiology (Table 7.5). Alternatively, magnetic resonance imaging (MRI) may be used.

Case history 5

A 55-year-old man was admitted to the Emergency Department where he presented with an episode of watery non-bloody diarrhea of 2 days duration accompanied by a moderate amount of lower abdominal cramping but no vomiting. The loose stools had greatly diminished in frequency, but what brought the patient to the Emergency Department was the fact that he had noted that the last two bowel movements he had had were coated with blood.

On examination the only positive finding was mild tenderness in the left lower quadrant. Ordinarily, such a patient would never have been admitted to the hospital, particularly since he was improving and was taking fluids by mouth, had it not been for his past history. Several years earlier the patient had received heart transplantation for severe cardiomyopathy that developed following a viral myocarditis. A few years thereafter, he developed chronic renal failure, attributed perhaps to toxicity from the immunosuppressive medication he had been on, and received a cadaveric renal transplantation. More recently he had developed an acute aortic dissection that required extensive vascular surgery. A graft from an iliac artery, and not from the inferior mesenteric artery, supplied his left colon. His wife mentioned that he had had a similar episode of 'gastroenteritis' a month or so earlier, although at that time he had not had blood in his stool. On examination he was hemodynamically stable, and except for the scars on his abdomen from previous surgery and the

Table 7.5 Causes of splenic vein thrombosis

Isolated splenic vein thrombosis
    Acute pancreatitis
    Chronic pancreatitis
    Pancreatic pseudocyst
    Pancreatic cancer
Splenic vein thrombosis associated with other venous thromboses
    Intraabdominal sepsis
    Hypercoagulable states
    Thrombocytosis
Polycythemia vera (hepatic vein thrombosis much more common)

transplanted kidney, the physical examination was unremarkable. The physicians who initially saw him in the Emergency Department felt he might be recovering from a bacterial gastroenteritis such as *Campylobacter jejuni* (it not being uncommon to have a predominantly non-blood watery diarrhea that later becomes bloody in such a case). However, in light of previous vascular surgery, the gastroenterologist who saw the patient felt strongly that ischemic colitis had to be excluded. Accordingly, a colonoscopy was done the next day which showed that the rectal mucosa was completely normal (Figure 7.14a). From 25 cm from the anal verge, for about 5 to 10 cm in the sigmoid colon, the mucosa showed patchy red blotches resembling ecchymoses (Figure 7.14b). From about 35 cm from the anal verge for the next 10–20 cm the mucosa was erythematous, slightly edematous and covered with exudate (Figure 7.14c). Thereafter the entire colon was normal until the cecum. The endoscopic appearance was consistent with colonic ischemia in the territory of the inferior mesenteric artery. Biopsies confirmed the diagnosis.

BLOOD SUPPLY OF THE GASTROINTESTINAL TRACT

The artery supply

Most of the arterial supply of the gut is through three unpaired arterial trunks: the celiac trunk; the superior mesenteric artery, and the inferior mesenteric artery.

Celiac trunk (Figure 7.15a & b) This is the artery of the foregut and it supplies:

(1) The stomach;

(2) The duodenum until the junction of the 2nd and 3rd parts;

(3) The pancreas, via the superior pancreaticoduodenal artery;

(4) The liver via the hepatic artery. On rare occasions the hepatic artery originates from the superior mesenteric artery. The liver, of course, in addition is supplied by blood from the gastrointestinal tract that ultimately reaches it via the portal vein.

Superior mesenteric artery (SMA) (Figure 7.15c) This is the artery of the midgut and it supplies the intestine from the junction of the second and third part of the duodenum to the junction of the proximal two-thirds and the distal third of the transverse colon. The SMA gives rise to:

(1) The inferior pancreaticoduodenal artery which contributes to the blood supply of the distal duodenum and a part of the pancreas;

(2) Jejunal branches that supply the jejunum and proximal ileum;

(3) The ileocolic artery that supplies most of the ileum, the cecum and appendix and some of the ascending colon;

(4) The right colic and its branches supply the remaining ascending colon;

(5) The middle colic artery supplies the transverse colon until the junction of the proximal two-thirds and the distal third where it anastomoses with the superior branch of the left colic artery, (the marginal artery of Drummond), which in turn is a branch of the inferior mesenteric artery.

Inferior mesenteric artery (IMA) (Figure 7.15d) This is the artery of the hindgut and it supplies the colon from the junction of the proximal two-thirds and distal third of the transverse colon to the upper rectum. The IMA gives rise to:

(1) The left colic artery which terminates into:

    (a) A superior branch, the marginal artery of Drummond, which supplies the upper part of the descending colon and the distal part of the transverse colon and anastomoses with the mid-colic artery at the junction of the proximal two-thirds and the distal third of the transverse colon, and

    (b) An inferior branch which supplies the lower descending colon and anastomoses with the sigmoid arcades.

(2) The sigmoid arteries which form arcades from which the sigmoid colon is supplied;

(3) The superior rectal (or superior hemorrhoidal) artery which is the name given to the last part of the IMA as it cross the pelvic brim where it divides into the anterior and posterior branches which supply the anterior and posterior aspects of the upper rectum. They end by forming loops around the lower rectum which anastomose with:

  (a) The middle rectal (or middle hemorrhoidal) artery, a branch of the internal iliac; and

  (b) The inferior rectal (or inferior hemorrhoidal) artery, a branch of the inferior pudendal artery.

Arteries of the distal and proximal ends of the gut

The distal (lower rectum and anus) and proximal (esophagus) ends of the gut have different arterial supplies:

(1) Lower rectum and anus:

  (a) The middle rectal (or middle hemorrhoidal) artery, a branch of the internal iliac; and

  (b) The inferior rectal (or inferior hemorrhoidal) artery, a branch of the internal pudendal artery.

(2) Esophagus:

  (a) Upper third: supplied by the paired inferior thyroid arteries;

  (b) Middle third: supplied by the bronchial arteries and the esophageal branches from the aorta; and

  (c) Lower third: supplied by esophageal branches of the left gastric artery.

Watershed areas

Watershed areas are parts of the intestine that are more prone to ischemic injury. There are two areas of the colon that are particularly at risk: the splenic flexure region (Griffith's point) and the rectosigmoid region (Sudeck's point). The vulnerability of these areas is a consequence of the anastomoses of the SMA with the IMA, and the IMA with the middle rectal and inferior rectal arteries. The watershed areas of arterial supply are illustrated in Figures 7.16 and 7.17.

Ischemic colitis

(NOTE: In this chapter we deal only with colonic ischemia. Ischemia in the small intestine, that is ischemia occurring in the superior mesenteric artery territory, is described in Chapter 9).

Pathogenesis of ischemic colitis

In the vast majority of cases, ischemic colitis occurs in patients over 50 years of age with atheromatous disease. Situations resulting in hypoperfusion, for example from systemic conditions resulting in even transient hypotension, can give rise to colonic ischemia. On occasion in the elderly, the degree of atheromatous disease is so advanced that ischemia may result even from relatively slight and not clinically obvious periods of hypoperfusion. Such cases generally involve the IMA territory. Most often the areas of the colon involved are the splenic flexure (Griffith's point) or rectosigmoid and sigmoid colon (Sudeck's point). The patient described in Case history 5 had advanced vascular disease and his left colon was being tenuously perfused via the anastomoses at Sudeck's point as shown on a previous angiogram. His previous aortic dissection had involved the root of the IMA.

Less frequently, colonic ischemia is seen in patients under 50 years of age who do not have atheromatous disease. Occasionally the reason for the ischemia is obvious, such as in a patient with systemic lupus or other known cause of vasculitis; however, in other cases the reason is not evident. The use of vasoconstrictive recreational drugs, such as cocaine, may be the cause in a few, and oral contraceptives have been blamed in others, but often the reason remains an enigma. In these younger patients the colonic ischemia may involve the IMA or the SMA territory.

Pathology of ischemic colitis

The pathology of ischemic colitis is shown in Figure 7.18.

Clinical presentation

The clinical presentation of ischemic colitis forms a triad; however, all three elements are not always present:

(1) Pain: lower abdominal, sudden in onset and usually mild, it may be colicky or steady pain. This is in contrast to the severe periumbilical pain without much tenderness in the early stages, experienced by patients with ischemia to the small bowel in SMA ischemia (see Chapter 9). In around

one-quarter of all patients there may be no pain felt (Figures 7.19 and 7.20).

(2) Tenderness in the lower abdomen occurs early and the condition may be mistaken for diverticulitis.

(3) Diarrhea: bloody in two-thirds of cases. The diarrhea may begin as a bloody diarrhea from the start, but often initially the stool is not grossly bloody although it often tests positive for occult blood. Bloody diarrhea usually occurs within the first day of the onset of pain.

Systemic symptoms of malaise and lethargy, often with a low-grade fever, are present. Fever is a late finding in small bowel ischemia from ischemic disease in SMA territory. An elevated white cell count is often present.

Diagnosis of colonic ischemia

When suspected on clinical grounds, a flexible sigmoidoscopy or colonoscopy is usually the first investigative step. Care is taken not to distend the colon too much during the procedure. As soon as the characteristic appearance of the mucosa is noted, and biopsies taken, the endoscopist is well advised not to attempt to complete the entire visualization of the colon.

The characteristic endoscopic features include mucosal edema, ecchymoses, erythema and often also a bluish appearance of the mucosa (see Figures 7.14, 7.19 and 7.20). Ulcerations may also be present. On occasion the lesion is contiguous, and at other times it is patchy with areas of normal mucosa intervening, much like that seen in Crohn's colitis. In fact, when the lesion occurs in the young or middle-aged, Crohn's colitis is the leading contender in the differential diagnosis.

The rectum, especially the lower rectum, is almost always spared in ischemic colitis, as it also often is in Crohn's colitis. Rectal involvement is seen more often in Crohn's disease and almost never in ischemia. The reason for the rectal sparing is evident from the anatomy of the blood supply of the colon (see Figure 7.15d). The lower rectum is supplied by the middle and inferior rectal arteries, which get their blood supply from the systemic and not the splanchnic circulation. Again, as mentioned earlier, the splenic flexure region or the rectosigmoid and sigmoid colon areas are the most frequently affected areas, although any area of the colon may be involved.

It is worth noting here that, whereas angiography is the gold standard for the diagnosis of ischemia of the small bowel, flexible sigmoidoscopy or colonoscopy is the study of choice in ischemic colitis. CT scans do have a role in the management of complicated ischemic colitis when the diagnosis is uncertain, as shown in Case history 6.

Case history 6

A 65-year-old man presented with right lower quadrant pain that had begun on the morning of admission. The pain had been in the right lower quadrant since its onset and was constant (i.e. not colicky). The pain was moderate in intensity, did not radiate to another region and there was no history of vomiting, fever, chills or dysuria. He had passed one bowel movement earlier that day and was passing flatus. The patient had a history in the past of passing renal stones and he likened the present episode to that he had experienced with his bout of renal colic. He was diabetic, had hypertension, and had had an aortic valve replacement, a coronary artery bypass graft, cholecystectomy and a perforated peptic ulcer over two decades earlier. When seen in the Emergency Department, his heart rate was 68 beats/min and blood pressure was 100/50 mmHg after receiving intravenous fluids. Salient features on examination were a systolic murmur in the heart, lungs clear to auscultation and an abdomen that was not distended. Guarding and tenderness were present on palpation in the right lower quadrant. Bowel sounds were present. His white cell count was elevated at 19 300/mm^3 with 83% segmented forms. Liver function tests and serum bilirubin were normal. A plain X-ray of the abdomen showed a stone in the right kidney. A CT scan was ordered and it showed no ureteral obstruction, but did show a markedly thickened wall of the ascending colon, hepatic flexure and proximal transverse colon. There was no evidence of appendicitis or diverticulitis, even though several diverticula were seen (Figure 7.21a). The patient then underwent a hypaque enema that showed thumbprinting in the region of the hepatic flexure (Figure 7.21b). A diagnosis of right-sided ischemic colitis was suspected and a colonoscopy attempted. For technical reasons it was not possible to advance the instrument beyond the sigmoid colon. The part of the sigmoid colon examined was normal except for several diverticula. The patient's condition gradually improved. A CT scan was repeated a few days later and showed evidence to suggest ischemia that was resolving (Figure 7.21c).

Comments   This patient's presentation generated a differential diagnosis that included diverticulitis, appendicitis and pancreatitis. These were excluded by laboratory and imaging studies. The marked thickening of the bowel wall suggested either ischemia or an inflammatory colitis localized to the right colon. The patient had been only on aspirin and had discontinued his warfarin. It is very likely that he experienced an embolism in a peripheral branch or branches of the SMA, thus leading to ischemic colitis involving the right colon.

The clinical course of ischemic colitis

For the most part, ischemic colitis is a self-limited disease. Symptoms generally subside in a few days. When symptoms become worse, especially if the pain increases with time, or if guarding or percussion tenderness develop over an area of involved bowel, the patient should be taken to surgery. Delay will inevitably result in infarction leading to gangrene and ultimately to perforation (Figure 7.22).

Colonic submucosal hemorrhage

Occasionally spontaneous bleeding from the colon may be seen in patients with a severe coagulopathy who develop submucosal hemorrhages. These hemorrhages are seen on endoscopy (Figure 7.23).

Rectal varices

Patients with portal hypertension on occasion develop rectal varices and these can be the source of massive rectal bleeding (Figure 7.24).

CHAPTER 8

Maladies due to gallstones and things that may mimic them

THE CONSTITUENTS OF BILE – UNDERSTANDING BASIC PRINCIPLES A MODERN-DAY PHYSICIAN WOULD DO WELL TO KNOW

Around 80% of gallstones encountered contain cholesterol and it is difficult to grasp how they are formed without a basic concept of the constituents of bile.

The parenchymal cells of the liver, called hepatocytes, secrete bile. The hepatocyte is a polar cell much like the cells that line the surface of the stomach, and small and large intestines, i.e. they have an apical and a basolateral domain. Bile is secreted from the apical domain, across the canalicular membrane of the cell, into the canaliculi. Canaliculi make up the meshwork of spaces between the apical domains of adjacent hepatocytes. From the canaliculi bile enters the smallest bile ductules (or canals of Herring) from whence the bile traverses bile ductules and ducts of increasing caliber, ultimately to emerge from the right and left hepatic ducts.

Hepatic bile

This is bile present in the common hepatic duct. It consists of bile that is secreted at the canalicular membrane of hepatocytes and modified somewhat as it makes its way through the bile ductules.

Gallbladder bile

This is bile present in the gallbladder. Hepatic bile enters the gallbladder whose epithelium is very active allowing for the transport of water and electrolytes across its wall, thus altering the concentration and electrolyte content of bile and rendering the bile more acidic.

Duodenal bile

This is a mixture of hepatic and gallbladder bile as it flows into the duodenum via the common bile duct. Its composition depends on the fed state of the individual. For example, after a meal rich in fat or protein, cholecystokinin, a gastrointestinal hormone, is released by the cells of the upper small intestine. Cholecystokinin contracts the gallbladder, and the composition of duodenal bile after a meal is essentially similar to that of gallbladder bile.

THE COMPOSITION OF BILE

Bile is composed of biliary lipids (bile salts, phospholipids and cholesterol), other solutes, water and electrolytes.

Bile acids

Primary bile acids are those synthesized in the liver by the biotransformation of cholesterol. They are cholic acid (a trihydroxy bile acid) and chenodeoxycholic acid (a dihydroxy bile acid).

Secondary bile acids are those modified by bacterial action in the lumen of the distal small intestine and colon, recirculated to the liver and secreted into bile. Examples of secondary bile acids are deoxycholic acid (a dihydroxy bile acid) and lithocholic acid (a monohydroxy bile acid).

Structure of bile acids

The structure of bile acids is illustrated in Figure 8.1. Both the primary and secondary bile acids possess a lipophilic ('lipid loving') sterol nucleus containing one to three polar hydroxyl groups and a carboxylic acid side chain. Almost all of the bile acids secreted into bile by the liver are in the conjugated form, i.e. their carboxylic acid side chain forms an amide bond with the amino acids glycine (NH_2-CH_2-COOH) or taurine (NH_2-CH_2-CH_2-SO_3H).

Properties of bile acids

Bile acids are detergent molecules that are amphipaths, i.e. they possess both polar groups that make them in part hydrophilic ('water loving') and lipophilic groups that make them in part hydrophobic ('water fearing'). Once they reach a critical concentration (that varies with the bile acid) of 0.5–5 mmol/l they spontaneously form macromolecular aggregates or simple micelles. Within each micelle the polar or hydrophilic groups are exposed to the aqueous solvent and the hydrophobic groups are oriented towards the middle, so that their exposure to the aqueous environment is minimized. The concentration of bile acids at which micelles form is termed the critical micellar concentration (CMC).

Synthesis of primary bile acids

The biotransformation of cholesterol (Figure 8.2) to primary bile acids occurs in hepatocytes. Two pathways of bile acid synthesis from cholesterol have been described: the classic and alternative pathways.

Classic or neutral pathway of bile acid synthesis   This is the major pathway in humans and here changes in the sterol nucleus of cholesterol antecede changes in the cholesterol side chain:

1) In addition to the hydroxyl (-OH) group at position 3 in cholesterol, the addition of more α-OH groups to the sterol nucleus (at position 7 in the chenodeoxycholic acid and at positions 7 and 12 in the case of cholic acid);

2) Saturation of the sterol nucleus of cholesterol;

3) Epimerization of the 3β-OH group of cholesterol to a 3α-OH group.

Only after changes in the sterol nucleus are made, is the side chain of cholesterol subjected to oxidation and truncation by three carbon atoms.

In this pathway cholic acid and chenodeoxycholic acid are synthesized in approximately equal amounts. The first enzymatic step, the 7α hydroxylation of the cholesterol nucleus by the enzyme 7α-hydroxylase (referred to as CYP7A), is the rate-limiting step. The

Table 8.1   Inborn errors of bile acid synthesis

Errors in steroid nucleus synthesis
Autosomal recessive
Cholelithiasis
Bile salt deficiency → deficiency in fat-soluble
    vitamins
Giant cell hepatitis → cirrhosis → portal hypertension
Side-effects avoided with early treatment with
    cholic acid

Errors in side chain synthesis
The important enzyme CYP27, which is the first step for bile
    acid synthesis in the acidic or alternative pathway, but is
    also a part of the neutral or classic pathway, is defective
No chronic liver disease
Defective cholesterol and cholestanol metabolism with their
    abnormal accumulation in:
    neural tissue → neurological disorders
    soft tissue → xanthomas
    arteries → premature atherosclerotic disease
    lens of the eyes → cataracts
Early detection can minimize complications using treatment
    with primary bile acids and 3-hydroxy, 3-methylglutaryl
    coenzyme A reductase inhibitors

activity of CYP7A is under feedback inhibition by bile salts. CYP7A has been isolated, purified, sequenced and cloned, and the feedback inhibition is controlled at the transcriptional level by hydrophobic bile acids, but not by hydrophilic bile acids such as ursodeoxycholic acid.

During ileal resection or disease, considerable amounts of bile acids are lost in the feces. The CYP7A gene receives a signal and ultimately more bile acids are synthesized (see the section on ileal resection in Chapter 4).

Alternative or acidic pathway of bile acid synthesis   In this pathway the side chain of cholesterol is modified before alterations in the sterol nucleus are made. The initial enzyme is CYP27. Only chenodeoxycholic acid is synthesized in this pathway. It is of little importance in humans during health, but in advanced chronic liver disease such as cirrhosis, this appears to be the pathway of preference.

Inborn errors of metabolism related to abnormal bile acid synthesis

Inborn errors can occur because of defects in either the classic or the alternative pathway. Errors may result from defects in the synthesis of the steroid nucleus or of the side chain. Each error is characterized by the identification in the urine of precursors of bile acid synthesis (Table 8.1).

Table 8.2 The pK_a of bile acids

Unconjugated: ~5.0
Glycine conjugates: ~3.8
Taurine conjugates: ~1.9

Since conjugated bile acids are strong acids, at the usual small intestinal pH they exist in the anionic form and are impermeable to the enterocyte membrane

Table 8.3 Bile acid pool and bile acid composition

Pool size: 1.5–4 g
Pool recirculates 6 to 15 times per day
2% of bile secreted by the liver is newly synthesized; the remainder is salvaged by the enterohepatic circulation
Composition
    cholic acid ~40%
    conjugated chenodeoxycholate ~40%
    conjugated deoxycholate ~20%
    conjugated lithocholate and ursodeoxycholate < 5%

Conjugation of bile acids

Both newly synthesized bile acids (only around 2% of the total bile acid pool), and those returned to the liver by the enterohepatic circulation, are conjugated in the liver to their glycine or taurine conjugates. This holds true for primary bile acids as well as the secondary bile acids, deoxycholic acid and lithocholic acid (see earlier section on Structure of bile acids). In the case of lithocholic acid, in addition to conjugation, it is also sulfated at the 3 position of the sterol nucleus.

Conjugation of bile acids results in a substantial fall in the pK_a (Table 8.2). Since the pK_a drops substantially below the usual pH of the small intestine, conjugated bile acids become impermeable to the enterocyte membrane. Therefore conjugated bile acids require a carrier (transporter) to transport them across the enterocyte membrane in order to be absorbed.

Secretion of bile acids from the hepatocyte

Bile acids within the hepatocyte are either synthesized *de novo* or enter the hepatocyte from the portal circulation via the sinusoids (basal membrane). Thye are delivered to the canalicular (apical) membrane either bound to a bile acid transport protein or by vesicle-mediated intracellular transport. They are then transported across the canalicular membrane via canalicular bile acid transporters.

Canalicular bile acid transporters   These are one or more ATP-dependent transport pumps that belong to the ATP binding cassette (ABC) gene superfamily. One such candidate is called sister of P glycoprotein (SPGP). Other transporters of the ABC superfamily may also be active in transporting bile acids against a concentration gradient into the canaliculus and thence into the biliary ductules. Another pump has also been identified on the canalicular membrane and is called multi-resistant protein 2, (MRP2), also termed multispecific organic anion transporter (cMOAT), which also belongs to the ABC superfamily. It transports a variety of organic anions such as sulfated

lithocholic acid, conjugated bilirubin and the antibiotic ceftriaxone (Figure 8.3).

Once bile acids are transported across the canalicular membrane they eventually find their way via the common bile duct into the duodenum, having undergone some modification during their travel through the bile ducts and the gallbladder.

Almost all of the bile acids secreted by the liver are conjugated with glycine or taurine (see earlier sections on Structure of bile acids and Conjugation). As seen in Table 8.2, conjugation lowers the pK_a of the bile acids and hence, at the physiological pH of the small intestine, for the most part they remain as anions (in their charged state) and are impermeable to cell membranes. Therefore, conjugated bile acids require a carrier (transporter) to transport them across the enterocyte membrane in order to be absorbed (Table 8.3).

Events in the jejunum   As noted above (Table 8.2), glycine- and taurine-conjugated bile acids, particularly the more hydrophilic trihydroxy conjugates of cholic acid, remain in the anionic (charged) form in the lumen of the intestine and cannot be absorbed passively. However, during the digestion of a meal, the pH in the duodenum may become fairly acidic and the glycine conjugates of the dihydroxy bile acids, chenodeoxycholic acid and deoxycholic acid, can become protonated (not charged). These protonated forms may be absorbed by passive non-ionic diffusion in the jejunum (Figure 8.4). A mechanism for the active absorption of conjugated bile acids is not present in the jejunum.

Events in the ileum   The vast majority of the conjugated bile acids in the distal ileum is actively reabsorbed by a carrier-mediated mechanism and returned via the portal circulation to the liver. A sodium-coupled transporter is located at the apical (luminal) border of the ileal enterocyte and is termed the ileal bile acid

Table 8.4 Extraction of bile acids from the portal circulation by the liver

Na⁺-coupled bile acid transporters

Hydrophilic glycine- and taurine-conjugated bile acids, especially cholic acid, are hydrophilic and charged (anionic), so that they cannot cross the liver sinusoidal membrane without a carrier-mediated mechanism. Coupling transport to Na⁺ provides the energy for the bile acid transport.

NTCP (~50 kDa glycoprotein). The rat equivalent gene is *Ntcp*. Conditions giving rise to cholestasis such as a mechanical bile duct ligation and lipopolysaccharide injection (model for sepsis), result in a reduction in *Ntcp* gene expression and protein production (Figure 8.3).

mEH (microsomal epoxy hydrolase). This is a rat microsomal enzyme also recently shown to be present on the sinusoidal membrane. In the latter location it serves as a Na⁺-coupled bile acid (sodium taurocholate) transporter. Its importance in the human is less certain as yet (Figure 8.3).

Na⁺-independent bile acid transporters

Non-conjugated secondary bile acids are the preferred substrates. They often function as antiporters, for example extruding a HCO_3^- anion for the entry of a bile acid anion.

OATP (Organic Anion Transport Protein, ~80 kDa glycoprotein). This is a family of transport proteins with specificity for various organic anions, bile acids among them.

Passive diffusion

Unconjugated bile acids, including secondary bile acids such as deoxycholic and lithocholic acids, have a pK_a much higher than conjugated bile acids and hence at physiological pH they can be protonated and diffuse through the sinusoidal membrane.

---

transporter (IBAT). Once in the cell, the conjugated bile acid is bound to the ileal lipid binding protein and is transported to the basolateral membrane of the ileal enterocyte. The exact mechanism of exit from the basolateral membrane is not well understood, but there is evidence for a bicarbonate exchanger (Figure 8.5).

Some of the conjugated bile acids may be deconjugated by bacteria in the distal ileum (i.e. bacterial enzymes remove the glycine or taurine moieties). These unconjugated bile acids have a much higher pK_a (Table 8.2) and can be protonated and thus reabsorbed into the portal blood by passive non-ionic diffusion, ultimately to reach the liver.

Events in the colon Some bile acids that escape reabsorption in the small intestine enter the colon, where bacterial enzymes mediate three separate processes:

(1) Deconjugation: The glycine or taurine groups are removed, forming cholic acid, chenodeoxycholic acid and deoxycholic acid;

(2) Dehydroxylated: The hydroxyl group in the 7α position is removed, thus: cholic acid → deoxycholic acid and chenodeoxycholic acid → lithocholic acid;

(3) Epimerization of the 7α-OH group to a 7β-OH group (occurs very little), thus: chenodeoxycholic acid (7α-OH group) → ursodeoxycholic acid (7β-OH group).

These deconjugated or deconjugated and dehydroxylated bile acids are absorbed by passive non-ionic diffusion and transported by the portal circulation to the liver.

Extraction of bile acids by the liver

At least three different mechanisms are known to exist for extraction of bile acids by the liver, these varied mechanisms being required on account of the different degrees of hydrophobicity/hydrophilicity of the different types of bile acid. They are depicted in Figure 8.3 and explained in detail in Table 8.4.

Serum bile acids

The liver extracts anywhere from 70 to 90% of the bile acids presented to it during the first pass, depending on the type of bile acid and whether it is conjugated or not. Bile acids not extracted spill over to the systemic circulation. Since the amount of bile acid presented to the liver after a meal is greater than in the fasting state, the postprandial bile acid concentration is two- to four-fold higher than the fasting value of approximately 3 μmol/l. In addition to the portal vein blood the liver receives, it has a further opportunity of extracting bile acids, as it receives about a third of its circulation from the hepatic artery.

Phospholipids

The major phospholipid in bile is phosphatidyl choline (lecithin) (Figure 8.6). The hydrophilicity of lecithin is limited and it is not soluble in water. However, its amphipathic nature enables it to enter simple bile salt micelles, forming complex micelles, thus ensuring its transport in the aqueous media of biological fluids such as bile (Figure 8.7). (See also discussion on micelles and vesicles in the section on Cholesterol transport in bile later in this chapter).

The transport across the canalicular membrane is a two-step process. First, translocation occurs of the phospholipid from the inner to the outer membrane of the canaliculus by a transporter termed MDR3, which thus serves as a 'flippase', flipping the lecithin from one side of the membrane to the other. MDR3 belongs to a class of proteins called P-glycoproteins (of which the canalicular bile acid transporter, sister of P glycoprotein, is also a member). The P glycoproteins in turn are members of the ABC superfamily (see section on Secretion of bile acids from the hepatocyte and Figure 8.3).

Second, phospholipids (mainly the phosphatidyl choline or lecithin and not other phospholipids that also make up the canalicular membrane) are then selectively released from the outer membrane of the canaliculus by the detergent action of bile acids within the canalicular lumen. The outer membrane of the canaliculus is the membrane facing the lumen of the canaliculus.

The major function of phospholipids in bile is that they form a crucial part of the mixed micelle, enabling the solubilization of cholesterol. They also protect the epithelium of the biliary tract from the damaging detergent effects of bile acids.

Cholesterol

Details related to the secretion of cholesterol into bile (transport across the canalicular membrane of the hepatocyte) and metabolism (biotransformation to bile acids) has been discussed earlier in this chapter. The present section is an integrated summary of these functions (Figure 8.8) and discusses, very briefly, the sources of hepatic cholesterol: endogenous synthesis; and uptake of lipoprotein particles from the circulation. Also discussed is the interplay between the two pools of cholesterol in the liver.

There are two pools of cholesterol in the liver that are in equilibrium (Figure 8.8):

(1) *Free cholesterol pool*   This contributes to both the cholesterol secreted into bile and that metabolized to bile acids. The cholesterol that constitutes the free cholesterol pool is derived from three sources:

    (a) Endogenous synthesis from acetyl CoA – the rate-limiting step (enzyme) in the synthetic pathway is 3-hydroxy, 3-methylglutaryl coenzyme A (HMG CoA) reductase, which converts HMG CoA to mevalonate (Figure 8.8)

    (b) Lipoproteins in the circulation – the sinusoidal side of the hepatocyte membrane has receptors for LDL, chylomicron remnants

and a special receptor, SR-B1 scavenger receptor for HDL (Figure 8.8)

    (c) From the storage pool of cholesterol ester (Figure 8.8). The enzyme cholesteryl ester hydrolase (CEH in Figure 8.8) generates free cholesterol whenever the need arises for secretion into bile or for the synthesis of bile acids.

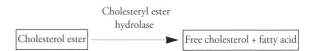

(2) *Esterified cholesterol pool*   This is a storage form of cholesterol. The hydroxyl group in the 3-position of the sterol nucleus of cholesterol is hydrolyzed with a fatty acid (fatty acyl-coenzyme A) forming a fatty acid ester. The enzyme responsible is acyl CoA-cholesterol ester transferase (ACAT in Figure 8.8).

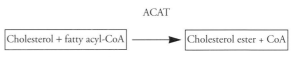

Transport of cholesterol in bile

The structural formula is shown in Figure 8.2. It is evident from the structure that cholesterol is not a polar molecule and is therefore insoluble in water. It is present in aqueous solutions (bile in the biliary tract or in the intestine) either in mixed micelles or in vesicles.

Simple micelles   Bile acids only, they form at critical micellar concentration (0.5–5 mol/l). Their size is 20–30 Å. They may solubilize tiny amounts of cholesterol.

Mixed micelles   These are bile acids and phospholipids, with or without cholesterol. They are more stable at high bile acid/phospholipid ratios. At low total lipid concentrations, they are rod shaped – size: several hundred angstrom units. At high total lipid concentrations, they are round – size: 40–80 Å.

Vesicles   These may be:

(1) *Unilamellar*   When the cholesterol concentration exceeds micellar solubility, unilamellar vesicles form. Unilamellar vesicles are single-membrane bilayers containing cholesterol, phospholipid and small amounts of bile acids. Their size is 500–1000 Å.

Table 8.5 Epidemiology of gallstones – in general for most populations

Overall prevalence: approximately 10%
  female : male ratio: 2–3 : 1
Incidence increases with age
The increased incidence in women is greatest between the ages of 30 and 40 years
By age 60 years the female preponderance is considerably diminished

Table 8.6 Epidemiology of gallstones – special populations

Cholesterol stone prevalence considerably increased in
  Pima Indians of Southern Arizona – 70% of females > 25 years
Cholesterol stone prevalence higher than elsewhere:
  American Indian populations in Canada and Alaska
Cholesterol stones decreased in
  African-Americans compared to Caucasians
  Sub-Saharan Africans
  Asians – low in South India but high in North India

(2) *Multilamellar* The cholesterol content of uni-lamellar vesicles is much more than that found in cell membranes. They are therefore thermo-dynamically unstable and tend to fuse to form multilamellar vesicles. When these vesicles become supersaturated cholesterol crystals may form.

Cholesterol is secreted from the liver into bile as uni-lamellar vesicles (see Figure 8.7). As mentioned in the legend to Figure 8.7, cholesterol is transported in bile either in mixed micelles or in vesicles, depending on its concentration relative to the concentrations of bile acids and phospholipids. Mixed micelles are thermo-dynamically much more stable than vesicles.

GALLSTONES

Epidemiology

In general for most populations, the epidemiology is summarized in Table 8.5. For special populations, it is summarized in Table 8.6.

Types of gallstone and their pathogenesis and risk factors

There are three principal varieties of gallstone: cholesterol stones, black pigment stones and brown pigment stones (Figure 8.9).

Cholesterol stones

Around 80% of all gallstones in Western populations are cholesterol stones.

Table 8.7 Cholesterol gallstones – composition

Major components
  cholesterol monohydrate crystals + mucin glycoprotein matrix
Minor components
  unconjugated bilirubin + calcium phosphate

Composition of cholesterol stones

The composition of cholesterol stones is shown in Table 8.7.

Risk factors for cholesterol stones

Estrogens
Mechanism:
  Up-regulation of hepatocyte LDL receptor → endogenous cholesterol pool↑ → cholesterol secretion into bile↑ → cholesterol saturation in bile↑
Examples:
  Female gender – puberty to menopause – is the single most important risk factor
  Oral contraceptives
  Administration of estrogens for medical reasons
  Pregnancy (incidence of : sludge↑ 30%, gallstones↑ 2%; much of this reverses)

Progesterone
Mechanism:
  Progesterone → gallbladder hypomotility
Example:
  Pregnancy: synergism between estrogen and progesterone effects

Age
Prevalence increases with age
Mechanism:
  Cholesterol 7α-hydroxylase activity ↓ → bile acid synthesis ↓ → cholesterol : bile acid ratio↑

Serum lipid profile
Serum HDL cholesterol Levels inversely related to cholesterol saturation in bile and gallstone prevalence.

Hypertriglyceridemia HMG-CoA reductase↑ → cholesterol synthesis↑ → cholesterol saturation↑ enterohepatic cycling of bile acids↓ → bile acid malabsorption → bile acid pool↓ → cholesterol : bile acid ratio↑ (seen with familial hypertriglyceridemia).

Obesity Gallstone incidence is proportional to the body mass index (BMI). When the BMI is > 45 kg/m^2, the incidence is increased seven times.

Table 8.8 Bile cholesterol supersaturation

Solubility of cholesterol in bile is dependent on:
   bile salt concentration
   phospholipid concentration
   total biliary lipid concentration
Cholesterol supersaturation is essential for cholesterol
   crystal nucleation to occur
Cholesterol supersaturation is not in and of itself sufficient
   to bring about nucleation

Table 8.9 Mucin glycoprotein secretion

Mucin secreted by the gallbladder mucosa is the major organic
   constituent of the gallbladder lumen
Hydrophobic oligosaccharide chains of mucin bind to
   hydrophobic portions of cholesterol, phospholipid and bile
   acid molecules
Aids in the formation of multilamellar vesicles from micelles
   and unilamellar vesicles
The addition of gallbladder mucin to supersaturated bile
   shortens the nucleation time

Mechanism:

HMG-CoA activity↑ → cholesterol synthesis↑ → endogenous cholesterol pool↑ → cholesterol secretion into bile↑ → cholesterol saturation in bile↑. The serum lipid profile is altered in obese persons (see above).

Rapid weight loss   The effect on cholesterol stones shows an incidence of 2.5% during obesity dieting and 50% for sludge or stones within 6 months of gastric bypass surgery.

Mechanism:

Secretion of cholesterol into bile↑ → cholesterol saturation in bile↑

Gallbladder hypomotility. Therefore, intake of a little fat with meals induces cholecystokinin (CCK) secretion and gallbladder contraction, preventing gallstone formation.

Total parenteral nutrition (TPN)   Approximately 40% develop gallstones over time and a much higher number develop sludge.

Mechanism:

Fasting → no CCK secretion → gallbladder hypomotility and failure of relaxation of the sphincter of Oddi (sludge/gallstones may be prevented by administration of small amounts of CCK-octapeptide).

Ileal resection or disease   (e.g. Crohn's disease)

Mechanism:

Active absorption of bile acids↓ → bile acid pool size↓ → biliary cholesterol : bile acid ratio↑

Spinal cord injury   There is a very high prevalence of gallstone formation in patients who have had spinal cord injury.

Mechanism:

Intestinal hypomotility → deconjugation of bile salts in ileum↑ → biliary deoxycholic acid concentration↑

Gallbladder hypomotility.

Drugs   Those involved are estrogens (as above); progesterone (as above); somatostatin analog (octreotide), leading to gallbladder hypomotility. Intestinal hypomotility → bile acid deconjugation → deoxycholate in

bile↑, which alters the concentration of bile in the gallbladder. Another drug is ceftriaxone. Quarter to half of patients develop sludge, and 20% develop symptoms. These are reversible after cessation.

Mechanism:

Secreted into bile as a divalent anion much like phosphate, carbonate or bilirubin → precipitated in bile as a calcium salt → forms sludge.

Pathogenesis of cholesterol gallstones (Figure 8.10)

Cholesterol crystal precipitation (nucleation) has to occur for sludge or gallstones to form.

Bile cholesterol supersaturation   Shown in Table 8.8.

Mucin glycoprotein secretion   Nucleation is the first step in gallstone formation. The process involves aggregation of cholesterol molecules from a supersaturated solution in which cholesterol is present in varied mixed micellar and vesicular states, through a series of thermodynamically unstable forms, which eventually go on to form cholesterol monohydrate crystals. Mucin glycoproteins secreted by the gallbladder mucosa are the most potent nucleating agents (pronucleators) (Table 8.9).

Accelerated nucleation   There are substances found in gallbladder bile that can hasten (pronucleators) or hinder (antinucleators) the nucleation process as assessed in *in vitro* experiments. As stated above, mucin glycoproteins are the most potent pronucleators known. It is not clear which of the other pronucleators and which of the antinucleators mentioned in Table 8.10 are important *in vivo*.

Altered composition of gallbladder bile   Altered by the following mechanism: deoxycholic acid is lithogenic and brings about cholesterol crystallization. Gallstone patients, as a group, have higher amounts of deoxycholic acid in bile.

Gallbladder hypomotility   (summarized in Table 8.11). Food, in the upper small intestine, especially long-chain

Table 8.10   Accelerated nucleation

Pronucleators

Mucin glycoproteins (discussed in text)
Other lower molecular weight glycoproteins, e.g. α_1-acid
   glycoprotein
Phospholipase C
Aminopeptidase N
IgG and IgM
Fibronectin
Calcium

Antinucleators

Apolipoproteins AI and AII
IgA
Other biliary proteins

Table 8.11   Regulation of gallbladder motility

Increased gallbladder contractility
   cholecystokinin (CCK) – most potent
   parasympathetic nerve supply
Decrease in gallbladder contractility
   gallbladder bile supersaturated with cholesterol
   sympathetic nerve supply

---

fatty acids and amino acids, is the natural stimulant for the release of CCK. Hence, patients on TPN have hypomotility of their gallbladders. In patients with spinal cord injury, gallbladder hypomotility is also present, probably as a result of the interruption of descending autonomic pathways.

However, gallbladder hypomotility is prevalent fairly universally in patients who harbor gallstones. Bile supersaturated with cholesterol diminishes gallbladder contractility. A vicious cycle is set up, since in the presence of gallbladder hypomotility bile remains longer in the gallbladder and becomes more concentrated, increasing total biliary lipid concentration, an important factor in the genesis of gallstones (Figure 8.11).

Altered gallbladder mucosal function   The mucosa of the gallbladder is one of the most active in the gastrointestinal tract (Table 8.12). In the event of malfunction of the gallbladder mucosa, several theoretical scenarios can occur, each of which can favor the formation of cholesterol crystals:

(1)   Increased mucin glycoprotein secretion $\rightarrow$ more rapid nucleation;

(2)   Increased secretion of other pronucleators $\rightarrow$ more rapid nucleation;

(3)   Less H^+ ion secretion $\rightarrow$ contents less acidic $\rightarrow$ solubility of calcium salts$\downarrow$ $\rightarrow$ precipitation of calcium salts providing a nucleus for gallstone formation.

Table 8.12   Functions of the gallbladder mucosa

Mucin glycoprotein secretion (discussed earlier)
Secretion of other pronucleators and antinucleators (Table 8.10)
Sodium-coupled water transport: 80–90% of water in hepatic
   bile is absorbed in the gallbladder
H^+/HCO_3^- exchange: H^+ ion secreted into the gallbladder lumen
   in exchange for bicarbonate absorption

Pigment stones

Pigment stones are of two distinct varieties – black pigment stones and brown pigment stones. Bilirubin is the major constituent of both these varieties and makes up on average around half of the dry weight of the stone.

A brief review of bilirubin and its transport aids in the understanding of the pathogenesis of pigment gallstones. Bilirubin is the breakdown product of heme and is formed outside the liver in the reticuloendothelial system of the bone marrow and spleen from whence it is transported to the liver.

The molecule is made up of: four pyrolle rings (hydrophobic); two propionic acid side chains (hydrophilic); and hydrocarbon side chains (hydrophobic). Overall, unconjugated bilirubin is a highly hydrophobic molecule. It is therefore conjugated in the liver with glucuronic acid to make it polar (hydrophilic) and water soluble. The enzyme responsible for the conjugation is UDP glucuronyl transferase. Around 80% is conjugated to form bilirubin diglucuronide (BDG) and approximately 20% to bilirubin monoglucuronide (BMG). Bile present in the bile ducts and gallbladder contains BDG and BMG in these proportions, but also contains a trace (about 3%) of unconjugated bilirubin.

The heme is converted ultimately to bilirubin (unconjugated) in the reticuloendothelial system and is transported to the liver tightly bound to albumin. A carrier-mediated system, the organic anion transport protein (OATP) transfers the bilirubin across the sinusoidal membrane. Unconjugated bilirubin is then conjugated to bilirubin diglucuronide and monoglucuronide in the hepatocyte (Figure 8.12).

Black pigment stones   These are characterized in Table 8.13 and Figure 8.13. It is not entirely certain how deconjugation of conjugated bilirubin occurs in the formation of black pigment stones. β-Glucuronidase is an enzyme present in several bacterial species that deconjugates conjugated bilirubin diglucuronide to bilirubin monoglucuronide and to unconjugated bilirubin. However, bacterial infection does not appear to be important in

Table 8.13   Black pigment stones

Distribution
  worldwide
Etiology
  chronic hemolytic anemias
  cirrhosis
  prolonged total parenteral nutrition
  normal people
Stone location
  gallbladder; *de novo* stone formation in the bile ducts not seen
Stone quality
  solid or powdery; not laminated
Constituents
  unconjugated bilirubin ~ 40% (calcium bilirubinate in polymeric
    and crystalline forms)
  calcium carbonate ~ 15%
  calcium phosphate ~ 5%
  mucins 25%
  lipid
    cholesterol < 5%
    saturated fatty acids ~ 1%

Table 8.14   Brown pigment stones

Distribution
  chiefly in Asia – Far East
Etiology
  infection (Enterobacteriaceae and anaerobic bacteria) –
    cholangitis
Stone location
  gallbladder and *de novo* stone formation in the bile duct
Stone quality
  laminated
Constituents
  unconjugated bilirubin ~ 50%
  calcium (chiefly as bilirubinate in monomeric form) ~ 5%
  calcium carbonate absent
  calcium phosphate < 1%
  mucins ~15%
  lipids
    cholesterol ~ 5–25% (increased hepatic cholesterogenesis)
    diminished hepatic bile acid synthesis
    diminished hepatic transport and secretion of phospholipids
    saturated fatty acids ~ 25%

the formation of black pigment stones as it is in the genesis of brown pigment stones. It is possible that β-glucuronidase is also secreted by the epithelial cells of the gallbladder, but this issue has not yet been resolved. Ordinarily, gallbladder bile contains a trace (about 3%) of unconjugated bilirubin. In patients with chronic hemolytic anemias, the level of bilirubin secreted by the liver is around ten-fold greater. Most of this is conjugated bilirubin. However, it is possible that the amount of unconjugated bilirubin that makes its way across the canalicular membrane of the hepatocyte together with the ten-fold excess of conjugated bilirubin is also proportionately increased. This would eventually precipitate out.

It has recently been shown that postprandial emptying of the gallbladder is delayed in patients with black pigment stones compared to control subjects. Hence, gallbladder stasis allows time for calcium salts and bilirubin to precipitate out. In fact, in patients on TPN and perhaps in those with cirrhosis, this may be the most important mechanism responsible for the formation of black pigment stones associated with these conditions.

Brown pigment stones   Brown pigment stones are mainly seen in the Far East. Patients present with recurrent bouts of cholangitis (Figure 8.14 and Table 8.14).

Gallstones and disease

Gallstones occur in 10–20% of people over the age of 50 years. In the event of their discovery during the investigation of an unrelated problem, as now frequently occurs with the ready availability of abdominal ultrasound, they should be left alone. Cholecystectomy should not be performed for asymptomatic gallstones.

The mechanisms by which gallstones cause disease are summarized in Table 8.15.

Case history 1

A 44-year-old woman complained to her physician of having had three distinct episodes of epigastric pain radiating to the back over the past 6 months, the last episode being a month earlier. Each time the pain came on fairly abruptly, on one occasion awakening her from sleep. It rose to its zenith in an hour or so, was continuous (i.e. not colicky) and very severe. She found no relief in any position she adopted in bed. She had tried taking antacids she had at home, and they provided her with no relief. On each occasion her pain subsided gradually after 2–4 h. She said she had not felt as if she had a fever. She did not have vomiting, but did feel nauseated. At the time the physician saw her, she was not in any discomfort, and her physical examination was entirely normal. The physician suspected biliary colic and ordered an abdominal ultrasound examination, which revealed several small gallstones with shadowing and which moved when the position of the patient was changed (Figure 8.15a). Her gallstones were symptomatic, having given rise to attacks of biliary colic on four occasions. The physician therefore recommended a cholecystectomy.

Table 8.15 Gallstones and disease

Stone impacted temporarily at the neck of the gallbladder or in the cystic duct or common bile duct → biliary colic

Stone impacted permanently at the neck of the gallbladder → mucocele of the gallbladder

Stone impacted permanently in the cystic duct → acute cholecystitis

Stone impacted permanently or for a prolonged period of time in the common bile duct → choledocholithiasis

   complications of choledocholithiasis
      cholangitis
      gallstone pancreatitis

Stone in gallbladder or cystic duct extrinsically compressing the common bile duct → Mirizzi's syndrome

Stone (large) penetrates gallbladder wall and enters intestine → gallstone ileus

Stone present for many years in the gallbladder may rarely cause carcinoma

---

Figure 8.15b shows an incidental finding from another patient who had gallbladder polyps. This is shown for comparison with the ultrasound scan in the previous patient that showed gallstones. Notably, polyps do not shadow, are adherent to the wall of the gallbladder and therefore do not move with change in the position of the patient.

Biliary colic

When do patients experience biliary colic? When the stone is lodged in the outlet of the gallbladder or in the cystic duct. What are the characteristics of biliary colic? The word 'colic', when used in the context of biliary colic or renal colic, is a misnomer. The pain in both these conditions is not colicky but steady. It is a severe ache that at least half the time is in the epigastrium (as in Case history 1); the other half of the time it is in the right upper quadrant or in both the epigastrium and the right upper quadrant. The pain frequently radiates to the back, to the subscapular region. Often, the patient is able to say that the pain radiates to the back along the lower right costal margin rather than burrowing through to the back, as it does in pancreatitis or pancreatic cancer. The pain may also be felt at the tip of the right shoulder. No position eases the pain. The patient may be seen moving in bed desperately, but unsuccessfully, trying to find a position that will provide relief. By contrast, pancreatic pain is often relieved somewhat by sitting up and leaning forward in bed.

The pain typically occurs about an hour after a meal or awakens the patient from sleep. In a given individual there is a tendency for the pain to begin around the same time of day during each recurrent attack. It generally progresses steadily to reach its zenith within an hour and is persistent until the stone either drops back into the gallbladder, if it was initially obstructing the outlet, or passes through the cystic duct or the common bile duct and then into the duodenum.

How long does an attack of uncomplicated biliary colic last? An attack of uncomplicated biliary colic does not generally last more than 4–6 h, most often less, but seldom if ever less than an hour. This is because the stone, initially lodged in the outlet (neck) of the gallbladder, drops back into the gallbladder, or the stone, obstructing the cystic duct, moves into the duodenum via the common bile duct. If the pain lasts longer than a day, it suggests strongly that the stone is not moving from the cystic duct or the gallbladder outlet and acute cholecystitis is developing.

Other gastrointestinal symptoms can be associated with biliary colic. Nausea is almost always present and some amount of vomiting is not unusual. The patient may also complain of bloating and belching.

How does one diagnose biliary colic? The presence of typical symptoms like those described above plus the presence of gallstones usually detected by an ultrasound examination aid the diagnosis. The sensitivity and specificity for the detection of gallstones by ultrasonography is over 95%.

What should be done for a patient who has experienced one or more attacks of biliary colic? All patients with symptomatic gallstones should undergo a laparoscopic cholecystectomy. In contrast, surgery should not be offered to patients with asymptomatic gallstones discovered by chance during an ultrasound examination performed for another purpose.

Mucocele of the gallbladder

Occasionally the gallstone in the neck of the gallbladder remains impacted (Figure 8.16). After an attack of biliary colic, on occasion a steady ache persists in the right upper quadrant and examination reveals a large, tense, palpable gallbladder. The gallbladder may reach an enormous size and necessitate a cholecystectomy.

Case history 2

A 52-year-old woman presented to the Emergency Department of a hospital with severe epigastric pain radiating below the costal margin to the back. She was awoken from sleep with pain that gradually increased over an hour to reach a steady level of intensity. The pain was constant and not colicky (i.e. did not come in spasms). She described the pain as a 'terrible ache', which had now lasted unabated for around 8 h. Over the past hour she also felt the pain over the tip of the right shoulder. She felt nauseated, was unable to eat because the pain was very severe and had upon arrival at the hospital vomited very small amounts of mucoid material a few times. Nothing in particular either exacerbated the pain or helped to relieve it. She was very nauseated and felt distended. On examination she was found to be hemodynamically stable, appeared a little dry and was seen to be rolling around in bed and even sitting up at times in an effort to find some relief, but without success. The abdomen was soft but she had guarding in the right upper quadrant and epigastrium. The tenderness was exquisite; Murphy's sign (momentary cessation of respiration during deep palpation below the right costal margin) was positive. The only abnormal blood test was the white blood cell count, which was elevated at $12.1 \times 10^9/l$ with 89% granulocytes. The serum levels of transaminases, alkaline phosphatase, bilirubin, amylase and lipase were all normal.

What is the leading contender in the differential diagnosis? The patient had a pain that strongly resembled that of biliary colic (see discussion that follows Case history 1). However, the pain had now lasted over 6 h, suggesting that we might be dealing here not merely with uncomplicated biliary colic, but much more likely with acute cholecystitis or choledocholithiasis. Soon the pain became intense in the right upper quadrant with guarding and marked tenderness in the same region. These physical findings together with the modestly elevated white blood cell count point much more to acute cholecystitis than to choledocholithiasis. However, they by no means rule out choledocholithiasis. A distended gallbladder consequent to a common bile duct stone may well result in right upper quadrant tenderness, or with the elevation in the white blood cell count one could postulate early cholangitis causing these symptoms and signs. The normal liver function tests in this patient clearly make acute cholecystitis much more likely.

Acute cholecystitis

What are the symptoms and signs of acute cholecystitis? Initially, the pain is identical to that of biliary colic. Thereafter, the pain continues but changes its character. The pain now acquires a characteristic that suggests involvement of the parietal peritoneum around the gallbladder, i.e. movement, coughing or straining causes a sharp increment in the pain. Also, tenderness develops over the gallbladder fossa. If the initial pain was epigastric, it now shifts to the right upper quadrant. When the pain lasts more than 6 h one must become suspicious that acute cholecystitis or choledocholithiasis is developing. At other times the pain of biliary colic eases or even disappears for a short while, only to return shortly thereafter. When it returns, its characteristics suggest parietal peritoneal irritation, i.e. made worse by movement, coughing or straining. Again, if the initial pain was in the epigastrium, when it returns it is more in the right upper quadrant. Murphy's sign is seen (palpation below the rib cage in the right upper quadrant as the patient takes a deep breath results in momentary cessation of respiration and sharp pain).

Other symptoms such as nausea, some vomiting and bloating may also be present in acute cholecystitis. Vomiting is bilious and may occur frequently. Fever is only infrequently over 101°F (38°C), but may be on occasion. Icterus is not a constant feature and when present is generally very slight. Deep jaundice must lead one to suspect choledocholithiasis, either alone or with cholecystitis (10% of cases of cholecystitis turn out to have choledocholithiasis simultaneously).

Gentle palpation of the gallbladder will often result in the clinician feeling a 'mass' in the right upper quadrant. This is the distended gallbladder. There is tenderness in this area and Murphy's sign is often positive (cessation of respiration on palpation below the right costal margin). Tenderness is much greater over an empyema of the gallbladder or over an emphysematous gallbladder (see below). The white blood cell count may be moderately elevated (12 000–14 000 cells/mm³).

What is the pathophysiology of acute acalculous cholecystitis? The pathophysiology in acute cholecystitis is illustrated in Figure 8.17. Acute cholecystitis could develop with the very first attack of biliary colic if the stone were permanently impacted in the cystic duct. Figure 8.18a shows a gross specimen of a gallbladder from a patient with acute cholecystitis. On the other hand, there are patients who experience several episodes of biliary colic over a fairly long period of time and do not undergo operation. Each time, the attack of biliary colic subsides and does not result in acute cholecystitis. Such patients develop chronic cholecystitis. The gallbladder in such patients has a thickened wall, owing to fibrosis below the epithelial layer and the serosa as well as from hypertrophy of the muscular wall. The mucosa is infiltrated by mononuclear cells and forms outpouch-ings called Rochitansky–Aschoff sinuses (Figures 8.18b and c).

Could liver function tests be normal in acute cholecystitis? To answer that question, let us consider the pathogenesis of acute cholecystitis. It is due to a stone in the cystic duct with subsequent inflammation and infection in the gallbladder. Therefore, since the common bile duct is ordinarily not obstructed, liver function tests should in theory be normal (see below). They were normal in the patient described in Case history 2.

Could liver function tests be abnormal in acute cholecystitis? Yes. Mild elevations in the serum bilirubin (almost always < 4 mg/dl) and mild elevations in the transaminases and alkaline phosphatase or combinations of such mild elevations may be seen. Acute cholecystitis is one of the causes of a mild elevation in serum amylase as well. The amylase may be elevated up to three times above normal and in such cases one does not have to invoke the diagnosis of acute pancreatitis.

What is the first test to order in a case where acute cholecystitis is strongly suspected? The answer is a right upper quadrant ultrasound examination. The ultrasound features of acute cholecystitis are: presence of gallstones with shadowing; thickening of the gallbladder wall by > 4 mm or edema ('double wall sign'); pericholecystic fluid; and sonographic Murphy's sign positive – i.e. tenderness of the imaged gallbladder under pressure from the transducer. Sensitivity for the detection of acute cholecystitis is 85%, and specificity for the diagnosis of acute cholecystitis is 95%.

Acute cholecystitis was the leading contender in the differential diagnosis in case history 2. The possibility of acute pancreatitis was very unlikely with normal serum amylase and lipase. An ultrasound scan of the right upper quadrant was obtained and showed evidence of acute cholecystitis (Figure 8.19a and b).

A computed tomography (CT) scan may also be used to diagnose acute cholecystitis; however, it should not be the imaging study of choice. At times the clinical picture may be confusing and a CT scan might be ordered to rule out other conditions. Figure 8.20 shows acute cholecystitis in another patient.

Another useful test to diagnose acute cholecystitis is technetium-99m radionuclide scintigraphy. Here the radionuclide is injected intravenously and normally within a few minutes it should be excreted into the biliary system, taken up by the gallbladder and excreted in the duodenum. Since, in acute cholecystitis, the stone is lodged in the cystic duct, the gallbladder does not fill. Non-filling of the gallbladder does not in itself establish a diagnosis of acute cholecystitis, although in the appropriate clinical setting and with the appropriate findings on physical examination (see Case history 2), it may be considered to be fairly definitive and would not warrant further investigation prior to surgery. Non-filling of the gallbladder could be a false-positive sign, particularly if the patient has not eaten for some time. In such a case the entire bile acid pool would be in the gallbladder, as a consequence of which the gallbladder would take up the technetium. Some nuclear medicine physicians would then reimage the area after administration of either morphine or CCK in the hope of filling the gallbladder. If the gallbladder still does not fill, it provides more confidence that the non-filling is due to a cystic duct obstruction and not due to fasting alone. On the other hand if the gallbladder fills with radionuclide, then one has definitively excluded an obstruction of the cystic duct, that is, excluded a diagnosis of acute cholecystitis (Figure 8.21).

Case history 3

A 71-year-old man with rheumatoid arthritis on oral prednisone and a previous history of two myocardial infarctions, and a partial colectomy with a colostomy for colonic cancer, presented with vague symptoms of malaise, fatigue and feeling cold. On examination he had a temperature of 100.2°F (37.9°C). The examination of his abdomen revealed very mild right upper quadrant tenderness with no guarding. Murphy's sign was not elicited. No masses were palpable, there was no evidence clinically of organomegaly and bowel sounds were normal. He had chronic changes in the joints of his hands due to the rheumatoid arthritis. His hemoglobin was 14.9 g/dl, hematocrit 46, white blood cell count 17.4×10^9/l with a shift to the left and a platelet count of 232×10^9/l. On account of his fever, blood cultures were obtained which grew *Escherichia coli*. He had no sediment on microscopic examination of his urine. Suspecting some intra-abdominal source for his fever and bacteremia, an abdominal CT scan with oral and intravenous contrast was requested. It revealed evidence of advanced cholecystitis (Figure 8.22).

Here was a clear-cut indication for a CT scan. The marked elevation in the white blood cell count, the elevated temperature, an *E. coli* bacteremia and the absence of Murphy's sign required that the differential diagnosis be broadened.

What is the optimal time to remove the gallbladder in acute cholecystitis? There have been two schools of thought in the antibiotic era; to operate within the first 2 days or to give a course of antibiotics and then remove the gallbladder after a month to 6 weeks. Recent studies suggest that there is no advantage in waiting.

What are the complications of acute cholecystitis? Complications of acute cholecystitis are shown in Figure 8.23. Empyema of the gallbladder is a gallbladder distended by pus. The patient is usually more toxic with a very elevated white blood cell count. Emphysematous cholecystitis occurs when air generated by bacteria (*E. coli*, *Klebsiella*, *Enterococcus*) is seen in the wall of the gallbladder or in the lumen on either plain radiograph of the abdomen or on CT scan. Patients complain of severe pain and bacteremia is common. Distension of the gallbladder results in ischemia to its wall and eventually in gangrene. A gangrenous gallbladder, if not operated on in time, will perforate. Perforation develops in close to 10% of cases of acute cholecystitis.

Case history 4

An 80-year-old man was admitted with septicemia following a urinary tract infection. He was not fully alert and developed bilateral aspiration pneumonia requiring intubation and placement on a ventilator. During the course of his illness he developed disseminated intravascular coagulation (DIC) and became hypotensive, requiring fluid resuscitation and for a while vasopressors. He was receiving TPN. His fever was gradually improving and his white blood cell count had returned to normal, until one morning when he developed high fever and an elevation in his white blood cell count which the following day rose to 22 000/mm^3 with a marked shift to the left. The patient was still on a ventilator, and his mental state, which had been rapidly improving until the recurrence of fever, deteriorated, the patient being more somnolent, though arousable. On palpation of the abdomen it was repeatedly noted that the patient winced considerably while the examiner was palpating the right upper quadrant. A mass was vaguely felt in the right upper quadrant as well. An imaging study was obtained (Figure 8.24). The appearance was that of acute cholecystitis, although no gallstones were seen.

The patient underwent surgery and the diagnosis of acalculous cholecystitis was confirmed.

Acalculous cholecystitis

How frequent is acalculous cholecystitis? It is infrequent. Around 5% of all attacks of acute cholecystitis

Table 8.16 Conditions that make patients prone to developing acalculous cholecystitis

Trauma
Burns
Septicemia
After major abdominal surgery of any kind
Coronary artery bypass graft
Long-term total parenteral nutrition

are due to acalculous cholecystitis. However, since cholecystitis is a common condition, acalculous cholecystitis is something every physician should be aware of, particularly those physicians who admit patients to intensive care units.

Which kind of patient is prone to developing acalculous cholecystitis? Acalculous cholecystitis occurs in patients who are critically ill and often in intensive care units. The patient described in Case history 4 had several of the risk factors shown in Table 8.16.

What is the pathophysiology of acalculous cholecystitis? The true answer is that it is unclear. Two factors, probably acting in concert, play a role:

(1) *Ischemia* Ischemia of the vessels of the gallbladder, instead of the usual picture of hyperemia seen with inflammation;

(2) *Gallbladder stasis* This is probably due to these patients not receiving enteral feeding, and the gallbladder being distended and storing much of the bile acid pool within it. Gallbladder distension should occur and this too can lead to further ischemia.

The clinical presentation of acalculous cholecystitis This is very similar to that of acute calculus cholecystitis. The diagnosis is generally made at ultrasonography. The criteria for diagnosis are similar to those for acute calculus cholecystitis except that no gallstones are seen on the ultrasound scan. The interpretation of a radiolabeled scintigraphic scan may be difficult, because the patient is fasting and so the gallbladder may not fill. The use of morphine along with cholescintigraphy may improve the sensitivity of the test.

What is the management of acalculous cholecystitis? Patients need to be taken to surgery for a cholecystectomy early.

Case history 5

An elderly man presented with epigastric pain that awoke him from sleep. The pain gradually increased in severity. He described it as being constant and said it felt 'like an ache'. Neither respiration nor movement affected the severity of the pain, and he had not found any position that provided him with comfort. The pain did not radiate to the shoulder, groin or scrotum. He mentioned that he had had a similar episode 6 weeks earlier that had brought him to the Emergency Room, but while he was waiting to be seen, the pain had abated and so he left. The total duration of the pain at that time had been for around 2–3 h. This time he remained at home, hoping that the pain would go away as it did the last time. It had been continuous for 6 h now. On examination he was a well-set elderly man in considerable pain. He was not jaundiced. He appeared a little dehydrated. His vital signs were stable. He was not febrile. His heart and lung examinations were normal except for a grade 2/6 mid-systolic murmur along the left sternal border and in the aortic area. The abdomen was soft, with minimal guarding in the epigastrium and right upper quadrant, with slight tenderness on deep palpation. Murphy's sign was negative. There was no tenderness in the costo-vertebral angle. His white blood cell count was not elevated and his urinalysis was normal, showing no crystals. The serum bilirubin level was 1.1 mg/dl, the serum ALT was 651 IU/l, AST 548 IU/l, alkaline phosphatase 89 IU/l and serum amylase and lipase were within normal limits. A plain radiograph of the abdomen did not show free air under the diaphragm and there were no dilated loops of bowel, nor were there any air–fluid levels.

The differential diagnosis included choledocholithiasis. The marked elevations in the serum transaminases support this diagnosis. Alkaline phosphatase and serum bilirubin are normal early on, and rise later only if the common duct remains obstructed by the stone. The similar attack of pain 6 weeks earlier that had lasted for 2–3 h was probably an attack of biliary colic. Whenever one thinks of choledocholithiasis one has to consider gallstone pancreatitis. The serum amylase and lipase levels are normal at this time, making that diagnosis unlikely. Other possibilities such as a perforated peptic ulcer and small intestinal obstruction were excluded on the basis of the physical examination of the abdomen and by the results of the plain radiograph. Acute cholecystitis must be considered. However, the lack of localized pain, tenderness and severe guarding in the right upper quadrant and the absent Murphy's sign make the diagnosis less likely, but do not exclude it. Abnormalities in the liver function tests are occasionally seen in acute cholecystitis

(see discussion above), but such high elevations in the serum transaminase levels as an isolated finding would be very unusual indeed in acute cholecystitis.

An abdominal ultrasound examination was performed which showed gallstones, a dilated common bile duct, but no dilated intrahepatic duct (Figure 8.25a). No stone was seen in the common bile duct. The gallbladder wall was not thickened and there was no pericholecystic fluid. These findings were compatible with choledocholithiasis because stones in the common bile duct are often missed on ultrasonography on account of bowel gas or body habitus. One expects dilatation of intrahepatic ducts to occur eventually with time. The patient underwent endoscopic retrograde cholangiopancreatography (ERCP) a few hours later which showed a dilated common bile duct, the gallbladder filled with contrast (thus eliminating cholecystitis from the differential diagnosis) and a large stone obstructing the bile duct in its distal third (Figure 8.25b).

Case history 6

A 60-year-old man with known alcoholic cirrhosis, portal hypertension and ascites presented with abdominal pain and fever, but no chills. According to the patient's family he continued to drink almost until the day prior to admission. On examination he had stigmata of chronic liver disease (i.e. palmar erythema and spider nevi), a temperature of 101°F (38°C) and a heart rate of 110 beats/min. He was slightly tachypneic. He had scleral icterus. There was no asterixis nor was he tremulous. The patient was somewhat confused. The examinations of the heart and lung were normal. Examination of the abdomen revealed distension and generalized tenderness with perhaps more tenderness in the upper abdomen, the spleen was not palpable and there was shifting dullness. He had a small amount of pitting edema around the ankles. He had an easily reducible umbilical hernia and no inguinal or femoral hernias. Bowel sounds were normal. Laboratory tests revealed hemoglobin 10.1 g/dl, hematocrit 30.0, white blood cell count 16 500/mm³ (segmented forms 76%, band forms 13%, lymphocytes 9%, monocytes 2%, eosinophils 0%), platelet count 76 000/mm³, prothrombin time of 18.0 s with control of 11.2 s, blood urea nitrogen 26 mg/dl, serum creatinine 1.2 mg/dl, serum total bilirubin 7.6 mg/dl, direct bilirubin 6.4 mg/dl, alkaline phosphatase 340 IU/l, AST 88 IU/l, ALT 20 IU/l, serum albumin 2.6 g/dl, and normal serum amylase and lipase. Urinalysis was normal. A chest radiograph was obtained and was normal.

Thus, the differential diagnosis was for a middle-aged man with known alcoholic cirrhosis and portal hypertension and who was still imbibing alcoholic beverages (according to his family), who now presented with fever, jaundice and abdominal pain and some confusion. The liver function test profile revealed an AST/ALT ratio of 4.4, a direct hyperbilirubinemia, an elevated alkaline phosphatase and a mild coagulopathy.

The presence of cirrhosis does not of course protect the patient from the usual causes of fever, such as urinary tract infection, pneumonia or skin or soft tissue infection. Pyelonephritis can certainly produce abdominal or flank pain and lower lobe pneumonias produce upper abdominal pain and tenderness. However, the history and physical examination as well as an examination of the urine and the chest radiograph ruled out all three of these common causes of fever and malaise. One of the conditions specific to patients with cirrhosis is spontaneous bacterial peritonitis. In any patient with cirrhosis who presents with a fever, it is important to rule out spontaneous bacterial peritonitis even if abdominal pain is absent. This patient's ascitic fluid was examined and did not reveal increased cells (> 250 polymorphonuclear leukocytes/mm^3 is required to make a diagnosis of spontaneous bacterial peritonitis) and the Gram stain was negative, thus ruling out that possibility. The ratio of serum AST/ALT of > 2 together with an elevated prothrombin time leads one to consider a diagnosis of alcoholic hepatitis. The direct hyperbilirubinemia and elevated alkaline phosphatase would be consistent with alcoholic hepatitis, since this condition is a cholestatic disease. Fever and abdominal pain are frequently present in moderately severe and severe alcoholic hepatitis. This patient certainly had alcoholic hepatitis based on clinical criteria. However, in such patients it is still essential to rule out an obstructive cause of cholestatic jaundice, since a delay in the diagnosis could have devastating consequences in patients with cirrhosis and/or alcoholic hepatitis. It is essential that such patients undergo a right upper quadrant ultrasound examination. This patient, in fact, underwent a CT scan (an ultrasound scan would have been just as effective an imaging modality and is much cheaper). The CT scan revealed a large gallstone in the gallbladder, a dilated common bile duct occupied by a large gallstone, dilated intrahepatic ducts and a normal-appearing pancreas. Blood cultures grew *E. coli*. The patient had choledocholithiasis with cholangitis. He underwent an emergency ERCP after receiving fresh frozen plasma to correct his coagulopathy which revealed large aglommerated filling defects in a very markedly dilated common bile duct (Figure 8.26).

Choledocholithiasis

This is a stone obstructing the common bile duct. Types of common bile duct stones are:

(1) *Secondary stones*   These are stones that originate in the gallbladder. They are occasionally seen even in people who have undergone cholecystectomy previously. By far the commonest cause of choledocholithiasis is a stone that leaves the gallbladder to find itself becoming impacted in the common bile duct.

(2) *Primary stones*   These are mostly brown pigment stones (see discussion on brown pigment stones earlier in this chapter and Table 14) that develop *de novo* within the common bile duct. They result from the stasis and infection of bile, the stasis often being due to:

(a) biliary stricture;

(b) papillary stenosis;

(c) dysfunction of the sphincter of Oddi.

Clinical presentation   The pain is similar to that of biliary colic but does not go away. The signs of peritoneal irritation are much less common than in acute cholecystitis. Icterus develops only if the stone remains impacted in the common bile duct. If it moves in a few hours into the duodenum, jaundice may never develop. However, in those cases where the gallstone remains in the common bile duct for a prolonged period, deep jaundice develops, much higher than in acute cholecystitis. Fever is an ominous sign and usually denotes the onset of cholangitis. In cholangitis the fever is very high and swinging temperatures with shaking chills are common. The jaundice also deepens.

Liver function tests   A variety of different patterns of elevation are seen in the liver function test profile in choledocholithiasis. The variations in the liver function tests seen in different patients with choledocholithiasis are due to two important facts:

(1) The time the stone remains in the common bile duct before it passes into the duodenum (or the stone never spontaneously passes into the duodenum);

(2) When in the natural history of the disease the patient is first seen.

The usual sequence of events as far as liver function tests are concerned is shown in Figure 8.27. It is evident from Figure 8.27 that the first abnormality in the liver function tests in choledocholithiasis is generally an elevation in the serum transaminases (ALT and AST). In animals, sudden ligation of the common bile duct results in a similar elevation in the transaminases. In contrast, transaminase elevations are not so prominent in patients who present with the consequences of a gradual obstruction of the common bile duct, as from a tumor. This can be either intrinsic to the bile duct (cholangiocarcinoma) or extrinsic to it (carcinoma of the head of the pancreas). The elevations in transaminases in choledocholithiasis are often very high. Values of 200–600 IU are frequently seen. The authors have on rare occasions seen values close to or above 1000 IU. These patients may be misdiagnosed as having acute viral or toxic hepatitis, particularly because early on the alkaline phosphatase and serum bilirubin may be completely normal or only slightly elevated.

It is also evident from Figure 8.27 that abnormalities in liver function tests may vary from being completely normal to high elevations in serum transaminases with or without elevations in the serum alkaline phosphatase and serum bilirubin. The following clinical scenarios will clarify the understanding of this important concept.

A patient develops the symptoms of severe biliary colic as a result of a stone obstructing the common bile duct and comes in a few hours later to see his physician. At this stage the serum transaminases (ALT and AST) would be elevated, but the alkaline phosphatase and serum bilirubin could be completely normal (Figure 8.27). If the stone continues to cause obstruction of the common bile duct, gradually the alkaline phosphatase and the serum bilirubin will rise and eventually the patient may develop a severe conjugated (direct reacting) hyperbilirubinemia. If, on the other hand, the stone spontaneously passes into the duodenum early after the onset of the obstruction, then the alkaline phosphatase and the serum bilirubin may never go up. In that case all that the physician would be left with would be the clinical history and the elevated serum transaminases. When serially followed for a few days, the serum transaminases will rapidly return to normal, quite unlike the case in a patient with hepatitis, in whom the decline in the transaminases would be gradual.

A stoical woman develops choledocholithiasis but remains at home for a day or two before coming in to see her physician. Let us say that her stone passes spontaneously into the duodenum. However, her husband insists that she take an urgent appointment with her physician even though her pain has almost completely subsided. Her liver function tests may be entirely normal at the time she first sees her physician. This is because the stone is no longer obstructing the common bile duct and the initial elevations in the ALT and AST that may well have occurred have now returned to normal (Figure 8.27). Because the stone spontaneously passed into the duodenum soon enough, the alkaline phosphatase and serum bilirubin never become elevated (Figure 8.27). Since the patient's pain had more or less subsided, the physician may miss the diagnosis of choledocholithiasis. A shrewd clinician, however, based on the history of the characteristics of the pain, would request a right upper quadrant ultrasound examination and make a diagnosis of biliary colic. The situation would be sufficient to warrant recommending an elective laparoscopic cholecystectomy.

Let us now consider a third scenario very similar to the one just described. A stoical patient has her common bile duct obstructed with a stone and soon thereafter develops acute gallstone pancreatitis. The pain is severe but the patient does not seek medical advice immediately. Soon thereafter the stone passes spontaneously into the duodenum. However, unlike in the previous case, the pain does not subside despite the passage of the stone into the duodenum, because of the pancreatitis. Finally, the raging pain brings this stoic in to see her physician a few days later. The serum amylase and lipase are still elevated (perhaps less than they might have been at the onset), but the liver function tests may be completely normal. The elevated transaminases that could have been detected had the patient come in sooner have now returned to normal, because the stone is no longer obstructing the common bile duct. Again, as in the previous patient, because the stone spontaneously passed into the duodenum fairly soon after the onset of the obstruction, the alkaline phosphatase and serum bilirubin did not become elevated. In such a case the etiology of the pancreatitis may not be evident.

Imaging and endoscopic tests for the diagnosis of choledocholithiasis Whereas right upper quadrant ultrasonography is very sensitive and specific in the diagnosis of gallstones, its sensitivity for the detection of stones in the common bile duct (i.e. the identification of shadowing from a stone in the common bile duct) is relatively poor, of the order of 65%. Spiral and helical CT scanning is a valuable tool and should be requested to exclude other intra-abdominal conditions if the diagnosis is not clear. The ERCP has for some time been regarded as the gold standard and indeed should be performed urgently to relieve obstruction in patients whose clinical picture suggests continued obstruction, in particular patients with cholangitis. At this time, a substantial amount of information is available using a relatively new technique, magnetic resonance cholangiography (MRCP). The sensitivity and specificity for the detection of common bile duct stones was 95% and 89%, respectively, in one study.

Let us consider a clinical scenario. A patient presents with an attack of acute pancreatitis, which for a variety of clinical reasons appears typical for gallstone pancreatitis. However, the right upper quadrant ultrasound scan and spiral CT scan do not show evidence for either common bile duct stones or even stones in the gallbladder. What would be the best method to rule out common bile duct stones in such a patient? ERCP would certainly be one choice. However, both MRCP and endoscopic ultrasonography (EUS) would be alternatives. In the right hands, EUS is extremely sensitive for the detection of stones in the common bile duct.

Management of choledocholithiasis   If evidence suggests that the stone is continuing to cause obstruction of the common bile duct, then an urgent ERCP is the procedure of choice. However, if there is clinical evidence that a stone has been passed into the duodenum, the patient's pain has subsided and the laboratory tests are steadily improving, one does not have to perform an urgent ERCP. An elective laparoscopic cholecystectomy should be recommended to such a patient.

Case history 7

A 66-year-old woman presented with right upper quadrant pain of 3 days' duration. She also noticed at that time that her eyes and skin had turned yellow. On examination she was jaundiced and had tenderness with some guarding but no rigidity in the right upper quadrant, and no mass was palpated. The liver span was normal and the spleen was not palpable. Normal bowel sounds were present. The white blood cell count was not elevated. She had a predominantly

conjugated (direct reacting) hyperbilirubinemia (total serum bilirubin 10 mg/dl), a serum alkaline phosphatase three times the upper limit of normal and only relatively mild elevations in the serum transaminases. A right upper quadrant ultrasound scan was interpreted as showing obstruction of the common bile duct by a large gallstone. There was sufficient disagreement among radiographers about the interpretation of the ultrasound scan to warrant a CT scan. The CT scan showed the large stone to be in the cystic duct, compressing the common hepatic duct and giving rise to dilatation of the biliary tree more proximally. An ERCP was performed (Figure 8.28a). It confirmed the CT scan findings. A stent was placed to decompress the obstructed biliary system prior to surgery (Figure 8.28b). A diagnosis of Mirizzi's syndrome was made. It was apparent that the obstruction to the common hepatic duct was of longer duration than just 3 days, to account for the marked elevation of the serum bilirubin and alkaline phosphatase. The patient's attention was probably drawn to her illness only when she developed right upper quadrant pain 3 days prior to admission.

Mirizzi's syndrome

A large stone in either the cystic duct or the Hartmann's pouch of the gallbladder can result in extrinsic obstruction of the common bile duct with the same sequelae as those seen in choledocholithiasis. The obstruction to the duct may be a consequence only of direct compression or it may be a combination of some compression and some inflammation around the area of the stone. By and large there are two types of Mirrizzi's syndrome described (although some surgeons have developed classifications that further subdivided the types resulting in either three or four different categories). For simplicity we shall describe only the original two types of Mirizzi's syndrome:

(1) *Type 1*   Here the stone is located within the cystic duct or the Hartmann's pouch.

(2) *Type 2*   Here the stone has wholly or partially eroded into the adjacent common hepatic duct, creating a partial or complete cholecysto-choledochal fistula.

In acute cholecystitis, hepatic duct occlusion can result from its entrapment within the inflammatory process surrounding the cystic duct. Obstruction of the hepatic duct in this instance is not due to the impingement of a stone within the cystic duct, but is totally a consequence of the adjacent inflammation. Some surgeons have termed this scenario also as Mirizzi's syndrome (type 4 in their classification). It is essential to obtain an ERCP in all patients with Mirizzi's syndrome in order to have anatomical information available on the exact nature of the obstruction and the presence or absence of a fistula prior to surgery, so that the operation may be tailored to the given patient.

Case history 8

An 80-year-old woman presented with colicky periumbilical pain of 2 day's duration. Initially she did not have abdominal distension but over the course of the 2 days the abdomen became very distended. She had one bowel movement a few hours after the onset of the pain, but none since. She has been belching. She developed bilious vomiting on the second day (i.e. the day of admission). She mentioned that over the past week or 10 days she had had two rather similar attacks of pain, but neither had lasted more than 6 or 7 h and the accompanying distension was trivial compared to this time.

During the physical examination there were periods when she would not permit the examination until an episode of pain that developed had subsided. Observed during one such episode, she was seen to have visible peristalsis around the umbilicus. The abdomen was fairly soft but distended and not with any specific area of tenderness. On percussion the abdomen was tympanitic and she had high-pitched bowel sounds in gushes. No umbilical, inguinal or femoral hernias were noted. A clinical diagnosis of intestinal obstruction was made and confirmed by a plain radiograph of the abdomen, which also showed air in the biliary tree. The air in the biliary tract without a previous history of biliary tract disease suggested a fistula between some portion of the biliary tract and either the duodenum or the stomach. That, coupled with symptoms and signs of intestinal obstruction, suggested a diagnosis of gallstone ileus.

Three options were available with regard to further management:

(1) Obtain a barium study with small bowel follow-through to confirm the above diagnosis;

(2) Obtain a CT scan with oral contrast to confirm the above diagnosis;

(3) Take the patient directly to surgery without wasting further time, since the old adage says that the sun must never set on an intestinal obstruction!

All three options have merit. In this case the patient underwent a CT scan (Figure 8.29). This confirmed the diagnosis of gallstone ileus.

Case history 9

The patient was a 90-year-old man who developed right upper quadrant pain while at home that lasted for 4 or 5 h. The pain was constant while it lasted and then gradually subsided. After a lapse of several hours the pain recurred, but this time it was in the periumbilical region, had an intermittent character to it and the patient began to vomit copious bilious fluid. On examination the patient was not febrile, the abdomen was not distended and bowel sounds were present but considerably diminished. There was no tenderness. A plain radiograph of the abdomen revealed air in the biliary tree. An upper gastrointestinal barium study was carried out (Figure 8.30). The diagnosis of gallstone ileus was made, this time the obstruction being at the ligament of Trietz.

Gallstone ileus

These two cases (Case history 8 and Case history 9) are examples of a rather uncommon manifestation of gallstone-related disease. There are similarities and differences in the clinical presentations between the two patients.

The similarities between these two patients are:

(1) Both were elderly;

(2) Both presented with intestinal obstruction resulting from a gallstone that had eroded through the gallbladder wall and the adjacent gut wall to enter the lumen of the gastrointestinal tract.

There are also striking differences between these two patients:

(1) The patient in Case history 8 had a more subacute presentation;

(2) The patient in Case history 8 had experienced two similar though milder events over the past 10 days. The patient in Case history 9 had not.

(3) Abdominal distension, while developing gradually, was marked in the patient in Case history 8. The patient in Case history 9 was not distended.

(4) Vomiting appeared later in the patient in Case history 8 and was not as severe. The patient in Case history 9 had vomiting early on and it was more copious.

Table 8.17 Gallstone ileus

The term 'ileus' is a misnomer. Gallstone ileus is not an ileus but an organic obstruction.
It is a disease of the elderly. Median age is 70 years.
Overall incidence in patients with gallstones is ~0.5%.
It is a rare cause of intestinal obstruction. When all causes and ages are taken together, the incidence ranges between 1 and 4%.
However, in the elderly, a quarter of the cases of non-hernia-related small intestinal obstructions are due to gallstone ileus.
Since gallstones are more frequent in women, so too, as anticipated, is gallstone ileus.
Sites of the fistula between the gallbladder and the adjacent gut are:
Duodenum: commonest site, > 70%
Gastric antrum: presentation like that of a pyloric obstruction (Bouveret's syndrome)
Colon
Clinical presentation:
Ileal obstruction. Patient may on occasion feel right upper quadrant pain at the time of the fistula formation which then often subsides. Such pain is frequently not reported by the patient. On a rare occasion the fistula formation in the stomach or duodenum may result in hematemesis.
The commonest site at which the small intestine becomes obstructed is the ileum, since the caliber of the ileum is narrower than the duodenum or jejunum. However, duodenal and jejunal obstruction does develop (Case history 8).
Patients who ultimately present with ileal obstruction fall into two groups:
Those whose initial symptoms are of ileal obstruction
Those who develop symptoms of partial small intestinal obstruction, albeit mild, one or more times before the final major occurrence. This is attributed to the stone obstructing the lumen of the small intestine at different levels until it finally lodges in the ileum, giving rise to total obstruction
Gastric outlet obstruction. Symptoms of gastric outlet obstruction develop in patients in whom the stone obstructs the pyloric channel or the first part of the duodenum. This syndrome is called Bouveret's syndrome.
Colonic obstruction. The stone is usually able to traverse the colon without giving rise to obstruction, but in patients with other causes such as a stricture from any cause or narrowing in the sigmoid colon after previous attacks of diverticulitis, the stone may become lodged behind a stricture.

The similarities in the symptoms in these two patients point out the hallmarks of this condition: it tends to occur more often in the elderly, and it is a consequence of the pathogenesis of gallstone ileus (Figure 8.31).

The differences in the clinical presentations of the two patients are those due to the differences between the presentation of a patient with a lower small intestinal (ileal) obstruction (Case history 8) and that of a patient with a high jejunal obstruction (Case history 9). Such differences are more fully described in Chapter 9, but briefly:

(1) Low small bowel obstructions result in gradually progressive distension that can become very marked, whereas in high jejunal obstructions the distension is much less;

(2) Vomiting begins somewhat later in low small intestinal obstruction and is seldom as copious, because the patient has been treated by then. Vomiting begins early in high small bowel obstruction and is copious.

Some important facts about gallstone ileus are summarized in Table 8.17.

Case history 10

A 77-year-old man was admitted with a history of recurrent episodes of postprandial right upper quadrant pain and weight loss. He had a history of hypertension, type 2 diabetes mellitus, coronary artery disease and peptic ulcer disease. On examination he had a blood pressure of 135/75 mmHg, a heart rate of 50 beats/min (the patient was on a β-blocker). The patient had marked tenderness in the right upper quadrant with some guarding but no rigidity or percussion tenderness. The rectal examination was normal. The abdomen was not distended. Bowel sounds were normal. Routine laboratory tests were normal; the white blood cell count was 7700/mm^3.

An ultrasound examination revealed a mildly distended gallbladder with diffuse thickening of the gallbladder wall, with several gallstones but no pericholecystic fluid. A CT scan of the abdomen was interpreted as being consistent with a complex cholecystitis (thickened wall with a small amount of pericholecystic fluid associated with what was thought to be a contained perforation related to the gallbladder fundus). The patient's white blood cell count was never elevated and this in many ways went against a diagnosis of acute cholecystitis (Figure 8.32). The patient underwent a laparotomy and a cholecystectomy. The pathology revealed a gallbladder that was thickened, gallstones and an adenocarcinoma infiltrating the gallbladder fundus.

Take home message The diagnosis of gallbladder carcinoma is frequently missed preoperatively. In this case the recurrent episodes of pain are not explained by the carcinoma. It is quite possible that he had recurrent bouts of biliary colic from his gallstones.

Gallbladder carcinoma

Gallbladder carcinoma is the commonest biliary tract cancer, commoner than cholangiocarcinoma and carcinoma of the ampulla of Vater. It is the fifth commonest cancer of the gastrointestinal tract.

Risk factors These are as follows:

(1) *Porcelain gallbladder* Gallbladder with calcification in the wall which may be seen on a plain radiograph of the abdomen or on ultrasound or CT scan done for another reason. All porcelain gallbladders should be removed.

(2) *Gallstones* Very few if any gallbladder cancers are detected in gallbladders that do not contain stones. The incidence of gallbladder cancer is nevertheless small, and so based on current data it is not recommended that asymptomatic stones be treated by cholecystectomy.

(3) *Polyps of the gallbladder* Most polyps of the gallbladder (cholesterolosis, adenomyomatosis, inflammatory polyps, etc.) are not premalignant conditions. Gallbladder adenomas are premalignant, but they are rare. The problem is that carcinomas appear on imaging studies like the benign polyps mentioned above. Ultrasound features have been described to distinguish benign polyps from adenomas and carcinomas, and while they may be valuable in centers with vast experience, overall the differentiation is not that simple. Therefore, all patients with gallbladders harboring polyps of > 1 cm in size require a standard cholecystectomy and those with polyps of > 2 cm require an extended cholecystectomy. Patients whose gallbladders contain polyps of < 1 cm should have them removed if gallstones are identified in the gallbladder by ultrasonography. When gallstones are not seen, then these patients require regular follow-up (initially in 6 months and later annually) to determine whether the polyp is increasing in size. If an increase in size is determined, surgery should be offered to the patient.

Clinical presentation May be asymptomatic (found during cholecystectomy for cholecystitis) or symptomatic (early non-specific symptoms of food intolerance, 'dyspepsia' → weight loss → right upper quadrant pain → jaundice → fever occasionally present).

Diagnosis Most gallbladder cancers are diagnosed incidentally at surgery for cholecystectomy for gallstone-related disease. In the case of the uncommon symptomatic cases, CT scan and MRPC are the most sensitive methods of diagnosis and provide information on the extent of local disease, and the extent of the involvement of the liver, lymph nodes, portal and hepatic veins and distant metastases. EUS may also be used to stage the carcinoma and to determine operability. In those patients who present with obstructive jaundice, an ERCP or a percutaneous cholangiogram is performed. A fairly long stricture of the common hepatic duct is the feature most often seen in gallbladder cancer. In contrast, the stricture in proximal cholangiocarcinomas (Klatskin tumor) is at the bifurcation in the perihilar region and in distal cholangiocarcinomas the stricture is much more distal, being located in the common bile duct.

Treatment When the lymph nodes and vascular structures are not involved and the liver is spared (or according to more aggressive surgeons the depth of liver involvement is < 2 cm), then surgery is the first option. When the extent of wall involvement does not go beyond the muscle layer, a simple cholecystectomy may be adequate. For other patients an extended cholecystectomy is indicated.

When lymph nodes, vascular structures or other distant organs are involved, or when there is extensive involvement of the liver, then the treatment is palliative. Radiation and chemotherapy by and large have not worked well for advanced disease and at this time should be offered only to patients on clinical protocols. Either endoscopic or percutaneous stenting with Wall stents should be placed to relieve itching and jaundice.

Case history 11

A 78-year-old man presented to the hospital because a friend told him that morning that his eyes and skin looked yellow. He had had more frequent bowel movements over the past month. The stools were bulky and pale and devoid of blood. When asked, he mentioned that he had lost 20 lb (9 kg) over the past month. He did not have abdominal pain, nausea, vomiting or fever. On examination his temperature was 97.6°F (36.4°C) heart rate 76 beats/min and blood pressure 130/75 mmHg. He was deeply jaundiced. The abdomen was mildly distended, soft, non-tender with no evidence clinically of organomegaly. Bowel sounds were present. The rectal examination was normal. There was no stool on the glove. His hematocrit was 37.6, mean corpuscular volume 86, total bilirubin 13.2 mg/dl, direct bilirubin 8.8 mg/dl, AST 163 IU/l, ALT 244 IU/l and alkaline phosphatase 1312 IU/l.

The patient thus presented with painless jaundice. The commonest causes are pancreatic cancer, cholangiocarcinoma, carcinoma of the ampulla of Vater or periampullary duodenal carcinoma.

While on rare occasions choledocholithiasis in the elderly patient may present with jaundice in the absence of pain, this is most unusual. Since neoplasm was suspected, a CT scan rather than an ultrasound examination was the first imaging study requested. The CT scan revealed extrahepatic biliary obstruction due to an ampullary tumor and a pancreas with no evidence of neoplasm (Figure 8.33a–d). The patient then underwent an ERCP. At endoscopy a 3-cm friable mass involving the ampulla was visualized at the ampulla and was biopsied. A stent was placed in order to decompress the biliary system prior to surgery (Figure 8.33e and f).

Carcinoma of the ampulla of Vater

These are less common than gallbladder cancers. They are almost always adenocarcinomas. It generally affects persons in the seventh decade.

The clinical presentation is as follows:

(1) Obstructive jaundice is the presenting symptom in over 80% of patients.

(2) Weight loss is seen in three-quarters of the patients.

(3) Abdominal pain is present in a half of the patients.

(4) Occult blood in the stool and iron deficiency anemia may occur as well. This distinguishes this tumor from cancer of the head of the pancreas.

(5) Acute pancreatitis occurs rarely but is much less common than in pancreatic cancer.

Helical CT (spiral CT) with oral and intravenous contrast is usually the first imaging test to obtain in patients presenting with obstructive jaundice. It provides evidence for the level of the obstruction and of local and distant spread. MRCP also provides excellent information. EUS gives excellent information that helps toward more accurate staging. ERCP enables identification of the tumor at the ampulla and provides an opportunity to obtain cytology and brushings. A stent may be placed to relieve obstruction.

CHAPTER 9

The acute abdomen – a pot-pourri

Acute abdomen is the abrupt onset of gastrointestinal symptoms (pain almost always being the predominant symptom), resulting from acute inflammation, perforation, obstruction or twist of an intra-abdominal viscus, or secondary to a traumatic or an intra-abdominal vascular event.

PAIN IN THE ACUTE ABDOMEN

The nature, location and time to maximal severity of pain is dependent on the pathogenesis of the event resulting in the acute abdomen.

Pain due to luminal obstruction

Pain secondary to obstruction reaches peak severity in hours (not minutes or days). Since the intestine and organs associated with the intestine (such as the biliary tree) arise in the midline, pain arising from distension resulting as a consequence of obstruction of the lumen of these structures is often referred to the mid-abdomen. The exact location depends on the segmental innervation of the viscus concerned. The nerves carrying visceral pain accompany the splanchnic sympathetic nerves to the spinal cord. Examples are as follows:

(1) *Small intestinal obstruction*   The pain is in the midline in the epigastrium or the periumbilical area, since the nerve supply is from thoracic segments 9–11. Pain is colicky.

(2) *Large intestinal obstruction*   The pain is in the midline in the hypogastrium. Occasionally when the cecum or ascending colon is obstructed, the pain may arise at the site of the lesion, if the mesocecum or mesocolon is very short.

(3) *Appendicitis*   The initiating event in appendicitis is obstruction to the lumen of the appendix, as by a fecalith. Therefore, the initial pain in appendicitis is in the midline and located in the epigastrium or in the periumbilical area, since the appendicular nerves are derived from thoracic segments 9–11. Pain is usually steady, but is occasionally colicky.

(4) *Biliary system*   Obstruction at the outlet to the gallbladder leads to biliary colic. Obstruction of the common bile duct leads to choledocholithiasis. In both these conditions pain is frequently in the epigastrium, although it can be in the right upper quadrant also. Despite being termed 'biliary colic', the pain is continuous and not colicky.

Pain due to inflammation

Pain secondary to inflammation reaches peak severity in hours (not minutes or days). Inflammation of a viscus involves the parietal peritoneum. Somatic nerves innervate the parietal peritoneum, leading to pain and tenderness at the site of the inflamed organ. Examples are as follows:

(1) *Appendicitis*   Once the wall of the appendix becomes inflamed, the nerves supplying the parietal peritoneum become involved and pain is present, localized to the site of the appendix, most often in the right lower quadrant.

(2) *Diverticulitis*   Pain is present over the inflammation in the sigmoid colon (left lower quadrant) following the mini-perforation of a diverticulum.

(3) *Acute cholecystitis*   The pain of biliary colic and the early phase of cholecystitis is due to distension of the gallbladder and is usually in the epigastrium or right upper quadrant and is relatively diffuse. When the gallbladder wall becomes inflamed, there is severe localized pain and tenderness and guarding over the gallbladder in the right upper quadrant.

Somatic nerves also supply the muscles on the anterior abdominal wall, resulting in these muscles contracting and producing guarding. The somatic nerves also supply the muscles on the posterior abdominal wall, resulting in spasm of these muscles. Examples are as follows:

(1) Psoas spasm elicited by the psoas test if the inflamed organ (e.g. appendix) lies on the muscle;

(2) Obturator internus spasm (e.g. appendix);

(3) Scoliosis with concavity facing the site of the lesion.

Pain due to perforation

Pain due to a perforated viscus reaches maximal severity at almost the instant the perforation occurs. This is particularly true of perforations of the stomach or duodenum, as from peptic ulcers in these locations, as hydrochloric acid immediately spills into the peritoneal cavity. Perforations of the lower small intestine and colon are often not as dramatic in onset, but particularly the latter are very sinister in that the peritoneum is instantly exposed to fecal bacteria.

In perforations, the parietal peritoneum is involved and hence guarding and rigidity are typical.

Pain due to a twist

Pain reaches maximal severity within minutes, and occurs at the site of the twist. Examples are as follows:

(1) Volvulus of the sigmoid colon or cecum;

(2) Twisting of an ovarian cyst;

(3) Torsion of a testis.

Pain due to intestinal ischemia

Pain reaches maximal severity in minutes. Examples are as follows:

(1) Thrombosis of the superior mesenteric artery or one of its branches;

(2) Embolism: this is classically seen when embolism from a heart valve or an intramural thrombus following myocardial infarction occludes a branch of the superior mesenteric artery;

(3) Strangulation, as of a hernia;

(4) Intussusception.

Testicular pain in the acute abdomen

The testes develop in the region of the kidney and migrate to the scrotum. They maintain their nerve supply from the 10th thoracic segment. That is why patients with renal colic due to stone disease frequently experience loin pain that radiates anteriorly to the testis of the same side. Another example of pain being referred to the testis is in acute appendicitis pain. Again, both the appendix and the testes are innervated by the 10th thoracic segment. In rupture of an abdominal aortic aneurysm, pain may also be referred to the testis.

Case history 1

A 44-year-old man presented with a complaint of abdominal pain of over a day's duration. It began as a 'gas pain' in the epigastrium and periumbilical area, which steadily grew worse. He developed anorexia and had not eaten. He became nauseated and vomited small amounts of bilious material on two or three occasions before he arrived at the hospital. After several hours the pain gradually became intense over the right lower quadrant. He had a history of hypercholesterolemia and drinking alcohol in binges. On examination he had a temperature of 99.2°F (37.3°C), a heart rate of 92 beats/min and a blood pressure of 125/82 mmHg. His heart and lung examinations were normal. Examination of the abdomen revealed no distension, his bowel sounds were present and the abdomen was soft to palpation, but clearly there was some guarding and tenderness localized to the right lower quadrant. The white blood cell (WBC) count was 15.6×10^9/l. Other routine laboratory tests were normal.

Acute appendicitis was suspected. A computed tomography (CT) scan with oral and intravenous contrast confirmed the diagnosis (Figure 9.1).

Acute appendicitis

The clinical presentation of acute appendicitis depends upon the stage in the pathology and the anatomical position of the vermiform appendix in the patient.

The stage in the pathology

Figure 9.2 depicts the stages in the pathogenesis of acute appendicitis. Obstruction of the lumen is the precipitating event, due to a fecalith in the majority of cases. The normal luminal capacity of around 0.1 ml is far exceeded by secretion into the lumen. With added distension, the venous outflow from the appendix becomes obstructed, whereas the thicker-walled arterioles are not compressed and arteriolar inflow continues unimpeded. This eventually results in infarction on the antimesenteric border. With bacterial multiplication, gangrene develops and perforation ensues. Perforation is frequently confined, with the development of a localized abscess. Rarely, the perforation may be generalized, with diffuse guarding and rigidity of the anterior abdominal wall, ileus and distension.

It is noteworthy that pain is initially periumbilical or even epigastric and without guarding or marked tenderness. This pain is caused by distension of the obstructed appendix (Figure 9.3). From a few hours to a day later, the pain becomes localized to the area of the anatomic location of the appendix.

The anatomical position of the vermiform appendix in the patient

The appendix may lie in a variety of different positions, depending upon the degree of rotation of the cecum during development. One of the commonest positions is in the right iliac fossa behind the ileocecal valve, with its tip pointing toward the spleen. However, it may lie retrocecally, lateral to the cecum or in several different positions, including in the true pelvis. In general it is worth considering the appendix as lying above the inlet of the true pelvis in the right iliac fossa (the iliac appendix), or partially or in its entirety within the true pelvis (the pelvic appendix).

The iliac appendix The clinical presentation is elaborated in Figure 9.4. Once the parietal peritoneum becomes inflamed, the pain will no longer be in the periumbilical or epigastric region, but pain and guarding are now present at the site where the appendix is located in the right iliac fossa. Rigidity in the right iliac fossa is felt especially with a localized perforation of the appendix. Owing to spasm of the iliacus and psoas muscles, the patient may lie in bed in pain, but with the right leg slightly flexed at the hip. The psoas sign may be present (resistance to and pain on attempting to extend the thigh. The test is best performed with the patient lying on the left side with the right leg extended at the hip).

Sometimes the appendix is retrocecal and very closely adherent to the posterior wall of the cecum. In such cases cecal ileus develops and the cecum becomes distended with air and lies between the inflamed appendix and the anterior abdominal wall in the right iliac fossa. Thus tenderness on percussion is less marked. There will be a tympanitic note on percussion in the right iliac fossa and guarding may not be present. Rigidity does not develop.

Irritation of the ureter as it crosses the pelvic brim might result in symptoms of dysuria. Lateral thigh pain and hyperesthesia may result from involvement of the right lateral femoral cutaneous nerve as it crosses the iliacus muscle.

The pelvic appendix The clinical presentation is elaborated in Figure 9.5. When the appendix is partially or wholly within the true pelvis, the initial symptoms are those due to distension of the obstructed appendix, and the patient complains of pain in the periumbilical region or in the epigastrium. In this regard, therefore, symptoms from an appendix located within the pelvis and one in the right iliac fossa are similar.

However, when the parietal peritoneum over the appendix becomes inflamed, the symptoms are different, The site of the pain does not then move to the right iliac fossa, but instead may remain periumbilical or epigastric for much longer. Later, the pain may become a little more diffuse. Guarding and tenderness in the right iliac fossa, so characteristic of appendicitis when the appendix is at a position in the iliac fossa, are not present. Even when the pelvic appendix perforates, and pelvic peritonitis sets in, there is still no rigidity present in the lower abdomen. In fact, at this point the epigastric or periumbilical pain is markedly relieved and for a while the patient may actually feel better. This is because the nerve segments that innervate the pelvic parietal peritoneum are not represented on the surface of the lower abdomen. The diagnosis of pelvic peritonitis may often be missed, until either a large pelvic abscess develops, if the peritonitis is contained, or generalized peritonitis develops when the pus fills the pelvis and spills out into the abdominal peritoneal cavity. In the latter instance, the fever rises and the patient becomes toxic and there is board-like rigidity.

When appendicitis develops with an appendix anatomically located in the true pelvis, the inflammation may involve the bladder, the rectum or the pelvic wall (Figure 9.6).

The nature of the bowels in appendicitis

Usually constipation is the rule. However, on occasion diarrhea may be present, because of ileal or rectal involvement from contiguous spread of the inflammation, usually from direct anatomic juxtaposition.

Vomiting in appendicitis

Pain almost always precedes vomiting. If it does not, one ought seriously to reconsider the diagnosis of appendicitis. Furthermore, the vomiting is usually not severe, although in children it can be.

Testicular pain in appendicitis

Pain from an inflamed appendix may sometimes be referred to the right (or less frequently to the left) testis, probably because the appendix and the testis are both supplied by the 10th thoracic nerve.

Intestinal obstruction in acute appendicitis

Inflammation from an adjacent inflamed appendix may rarely result in the involvement of an adjacent loop of ileum or sigmoid colon, to the extent that the intestine may become obstructed. The clinical presentation in such cases is complicated, with signs of inflammation and obstruction occurring at the same time.

The differential diagnosis in acute appendicitis

The differential diagnosis varies according to the stage of the appendicitis and its later presentation, which, as discussed above, is due to its anatomic location.

EARLY on, at the stage of distension of the appendix and before the involvement of the parietal peritoneum in the appropriate clinical setting, one may need to consider **exacerbation of peptic ulcer disease or biliary colic** in the differential diagnosis.

LATER, once the parietal peritoneum is involved, **sigmoid diverticulitis** might become a consideration in the middle-aged and elderly. It must be remembered that appendicitis is much more common in the young, when sigmoid diverticulitis is not a consideration in the diagnosis. However, older persons are not immune from developing appendicitis. Occasionally, in sigmoid diverticulitis, the loop of sigmoid is long and may swing out of the pelvis and veer to the right lower quadrant before returning to the left side. In such cases, the pain, guarding and tenderness may occur in the right iliac fossa. **Cecal diverticulitis** may occur in an isolated cecal diverticulum. It is uncertain whether such diverticula are congenital or acquired, but they are seen in young subjects, and isolated cecal diverticulitis is a disease of the young. Most patients are taken to the operating room with a diagnosis of a ruptured appendix. In older patients, penetration of a **cecal cancer**, or even a perforation of one, may present with symptoms very similar to those of acute appendicitis. On a rare occasion a cecal cancer at the apex of the cecum may in fact obstruct the lumen of the appendix, and acute appendicitis may result from it. In young sexually active women, **pelvic inflammatory disease** is a very important differential. Cervical motion tenderness, while always present in pelvic inflammatory disease, may be present with any cause of pelvic peritonitis, and may be seen therefore in the later stages of pelvic appendicitis. In pelvic inflammatory disease the epigastric and periumbilical pain of early appendicitis is not seen, the pain is not confined to the right lower quadrant but more typically is bilateral, a vaginal discharge is frequently present and cervical swabs must always be Gram stained and cultured. Vomiting, while later in onset after the pain and seldom very pronounced in appendicitis, is usually absent in pelvic inflammatory disease. A **twisted ovarian cyst** usually causes severe lower abdominal pain of fairly dramatic suddenness, often associated with vomiting. On occasion the rupture of a right-sided **follicular cyst** or right-sided corpus luteum cyst may result in pain very similar to that of appendicitis, in that right lower quadrant pain may be intense with tenderness in the right iliac fossa. The initial epigastric or periumbilical pain is not felt and the association with the menstrual cycle is characteristic. With the former condition the pain occurs mid-cycle and with the latter at the time of the menses. **Rupture of a tubal gestation** must always be considered in women of childbearing age. The pain is sudden in onset. While the pain is generally in the suprapubic region, it may also be in the upper abdomen. A shock state and intense pallor are generally associated. Acute onset of **Crohn's disease**, the first attack, may frequently mimic acute appendicitis. Prior to the days of imaging, several of these patients were operated upon with a preoperative diagnosis of acute appendicitis. In teenagers and young adults, infection with *Yersinia enterocolytica* often presents almost identically to an attack of appendicitis. Diarrhea is frequently but not always present, right iliac fossa pain, guarding and tenderness are characteristic and frequently occur. The onset very often is more gradual than in appendicitis, the patient complaining of milder symptoms for several days. In contrast, in young children and infants, the infection gives rise to a more typical gastroenteritis with loose stools and fever. The diarrhea in such cases is generally non-bloody, but a bloody diarrhea is occasionally seen. *Yersinia* is usually spread through contaminated food or water. The organism attaches to the surface epithelial cells of the terminal ileum, penetrates the mucosa, settles in the Payer's patches and then reaches the local mesenteric lymph nodes, before entering the systemic circulation. Diagnosis is usually established by stool examination (warning the laboratory in advance of one's interest in this organism). The organism can be cultured from stool for quite some time after symptoms have abated. It may on occasion grow in blood culture as well. An enzyme-linked immunosorbent assay (ELISA) is now available that tests positively for IgG, IgM and IgA antibodies. In countries where *Yersinia* is much commoner than in the USA, such as Scandinavian countries and Japan, sera may be positive for IgG antibodies in the normal population. Therefore, IgM antibodies or a serial rise in IgG titers is required to make a serological diagnosis. Stool culture remains the gold standard.

Imaging studies

When are imaging studies necessary? In the days before abdominal ultrasonography and CT scanning were available, the diagnosis of acute appendicitis was a clinical one. It is believed that at least 10% of patients operated on for a clinical diagnosis of acute appendicitis had normal appendices. Did, for example, the patients described in Case history 1 require an abdominal CT scan? Older clinicians would scoff at the need for a CT scan in that particular patient. Yet others would argue that if a CT scan were rapidly available, as it is in most urban emergency departments in the West, then it ought to be performed to save the patient needless surgery. The following story occurred in the recent experience of one of the authors.

> A 26-year-old medical intern developed vague abdominal pain that was initially crampy, but soon thereafter was continuous and localized to the right lower quadrant. On examination the young doctor had a temperature of around 100 °F (38 °C), and the salient features on physical examination were marked tenderness and guarding in the right iliac fossa. Bowel sounds were present. No masses were palpable. He had a history of occasional episodes of mild to moderate diarrhea for the past year. During such episodes (which seldom lasted beyond 2 days), he would pass three to five mushy or watery non-bloody stools over a 24-h period. Pain was not a major feature during those

earlier episodes. It was felt that he had irritable bowel syndrome, the ailment being exacerbated by the stresses of internship. The present attack of acute abdominal pain was quite unlike what he had previously experienced. A clinical diagnosis of acute appendicitis was entertained. The gastroenterologist who saw him decided to request a CT scan with oral contrast. The appendix appeared normal, and no enlarged mesenteric lymph nodes were evident, but the terminal ileum appeared uniformly thickened. A colonoscopy was performed 2 weeks later, and revealed ileal ulcerations consistent with Crohn's disease. This was a classic example of a situation when, in the absence of a CT scan, the patient might have been taken for surgery.

In women, imaging is even more important to distinguish acute appendicitis from many of the clinical entities mentioned above in the differential diagnosis. In a younger female abdominal ultrasonography is a suitable first test to consider, if negative to be followed by transvaginal ultrasonography. In older women, depending on the clinical presentation, an ultrasound or CT scan could be considered as the imaging modality of choice. Obesity, of course, is a limitation for the use of ultrasonography. Both pelvic ultrasonography and a CT scan may be used in the diagnosis.

Pelvic ultrasonography　Pelvic ultrasonography is frequently the imaging modality of choice, particularly in people with a slender body habitus. Figure 9.7(a, b) shows typical ultrasonographic findings in a patient with acute appendicitis.

Computed tomography scanning for the diagnosis of acute appendicitis　Oral contrast must be administered in sufficient quantity, via a nasogastric tube if need be, to fill ileal loops and the cecum so that inadequately filled ileum is not misidentified as appendix. Unless the patient has a contrast allergy or is in renal failure, intravenous contrast should also be used. An inflamed appendix enhances with intravenous contrast, thus making its identification easier. An example of inadequate visualization of the appendix when intravenous contrast was not initially administered is shown in Figure 9.7c. This was an unusual case of a young man who presented with minimal abdominal pain and Gram-negative sepsis. When CT scanning was repeated with intravenous contrast, the diagnosis of acute appendicitis became evident (Figure 9.7d). In the vicinity of the appendix, thin slices at 5-min intervals or less should be obtained.

CT criteria for the diagnosis of acute appendicitis are as follows:

(1) Distension > 6 mm;

(2) Wall thickened circumferentially, sometimes giving rise to the so-called 'target' appearance;

(3) Periappendiceal inflammation and edema ('dirty fat') leading to phlegmon and abscess.

The presence of a fecalith with one or more of the above features increases the likehood.

Case history 2

A 68-year-old man presented with a 1-day history of marked constant pain in the right lower quadrant. He had no previous gastrointestinal symptoms. He was not febrile. The abdomen was soft, and there was guarding, tenderness and slight tympany on percussion in the right lower quadrant. He had no hernias evident on examination. Bowel sounds were present. His WBC count was 15.3×10^9/l. The results of other routine laboratory tests were normal. A diagnosis of appendicitis was suspected despite the patient's age. A CT scan was obtained. This showed pericecal inflammation and mesenteric stranding and slightly enlarged (approximately 0.8 cm) pericecal lymph nodes. The appendix was visualized and was of normal diameter. At surgery a cecal carcinoma (4×4 cm) was noted. On pathological examination the tumor was shown to extend through the muscle and serosal layers, penetrating into the pericecal fat (Figure 9.8).

In the elderly, cecal cancers that either have penetrated into the surrounding mesentery or have perforated will frequently present with symptoms that mimic an acute appendicitis.

Case history 3

A 43-year-old man with a known history of diverticulosis and one previous attack of diverticulitis presented with left lower quadrant abdominal pain of 2 days' duration. The pain had come on fairly gradually, was continuous and had grown worse. He had not eaten any food and felt he had no appetite. He had three loose bowel movements at the onset and developed chills a few hours prior to admission. On examination he was clearly in pain, lying fairly still in bed, had a temperature

of 101°F (38°C), a heart rate of 96 beats/min, a respiratory rate of 16/min with shallow breathing and a normal blood pressure. His breathing was more thoracic than abdominal. He had some diffuse tenderness all over the abdomen, but this was maximal over the left lower quadrant. Percussion tenderness was present over the left lower quadrant. Bowel sounds were present but markedly diminished. Rectal examination was normal. His heart and lung examinations were unremarkable.

Despite the fact that the patient was only in his forties, with previous knowledge of diverticular disease and pain, tenderness and percussion tenderness maximal over the left lower quadrant, sigmoid diverticulitis was the leading diagnosis. The CT scan ordered showed typical features for diverticulitis (Figure 9.9).

Case history 4

A 75-year-old man presented with fever and chills of around a week's duration. At the time of admission he did not complain of abdominal pain, although on asking him a leading question, he did admit to a rather vague steady but not severe pain over the left side of his abdomen of a few weeks' duration. He did not indicate any radiation of the pain and was not able to describe aggravating or relieving factors. He did, however, have symptoms of dysuria and some frequency of micturition. He had a history of hypertension and benign prostatic hypertrophy. He had had his gallbladder removed 4 years previously. He had a temperature of 102.2°F (39°C), heart rate of 87 beats/min and blood pressure of 120/75 mmHg. He was tachypneic with a respiratory rate of 32/min. He did not appear jaundiced. His heart and lung examinations were normal, other than for the rapid respiratory rate. His abdomen was not distended, there was no guarding, it was soft to palpation, no masses were palpated, there was no evidence clinically of organomegaly and there was no percussion tenderness. No tenderness was elicited in the renal angles. A clinical diagnosis of a urinary tract infection with probable sepsis was made prior to obtaining the results of investigations. His WBC count was 13 200/fl with a marked shift to the left. Serum electrolytes were normal. His urinalysis was also normal, effectively ruling out a urinary tract infection as the cause of the fever. Liver function tests were ordered and revealed very mild elevations in the serum transaminases (serum ALT 58, serum AST 47) and an alkaline phosphatase elevated at 227 IU (normal level 100). Serum amylase and lipase were normal. With the history of fever and abdominal pain, even though it was fairly mild, a CT scan of the abdomen with oral contrast was ordered. Intravenous contrast was not used, as the patient had a mild degree of renal insufficiency (blood urea nitrogen (BUN) 45, serum creatinine 2.2 mg/dl). The CT scan revealed extraluminal contrast communicating with the sigmoid colon, which was also greatly thickened and with numerous diverticula present. The liver showed numerous small liver abscesses and thrombosis of a branch of the left portal vein (Figure 9.10).

The most important feature in this case is the fact that, despite such advanced disease following a diverticular perforation, the patient did not complain of much abdominal pain. Abdominal pain is frequently mild and occasionally absent in elderly patients with acute abdomen. The elevated alkaline phosphatase was most likely due to the liver abscesses. The portal vein thrombosis was almost certainly due to pyleophlebitis occurring as a result of ascending infection from the colon via the mesenteric and ultimately the portal vein.

Case history 5

A 78-year-old man presented to the Emergency Department with malaise of 3–4 weeks' duration which he attributed to a cold he had recently acquired. He had seen another physician earlier who had prescribed antibiotics, which the patient had taken for 10 days. He also developed mild to moderate pain in the lower abdomen and back a few days prior to the current visit. He had a temperature of 100.2°F (37.9°C) and a normal physical examination except for tenderness in the lower abdomen, mostly in the left lower quadrant. A clinical diagnosis of diverticulitis was considered in the Emergency Department and he was sent home on antibiotics. He returned with urinary tract infection a week later and the antibiotic was changed. A month or so after his initial symptoms began, he presented once again to the Emergency Department, this time not only with frequency of micturition as before, but also with the symptom of recent pneumaturia. A diagnosis of colovesical fistula resulting from diverticulitis was considered. He underwent a CT scan with oral and intravenous contrast, which revealed a diverticular abscess and a communication between the bladder and the sigmoid colon (Figure 9.11).

Take home message In the elderly, acute intra-abdominal disease often presents in more subtle fashion. Even though a diagnosis of acute diverticulitis was suspected at an earlier visit, he had none of the usual symptoms and signs of severe pain, tenderness and guarding. Older patients with diverticulitis, appendicitis, cholecystitis and at times even with perforations of abdominal viscera present in less dramatic fashion than do younger patients.

Diverticulitis

By definition diverticulitis is a perforation of a diverticulum and not merely infection or inflammation. The majority of attacks of diverticulitis involve the sigmoid colon. Milder attacks of diverticulitis result in confined perforations with surrounding soft tissue inflammation and phlegmon formation that resolve with rest and antibiotics. However, in more severe cases abscess formation may occur, requiring surgery. On occasion pyleophlebitis and liver abscesses may develop. Rarely, free perforation may occur with generalized peritonitis.

Abscesses may adhere to and penetrate adjacent viscera, giving rise to colovesical fistulae, colovaginal fistulae, colocutaneous fistulae and enteroenteric fistulae (Figure 9.12).

Just as a perforated cecal cancer can mimic acute appendicitis (Case history 2), on occasion a sigmoid colon cancer can perforate and mimic acute diverticulitis. An example of a particularly devastating case is shown in Figure 9.13.

Case history 6

A 72-year-old man with history of extensive drinking for decades presented with severe epigastric pain. The fortnight prior to this episode, he had been drinking particularly heavily. The pain began rather abruptly a few days ago. Initially the pain was epigastric but after a day also involved the right side of the abdomen, especially the right lower quadrant. The pain radiated to the back. He was very nauseated, could not eat, initially tolerated oral fluids but soon thereafter vomited the little he drank. On examination he was sitting in bed in agony, the pulse was 110/min and of small volume, and his blood pressure was 95/75 mmHg. He had poor intensity of breath sounds at both lung bases and an ejection systolic murmur along the left sternal border. There was marked generalized guarding of his abdomen. The abdomen was excruciatingly tender even to superficial palpation. Initially he had a few bowel sounds heard, but soon thereafter the abdomen was silent.

What is the differential diagnosis and how does one approach the diagnosis? The nature of the abdominal pain, the long history of alcoholism, the marked abdominal tenderness, the absent bowel sounds and the recent binge drinking suggested alcoholic pancreatitis. Acute cholecystitis or choledocholithiasis with or without acute pancreatitis were other possibilities. The pain, while sudden in onset and becoming intense fairly quickly, did not reach peak intensity quite as rapidly as one would have expected from a perforated peptic ulcer. Nevertheless, a perforation needed to be excluded.

His hematocrit was 45%, WBC count 14 100/mm³, he had normal electrolytes, serum creatinine of 1.8 mg/dl and serum calcium of 9.9 mg/dl. His serum amylase was 2916 U/dl (normal < 100 U/dl) and serum lipase 850 U/dl (normal < 200 U/dl). Liver function tests revealed a mild elevation in the serum AST compatible with his history of heavy drinking. The serum ALT, alkaline phosphatase and serum bilirubin were within normal limits. A diagnosis of acute pancreatitis was thus established.

What is the etiology of the acute pancreatitis in this patient? He had a history of heavy drinking for years that cannot be ignored. However, the serum amylase value of 2916 U/dl in this patient should raise a red flag while considering a diagnosis of acute alcoholic pancreatitis. While this was certainly possible, experience has shown that the serum amylase is seldom over 1000 U/dl in alcoholic pancreatitis. Elevated levels of amylase, in the vicinity of 1000 U/dl or above, should lead one to consider alternative etiologies despite a history of alcoholism. Alcoholism does not protect one from other etiologies of acute pancreatitis! Among the other causes of acute pancreatitis (Table 9.1), gallstone pancreatitis is by far the commonest cause. The patient was not on any drug known to cause pancreatitis. His serum calcium was normal (in any event hypercalcemia is seldom a cause of pancreatitis) and acute pancreatitis resulting from very high serum triglyceride levels is characterized by normal or relatively mild elevations of the serum amylase. This is because hyperlipemic serum interferes with the assay for amylase. Therefore, gallstone pancreatitis is a leading contender. Ultrasonography is certainly more sensitive than CT scanning in the diagnosis of gallstones present in the gallbladder. However, ultrasonography is not nearly as sensitive as CT scanning in the detection of acute pancreatitis, nor does it help as much in assessing the extent of

Table 9.1 Causes of acute pancreatitis

Congenital
   mechanical: choledochocele type V
   genetic: (see Chapter 5) α_1 antitrypsin deficiency
Alcoholism
Gallstone disease
Gallbladder sludge
Hypertriglyceridemia
   inherited disorders associated with serum triglyceride
     > 1000 mg/dl
   acquired (often additive with milder forms of the inherited
     variety)
     alcoholism
     type 2 diabetes mellitus
     obesity
     nephrotic syndrome
     hypothyroidism
     cholestatic liver disease
Hypercalcemia – uncommon
Trauma – blunt or penetrating
Drugs
   6-mercaptopurine, azathioprine, didanosine, pentamidine,
     sulfonamides, including trimethoprim/sufamethoxazole,
     sulfasalizine, valproic acid, furosemide,
     thiazides, 5-amino salicylates, sulindac
   toxins – methanol, scorpion venom
Infections
   viral: Coxsakie, mumps, herpes simplex, herpes zoster,
     cytomegalovirus, hepatitis B
   mycoplasma
   bacteria: *Legionella, Salmonella*
   fungal: *Aspergillus*
   parasitic: cryptosporidium, toxoplasmosis
Postoperative – post-intra-abdominal surgery or surgery not
   involving the abdominal cavity
Post-ERCP – common post-sphincterotomy in patients
   with sphincter of Oddi dysfunction
Obstructive – obstruction of ampulla of Vater or pancreatic duct
   mechanical obstruction
     carcinoma of the head of the pancreas
     perimpullary carcinoma
     periampullary (duodenal) diverticulum
     ampullary stenosis – fibrosis
   functional
     sphincter of Oddi dyskinesia
Vascular
   vasculitis
     systemic lupus, polyarteritis nodosa, Sjögren's syndrome
   severe acute mesenteric ischemia – uncommon
Autoimmune:
   Sjögren's syndrome, primary sclerosing cholangitis,
     primary biliary cirrhosis, thyroiditis
Idiopathic

ERCP, endoscopic retrograde cholangiopancreatography

intra-abdominal and retroperitoneal damage. In this patient the history, physical examination and laboratory studies have established the diagnosis of acute pancreatitis. Therefore, it would be more cost effective to obtain a CT scan, as this would enable both the staging of the severity of the acute pancreatitis and the detection of gallstones in the majority of patients. It is also more sensitive than ultrasonography in the identification of gallstones in the common bile duct.

A CT scan of the abdomen with oral and intravenous contrast (Figure 9.14) revealed swelling of the pancreatic head, peripancreatic edema and areas of low attenuation within the body and tail of the pancreas suggestive of focal pancreatic necrosis.

Case history 7

A 78-year-old man in otherwise good health except for a history of well controlled hypertension, diabetes mellitus and congestive heart failure went to see his physician with a complaint of weakness of recent onset. His medical condition had been very stable and he was reasonably active, and able to take gentle walks for up to a mile without feeling tired. The weakness had come on gradually a few days previously and just prior to hospitalization he had found it a major effort to make it to the bathroom, which was adjoining his bedroom. He was able to lie flat in bed, perhaps with a little low back pain, but no shortness of breath. He had no history to suggest paroxysmal nocturnal dyspnea. His physical examination was reported to be normal. Blood was also drawn for complete blood counts and serum chemistries and the patient was sent home with a follow-up visit scheduled.

However, he returned to the Emergency Department of the hospital three days later complaining of very severe fatigue. This time, when questioned, he admitted to having mild continuous low back pain and a little upper abdominal discomfort of 2 days' duration. This time on physical examination he appeared to be comfortable lying on one pillow, he was dehydrated and had a supine blood pressure of 105/60 mmHg which fell to 70/40 mmHg when he sat up in bed. His heart rate was 100 beats/min. He had decreased breath sounds at both infrascapular regions with slight dullness on percussion. He was not in congestive cardiac failure and his jugular venous pressure was not elevated clinically. Bowel sounds were present but decreased. The abdomen was slightly distended, but as he was a moderately obese man, this did not draw the clinician's attention at the time. The abdomen was not tender.

No masses were palpated and no organomegaly was clinically evident. Examination of the nervous system was normal, muscle strength was not diminished and the joint examination and examination of the spine were normal. Laboratory test results were: hemoglobin 15.8 g/dl, hematocrit 49.3, BUN 88 mg/dl, serum creatinine 1.8 mg/dl, serum glucose 130 mg/dl and serum electrolytes, other than for mild hypernatremia, were normal, there being no anion gap. His serum total calcium was 5.3 mg/dl, serum albumin 2.7 g/dl (corrected serum calcium 6.3 mg/dl), serum phosphate 2.6 mg/dl and serum magnesium 1.1 mg/dl. Serum alkaline phosphatase was within normal limits. His serum calcium measured at the medical visit just 3 days previously was 9.2 mg/dl and his serum albumin was 4.0 g/dl at that time. No ketones were detected in the urine. The patient's electrocardiogram (ECG) was similar to his baseline ECG.

What is the cause of the severe fatigue, dehydration and sudden drop in serum calcium and albumin? One had to view the recent onset of severe fatigue in the context of two separate, yet possibly related, constellations of findings. The evaluation initially focused on trying to find explanations for these two sets of findings. The first constellation of findings was a sudden drop in serum ionized calcium together with a drop in the serum albumin within the span of 3 days. The second was the profound dehydration sufficient to cause hemoconcentration, prerenal azotemia and hypotension in the absence of overt blood or fluid loss from diarrhea, vomiting or polyuria. Furthermore, the fatigue could not be attributed to dyspnea of cardiac or pulmonary origin.

Could the patient be collecting fluid in a 'third space', i.e. his abdomen? What condition could allow accumulation of fluid in the abdomen and simultaneously rapidly lower the serum calcium and serum albumin? Of all acute abdominal conditions acute pancreatitis could certainly do so. The drop in serum calcium in acute pancreatitis is due to the formation of calcium soaps with the free fatty acids available in the abdomen from the action of pancreatic lipase on mesenteric and omental fat. Serum albumin can drop rapidly on account of exudation of fluid from 'leaky' capillaries resulting from the action of inflammatory mediators and cytokines. This fall in the serum albumin can lower total serum calcium; the ionized calcium may remain normal, hence the importance of either correcting the serum calcium for the level of the albumin or, better still, obtaining an ionized serum calcium level. The serum calcium level can be low in acute pancreatitis also because of a low serum magnesium level, as was the case in this patient. Magnesium was constantly repleted. The patient had developed some back and upper abdominal discomfort, but it appeared not to be severe, as might be expected in a patient with acute pancreatitis. Despite the absence of severe abdominal pain or tenderness, acute pancreatitis was suspected and serum amylase and lipase levels were obtained. His serum amylase was 209 U/l (normal: < 100 U/l) and serum lipase 3.6 U/ml (normal: < 1.5 U/l). With these moderately elevated levels of serum pancreatic enzymes it was felt that he might well have acute pancreatitis. A CT scan was ordered which revealed severe pancreatitis. There was enlargement of the entire gland peripancreatic stranding and inflammatory changes around the splenic hilum, retroperitoneum, right paracolic gutter, the root of the mesentery and the right psoas muscle. He had evidence of pancreatic calcification suggesting that he had had silent chronic pancreatitis of unknown etiology. The fact that the serum amylase and lipase were only modestly elevated could have two explanations. The first is that this appeared to be an acute pancreatitis occurring in a patient with hitherto silent chronic pancreatitis. The second explanation is that pancreatic enzymes were obtained several days into the course of the episode of acute pancreatitis. In any event, the degree of the elevation of serum amylase and lipase does not correlate with the severity of pancreatitis. The relatively mild symptoms in the presence of striking findings on the CT scan were quite unusual. However, the authors have always been impressed how commonly abdominal symptoms and signs are altered in the elderly, particularly in pancreatic–biliary disease and in diverticulitis.

The patient's fatigue improved remarkably upon repletion of his serum calcium. However, after a few days his condition declined. His abdomen became severely distended and he had ileus. He developed pleural effusions, became hypoxic and required ventilation on a respirator. A CT scan obtained later in the course of his disease revealed that he had developed necrosis of his entire pancreas and had large fluid collections in the abdomen and retroperitoneum with dissection into the right thigh (Figure 9.15). A sample of

the fluid was obtained under CT guidance. Gram stain was negative, as were the cultures. A diagnosis of sterile necrosis was made and the patient was placed on antibiotics. His general condition continued to decline with staphylococcal pneumonia and he did not recover.

Acute pancreatitis

This is defined as acute inflammation of the pancreas (see Table 9.1 for etiology). Types are as follows:

(1) *Interstitial or edematous pancreatitis:* The gland is swollen with intra- and/or peripancreatic fluid accumulation, fibrin and polymorphonuclear leukocyte infiltration, often with thickening of the pararenal fascia. The edematous pancreas, like normal pancreatic tissue, enhances on dynamic CT with intravenous contrast (from 40–50 Hounsfield units (HU) to 80–90 HU).

(2) *Necrotizing pancreatitis:* Focal, segmental or total necrosis of the pancreas may occur. The pancreas does not enhance on dynamic CT with intravenous contrast (< 80 HU after intravenous contrast, highly suggestive of necrosis; < 50 HU definitive).

The course of the disease is shown in Figure 9.16.

Even in interstitial pancreatitis, endocrine or exocrine dysfunction may develop during the acute attack, but eventually, rarely after as much as several months, full recovery occurs. In contrast, when necrosis occurs in the pancreas, full recovery of endocrine or exocrine function often does not occur.

By definition, fibrosis does not occur in acute pancreatitis. However, it is impossible to know during an acute attack whether in time chronicity (fibrosis and eventually calcification) will or will not develop.

Many of the causes of acute pancreatitis go on to produce recurrent attacks, particularly if the cause is not eliminated. Examples are:

(1) Continued consumption of alcohol in alcoholic pancreatitis. Note, patients with alcoholic pancreatitis may continue to have recurrent attacks despite cessation of drinking. In many patients the changes of chronic pancreatitis have already developed prior to the first bout of 'acute' pancreatitis.

(2) Gall bladder not removed after initial attack of gallstone pancreatitis may result in recurrent attacks, but not pancreatic fibrosis.

(3) Lack of control of serum triglyceride level in hyperlipidemic pancreatitis.

(4) Failure to eliminate the offending drug or toxin in drug or toxin induced pancreatitis.

(5) Failure to eradicate the cause of hypercalcemia etc.

Patients with pancreatitis due to genetic defects, continue to have recurrent attacks.

Several of the causes have been eluded to above (Table 9.1). Alcoholism and gallstone disease together contribute to 75% of the cases of acute pancreatitis encountered in clinical practice. Hypertriglyceridemia makes up about 4%.

Pathology

See Figure 9.17.

Pathogenesis

Irrespective of the etiology (e.g. gallstone, alcoholic, trauma), it appears that the final common pathway is the intrapancreatic activation of pancreatic enzymes, e.g. trypsinogen, phospholipase A$_2$. Endothelial damage, ischemia–reperfusion, generation of oxygen radicals, arachidonic acid metabolites and proinflammatory cytokines all play a role in the perpetuation of both local damage and systemic complications, e.g. adult respiratory distress syndrome (Figure 9.18).

Clinical presentation

Onset This is fairly dramatic as a rule, with severe abdominal pain, the severity being doubtless related to the organ's close proximity to the celiac plexus.

Pain The site of pain is shown in Figure 9.19. Pain most often develops in the epigastrium and in one or both loins. The pancreas is a retroperitoneal structure and hence may produce loin pain. If only the body of the pancreas is involved in the inflammatory process, the pain may occur in the left upper quadrant only. When the tail is involved, left loin pain is also present, since the tail is in the left loin, and abuts the splenic hilum. If there is substantial parapancreatic inflammation or fluid collection, the diaphragm can become irritated, with pain being radiated to the tip of the left shoulder. Pain may also be felt over the left scapula. Later, pain may be felt in the right iliac fossa, owing to fluid collections in this region.

Vomiting Vomiting generally follows pain and may at times be incessant. However, the patient generally does not bring up much in the way of vomitus and at times only retches continuously. Nausea may be absent. On rare occasions, a swollen pancreatic head or more often a pseudocyst may compress the duodenum or proximal jejunum, effectively giving rise to an upper small bowel obstruction. In such cases the patient will vomit copious amounts of clear or bilious fluid.

Temperature Patients with mild attacks of pancreatitis may not be febrile, but with moderate and severe attacks it is not uncommon to have a temperature of 101°F (33°C). On occasion, even in the absence of infection, the temperature may be as high as 102°F–103°F (38–39°C). A higher temperature should alert one to an infections complication.

Hypovolemic shock As in the case of the patient described above in Case history 7, 'third spacing' of fluid is common in acute pancreatitis. In fact, the more severe the attack the greater the inflammation and digestion of intra-abdominal and retroperitoneal structures, resulting in large fluid collections. The more severe the pancreatitis the more difficult it is to maintain a normal blood pressure, often requiring liters of intravenous fluids in order to do so.

Icterus Mild jaundice is seen often and is due to compression of the common bile duct by an edematous pancreas. Of course, one always has to rule out the possibility of continued obstruction of the common bile duct by a gallstone in patients with gallstone pancreatitis.

The abdominal examination Regarding bowel sounds, the more severe the pancreatitis the more likely there is to be paralytic ileus. Prolonged ileus is a bad prognostic sign. Epigastric tenderness is almost always present. It is rare not to have epigastric tenderness, as was seen in the patient described in Case history 7. The tenderness may be more diffuse at times. The pancreas is a retroperitoneal structure and hence, even when it is very swollen, it is seldom palpable. However, large fluid collections and pseudocysts are often palpable. Large fluid collections may at times be identified by percussion; often dullness that does not shift may be detected in one loin or flank. Rigidity may often be seen, especially in the early hours following the onset of pancreatitis. However, more often, the abdominal wall is fairly lax, much more so than in perforation. Inflammation during an acute attack of pancreatitis may be so severe

Table 9.2 Unfavorable prognostic features of acute pancreatitis

Hypovolemia
    postural hypotension→ hypotension supine→ shock
    features that provide an early clue
        fluid sequestration ('third spacing')
            large fluid requirements to maintain blood pressure
            > 90 mmHg
        hemoconcentration – a rising hematocrit without transfusion
        oliguria (output falls, below 30 ml/h)
        heart rate > 110 beats/min or proportionately higher
           if febrile
        BUN/serum creatinine ratio > 20 or BUN rising
           > 5 mg/dl over 48 h
        Fractional excretion of sodium < 1.0
Fall in hematocrit
    a fall in hematocrit of > 10 mg/dl over 48 h suggests severe
        pancreatitis
Hypoxia
    pulse oximetry: oxygen saturation (SaO_2) < 90% or a falling
        SaO_2 requiring checking of arterial blood gas is a
        particularly bad prognostic sign. A falling SaO_2 and a
        falling PaO_2 require prompt action and observation in an
        intensive care unit even as ARDS might be impending.
        One should not wait for the 'magical' PaO_2 value to fall
        below < 60 mmHg, the value mentioned in several of the
        prognostic criteria frequently used
Hypocalcemia
    fall in ionized calcium is a poor prognostic sign. Two factors
        contribute: the formation of insoluble calcium soaps in
        the extracellular compartment and concomitant
        hypomagnesemia
Prolonged paralytic ileus
Rising leukocyte count after correction of dehydration to
    > 15.0×10^3/l
Serum lactate dehydrogenase > 600 IU/l
Serum aspartate aminotransferase > 200 IU/l
Serum glucose > 200 mg/dl in the absence of a history of
    diabetes mellitus
Bad prognostic signs obtained at CT scan, particularly
    pancreatic necrosis
    infected necrosis worse than sterile necrosis

BUN, blood urea nitrogen; ARDS, adult respiratory distress syndrome

as to give rise to hemorrhage. Blood may find its way via tissue planes to the anterior and lateral abdominal walls. Ecchymoses, red, green or yellow, may be evident as Cullen's sign when present around the umbilicus, or as Gray Turner's sign when present in the loin. These signs are very uncommon and, when seen, signify severe pancreatitis.

Staging and prognosis of an attack of acute pancreatitis

A great deal has been written about different criteria used to differentiate a mild attack of acute pancreatitis from a severe one. Most of these, such as the Ranson's criteria, Glasgow criteria and the Acute Physiologic and Chronic Health Evaluating Scoring System, versions II or III (APACHE II or III) grading system, require the grouping together of clinical features with laboratory test results at the time of presentation of the patient and again at 48 h after admission. In the opinion of the authors, while such grading systems may be useful, almost as much information can be obtained by careful and frequent clinical examination and assessment of a few laboratory test results without slavishly calculating scores. Table 9.2 provides guidelines that will help the clinician decide how well his or her patient is doing.

CT scanning also provides for excellent prognostication. The appearance of the pancreas is first assessed on the unenhanced CT scan: normal → enlargement of the pancreas often with irregular borders → peripancreatic inflammation → intrapancreatic and/or extrapancreatic fluid collections → large collections of gas in the pancreas or retropancreatic area. The enhanced or dynamic CT scan is then assessed with intravenous contrast. The normal pancreas has a density of around 40–50 HU. On a dynamic CT scan it enhances substantially to > 80 HU. Enhancement of < 80 HU is suspicious for necrosis and < 50 HU is characteristic. The prognosis varies with the amount of necrosis noted with the organ.

Furthermore, CT scanning provides more than just prognostication. It provides information as to intra-abdominal or chest complications of acute pancreatitis. For example, if pancreatic necrosis is identified, then it has major consequences for management. Presently, all authorities on the subject would agree that the detection of necrosis requires aspiration of the necrotic area under CT guidance to determine whether the necrosis is sterile or infected. Sterile necrosis can be followed carefully with the patient on antibiotics, but infected necrosis requires surgery.

Complications

Complications are listed in Table 9.3.

Case history 8

A 67-year-old man presented with colicky mid-abdominal pain of several hours' duration. He claimed the pain began after he had eaten a steak sandwich at dinner. He felt nauseated and induced vomiting. However, his symptoms were not relieved. Thereafter, he vomited a few more times, bringing up undigested food and bilious material each time. When asked, he said he was not passing flatus and had not had a bowel

Table 9.3 Complications of acute pancreatitis

Intra-abdominal
Fluid collections
Necrosis
  sterile
  infected
Pseudocyst – sterile
Abscess
Ascites

Extra-abdominal
Circulatory collapse
Pulmonary
  atelectasis
  pleural effusion
  adult respiratory distress syndrome
  nosocomial pneumonia
Renal
  prerenal azotemia
  acute tubular necrosis

Table 9.4 Types of intestinal obstruction

Mechanical obstruction
Extrinsic
  adhesions
  hernias: inguinal, umbilical, femoral, incisional, internal
  tumor from an adjacent viscus compressing intestine
  abscess adjacent to a loop of intestine – diverticulitis,
    appendicitis, etc.
  acute pancreatitis: compression of duodenum by inflamed
    swollen head
  congenital bands
  anomalous arteries

Intrinsic
  lesion in the wall
    inflammatory – Crohn's disease, tuberculosis
    primary tumor – carcinoma, lymphoma, carcinoid
    metastatic tumor – breast, melanoma, colon, stomach,
      ovary
    radiation stricture
    ischemic stricture
    intussusception
    volvulus
  lesion in the lumen
    fecal impaction
    gallstone – gallstone ileus
    foreign body
    enteroliths
    bezoar – gastric bezoar that traversed the pylorus
    Ascaris worms obstructing the lumen in little children

Functional obstruction or ileus or pseudo-obstruction
Acute
  paralytic ileus with peritonitis
  paralytic ileus due to hypokalemia, hypercalcemia
  Ogilvie's syndrome
Chronic
  secondary
    myxedema
    amyloidosis
    scleroderma
  primary
    idiopathic pseudo-obstruction – neurogenic
    idiopathic pseudo-obstruction – myogenic

movement since the onset of the pain. He had a history of two previous myocardial infarctions and emphysema, and had undergone repair of an abdominal aortic aneurysm 11 years previously. A year after surgery for the aneurysm he had developed similar symptoms as at present and had undergone lysis of adhesions. On examination his abdomen was mildly distended, bowel sounds were present with low-pitched tinkles. No masses were palpated, there was only minimal diffuse tenderness and no organomegaly was clinically evident. No hernias were detected on careful examination. A small bowel obstruction due to adhesions was suspected, and supine and upright films of the abdomen were ordered to confirm the diagnosis. These plain radiographs showed dilated loops of small intestine and air–fluid levels (Figure 9.20a and b). A better example of a plain radiograph of the abdomen with air–fluid levels in another patient with small intestinal obstruction is shown in Figure 9.20c. A CT scan of the abdomen was ordered to help localize the site of obstruction (Figure 9.20d and e).

It may not always be necessary to localize exactly the site of the obstruction prior to surgery. Before CT was available, this patient would have been taken to surgery based on the clinical presentation and plain films of the abdomen. Serious consideration should be given to doing so even today. If for any reason, depending on the individual circumstances of the case, the surgeon wishes to localize the site of the obstruction or to consider other etiological possibilities, then either a CT scan with oral contrast or barium studies may be requested. Depending on what information is being sought,

barium studies may provide more valuable information than a CT scan. It is perfectly safe to put barium proximal to a small bowel obstruction, but not proximal to a large bowel obstruction. Therefore, if a barium upper gastrointestinal small bowel follow-through study is requested in a suspected case of intestinal obstruction, it is mandatory to rule out a colonic obstruction. This may be done clinically, given the patient's history; if not, then by colonoscopy or barium enema.

Intestinal obstruction

The classification shown in Table 9.4 divides intestinal obstruction into mechanical and functional obstructions.

Mechanical obstruction

Mechanical obstruction to the bowel is best looked upon as being due to lesions outside the bowel, in the wall of the bowel or in the lumen of the bowel.

Causes due to lesions outside the bowel, although adjacent to it   Adhesions and hernias, the commonest causes of intestinal obstruction, belong in this category. Prior to World War II, most of the large series describing intestinal obstruction described hernias as the commonest cause. Since then, in the developed world, hernias tend to be repaired early on and the total numbers of operations on the abdomen for various reasons have increased considerably. As a consequence, adhesions are now the commonest cause of obstruction in the developed world. In developing countries, however, hernias remain by far the commonest cause of intestinal obstruction. Unlike obstructed hernias, which give rise to symptoms instantly, adhesions may give rise to an acute obstruction, as it did in the patient described in Case history 8, or they may give rise to subacute episodes of obstruction. Adhesions may develop shortly after surgery or at times years after. An inflammatory or pyogenic complication in the abdomen, such as a perforation of a viscus or an abscess, is more prone to the development of adhesions. Talc, used in surgical gloves in the old days, when spilled in the peritoneal cavity, has been known to give rise to a very aggressive and chronic form of adhesive 'peritonitis' that in effect causes bowel obstruction in much the same way as do adhesions.

Causes due to lesions in the wall of the bowel   Crohn's disease would be the commonest cause in this group in the West and tuberculosis in many developing countries. Crohn's disease may cause either subacute or acute obstruction. It is worth remembering that both ischemic and post-radiation strictures may occur many years after the initial ischemic or radiation injury. Both intussusception and volvulus may be regarded as 'lesions' in the wall. Intussusception is much commoner in children. However, occasionally a lymphoma or carcinoma may be at the leading edge of an intussusception in adults. Intussusception of a Meckel's diverticulum may also occur, patients presenting with intermittent pain and gastrointestinal hemorrhage. Volvulus in the West is less common than in several developing countries and almost always involves the colon, the sigmoid colon being much commoner than the cecum (see Case histories 9 and 10, below).

Table 9.5   The more common causes of small bowel obstruction

Adhesions (60% of small intestinal obstructions)
Crohn's disease
Tuberculosis in developing countries
Hernias
Gallstone ileus
Metastases to the small intestine from:
   breast cancer
   ovarian cancer
   melanoma
   gastric cancer
   colonic cancer

Causes due to lesions in the lumen of the bowel   Bowel obstruction resulting from material in the lumen of the intestine is called obturation. Fecal impaction, particularly in the elderly, is the commonest cause. Symptoms tend to be more chronic than acute, the patients presenting initially with spurious 'diarrhea' (see Chapter 4) and later developing distension. If not treated soon enough, these patients will eventually develop distension of the colon, and if the ileocecal valve is patent, than distension of the small intestine as well. If the impaction is in the rectum, these patients will need digital evacuation prior to enemas ('milk and molasses' enemas work particularly well in these cases). On occasion the impaction may be in the sigmoid colon, and thankfully rarely, patients have required surgery for removal of the impacted feces. Gallstone ileus (the term 'ileus' is incorrectly used, as this is a true mechanical obstruction), occurs not too infrequently in the older population (see Chapter 8). An enterolith may on occasion cause an acute obstruction when it lodges behind a small intestinal stricture (Figures 9.21 and 9.22).

The more common causes of small bowel obstruction as shown in Table 9.5, and the more common causes of colonic obstruction in Table 9.6. In parts of Eastern Europe, Central Africa and Asia, sigmoid volvulus is the commonest cause of colonic obstruction.

There are three types of mechanical obstruction: simple obstruction; strangulated obstruction; and closed loop obstruction.

Simple obstruction   Here the obstruction is at a single point in the intestine and the blood supply to the intestine proximal to the obstruction is not compromised. The intestine proximal to the obstruction becomes dilated, initially by swallowed air and much later by gases produced by bacterial fermentation (CO_2, H_2 and

Table 9.6 The more common causes of colonic obstruction in Western Europe and the USA

Colon cancer (65%)
Diverticulitis (10%)
Volvulus (5%)
Miscellaneous (20%)
    includes ischemic and post-radiation strictures and impaction

Table 9.7 Symptoms and signs suggestive of strangulation

Strangulation must be suspected when the colicky pain of intestinal obstruction becomes constant at a specific site. The pain now is due to involvement of the parietal peritoneum as a consequence of ischemia/infarction of the obstructed segment of bowel.
    guarding
    tenderness over the specific area of pain
    percussion tenderness (or rebound tenderness)
    if a tender mass is palpated in this setting, it clinches the diagnosis
    plain rediograph shows separation of adjacent loops of bowel (late sign)
    thumbprinting of the involved segment of bowel indicating ischemia to the obstructed segment may be seen
    very late in the course, air in the wall of the bowel and mesenteric and portal veins may be seen
    finally, if perforation occurs, free air under the diaphragm would be seen

methane). Fluid secretion also contributes considerably to the distension. The intestine proximal to the obstruction secretes a large amount of fluid into the lumen, and the secreted fluid is not adequately reabsorbed, hence the 'air–fluid level' seen on plain X-rays of the abdomen.

The three cardinal features of a simple mechanical obstruction of the intestine are:

(1) Abdominal pain

    (a) colicky periumbilical pain in small intestinal obstruction,

    (b) colicky, occasionally steady, pain located in the hypogastrium;

(2) Vomiting;

(3) Distension;

(4) Patient not passing stools or flatus.

All three of these symptoms are frequently present at some point in the course of the obstruction. However, depending on the level of the obstruction, one or other of these symptoms may develop late or not at all:

(1) *Upper small intestinal obstruction* Obstruction is at the duodenum or upper jejunum. Vomiting occurs early. Distension may appear of the stomach only, mimicking a gastric outlet obstruction or, if vomiting is brisk, no distension may develop at all. The intestine may evacuate its contents for a while before constipation eventually sets in.

(2) *Lower small intestinal obstruction* Obstruction is at the level of the lower jejunum or ileum. All four of the cardinal symptoms occur in mid and lower small intestinal obstruction. The higher the obstruction the earlier vomiting begins, and the lower the obstruction the greater the distension.

(3) *Colonic obstruction* Obstruction is anywhere in the colon. Distension occurs early and can become massive. The classic example is with sigmoid volvulus (see Case history 9, below). Pain in colonic obstruction is usually colicky early on, but occasionally may be steady. It is generally present in the hypogastrium.

Strangulated obstruction Here the blood supply to and from the obstructed segment of bowel is compromised. This is a feared complication and will result in infarction and gangrene of the bowel. Examples are hernias, volvulus, intussusception and a closed loop obstruction (see Figure 9.23 and Table 9.7).

Closed loop obstruction Here the intestine is obstructed at two points, distally and proximally, so that a segment of bowel is obstructed ('closed') at both ends. Since the intestine is obstructed proximally as well, it does not become dilated by swallowed air as it does in a simple obstruction. However, as in a simple obsruction, the intestine becomes a secreting organ and the loop fills up with fluid. If not diagnosed early, it may overdistend and become ischemic, as the venous outflow becomes obstructed (pathophysiology similar to strangulation, see Figure 9.23). The pain becomes intense and localized over the 'closed' segment. Tenderness is detected on palpation. A rapid diagnosis is essential to avoid an intra-abdominal catastrophe. The condition is often not diagnosed, since the plain radiograph of the abdomen may not show bowel dilated by air, since it is distended by fluid.

Examples of closed loop obstruction would be a colonic obstruction, for example from a volvulus (the distal site of the obstruction), with an ileocecal valve that

Table 9.8 Causes of Ogilvie's syndrome

After surgery
   orthopedic surgery
   spinal surgery
   abdominal and pelvic surgery
Obstetrical procedures
Trauma
Neurological conditions
Metabolic disorders
Sepsis

remains competent (the proximal site of the 'obstruction'). Another example would be where a loop of bowel becomes entrapped between two adhesions or bands.

Functional obstruction (ileus, pseudo-obstruction)

Functional obstruction of the bowel is due to impaired gut motility in the absence of a mechanical obstructive lesion and may involve the small or large intestine (Table 9.4). As shown in Table 9.4 functional obstruction may occur acutely as with peritonitis or secondary to an electrolyte disorder.

A poorly understood cause of acute functional obstruction is the so-called Ogilvie's syndrome. Here colonic motility is impaired and the patient develops distension that can become quite massive. It tends to occur mostly in middle-aged or elderly persons with other medical or surgical conditions (see Table 9.8). For some reason, it is common after orthopedic surgery and spinal surgery (Table 9.8). Abdominal distension can be so marked that it can make breathing in the supine position difficult. On examination the abdomen is tympanitic and bowel sounds are generally heard. Bowel sounds may even be very active as a consequence of the normally functioning small intestine making an effort to move contents stagnating in the paralyzed colon. The cecum is the most vulnerable part of the large bowel and is always at risk for perforation. Most gastroenterologists will agree that in acute functional obstruction a cecal size of 12 cm or greater warrants colonoscopic decompression. More recently prostigmine has been shown to be of benefit in this setting and may be tried first in patients who do not have a contraindication to the drug.

Case history 9

A 65-year-old man with chronic obstructive pulmonary disease requiring oxygen at home presented to the hospital with acute bronchitis. During the course of his treatment he acutely developed a very distended abdomen and constipation. He felt uncomfortable on account of the distension, but did not have pain. On examination his abdomen was very dilated, non-tender and tympanitic, and his bowel sounds were active. A rectal examination revealed neither masses nor impacted stool. A plain radiograph of the abdomen revealed massive dilatation of the descending, transverse and ascending colon with a cecal size of 10 cm (Figure 9.24). Since there was only a minimal amount of air in the sigmoid colon and rectum, a distal organic colonic obstruction required to be excluded by a watery soluble contrast enema. No distal obstruction was seen. Colonic decompression was then carried out. Water-soluble contrast enemas, being hyperosmolar, achieve excellent cleansing prior to colonoscopy. On occasion gastroenterologists will proceed directly to colonoscopy, hoping to rule out a distal obstruction directly.

Case history 10

A 76-year-old man who lived in a nursing home was noted by the nurses to have developed sudden abdominal distension. This was associated with mild abdominal pain. He had lost his appetite and felt a little nauseated, but had not vomited. He had not passed a bowel movement in 5 days, but he gave a history of constipation for many years. He denied passing flatus. He had no past history of previous abdominal surgery. The temperature was 97.4°F (36.3°C), his heart rate was 68 beats/min, blood pressure 140/85 mmHg and an oxygen saturation of 98%. The abdomen was very markedly distended, the distension involving the entire abdomen. There was no guarding or rigidity, nor was there tenderness on palpation. There was no percussion tenderness, but the abdomen was tympanitic on percussion. Frequent high-pitched tinkles were heard upon auscultation.

Clinically he was felt to have an intestinal obstruction. The large amount of abdominal distension and the absence of vomiting made it more likely to be colonic obstruction. An abdominal plain radiograph showed distended loops of large bowel, with a small amount of air within the rectum (Figure 9.25a). Multiple air–fluid levels were noted on the left lateral decubitus film. An abdominopelivc CT scan was ordered to evaluate the possible cause of the distal obstruction. This showed evidence for a sigmoid volvulus (Figure 9.25b–e). The patient refused colonoscopic decompression. He was then offered an enema performed with a water-soluble contrast agent (Hypaque®).

The site of the volvulus was again identified (Figure 9.25f and g). It was possible to reflux the contrast beyond the obstruction and this resulted in decompression of the volvulus. Colonoscopic decompression is the procedure of choice, but a barium or water-soluble contrast enema may also be used to achieve decompression of the volvulus. If these conservative methods fail or if peritoneal signs have developed before the patient seeks help, then urgent surgery is indicated.

Sigmoid volvulus

This condition is much less common in the West (approximately 4% of intestinal obstructions) than in Africa (Uganda), Iran and Eastern Europe (Russia). The common age of occurrence is the fifth to sixth decade.

The development of a sigmoid volvulus is outlined in Figure 9.26.

Clinical presentation

Many patients have a history of chronic constipation. It is not uncommon in the demented or senile patient. Patients present with an acute onset of pronounced abdominal distension and accompanying pain, nausea and constipation. Vomiting is late. The twisted sigmoid may be palpable and after some time becomes tender. The abdomen is tympanitic. Colonoscopic decompression should be attempted. If unsuccessful, then surgery is performed.

Case history 11

A 65-year-old man presented with severe mid-abdominal pain of less than a day's duration that was progressively worsening. There was no history of previous abdominal surgery. Examples of a plain radiograph and CT scans of the abdomen in a patient who had a cecal volvulus are shown in Figure 9.27.

Cecal volvulus

Cecal volvulus is much less common than sigmoid volvulus (< 1% of all intestinal obstructions). Again, abdominal pain and distension, often with vomiting, are the symptoms. The abdomen, though distended, is usually less so than with a sigmoid volvulus, because the colon distal to the cecum does not contain air. The twisted cecum is frequently seen and palpated centrally, a little to the left of the midline, and has a tympanitic note on percussion. The right iliac fossa on palpation feels empty.

It is important to make an early diagnosis, since on occasion the ileocecal valve is very competent and a closed loop obstruction may result. When that happens, the cecum proximal to the torsion becomes filled with fluid, and gaseous distension will then not be evident on a plain radiograph. Closed loop obstructions are dangerous, since the venous flow to the bowel is impeded by the compression from the distended bowel and ischemia and gangrene result ultimately in perforation. When peritoneal signs develop in a patient with intestinal obstruction, a closed loop obstruction must be suspected.

Case history 12

A 72-year-old man began vomiting after a corned beef and cabbage dinner on St Patrick's day. His vomitus contained food eaten at the previous meal and toward the end had the appearance of 'coffee grounds'. He had no abdominal pain. He said he had a 'hiatus hernia' and gave a history of drinking a pint of spirits daily for many years. He was afebrile, his blood pressure was 155/95 mmHg supine and 145/100 mmHg sitting up. His pulse rate was 84/min lying down and 100/min sitting up. His heart and lung examinations were normal. His abdomen was soft and non-tender, with no distension, and with no masses clinically evident. His bowel sounds were normal. A chest X-ray was obtained (Figure 9.28a and b) and showed two air–fluid levels in the left hemithorax and the absence of a gastric bubble in its anticipated position. This was highly suggestive of a gastric volvulus. The patient underwent a CT scan, which revealed a gastric mesoaxial (or mesentericoaxial) volvulus with the entire stomach located in the chest (Figure 9.28c–e).

At surgery the patient was shown to have a paraesophageal hiatus hernia with a mesoaxial gastric volvulus.

Paraesophageal hiatus hernia and gastric volvulus

A sliding hiatus hernia (described in Chapter 2) is a very common entity and occurs as a result of a laxity of the phrenoesophageal membrane. The phrenoesophageal membrane surrounds the lower end of the esophagus and anchors it to the diaphragm. Heartburn is the commonest symptom that patients with a sliding hiatus hernia complain of. In contrast, a paraesophageal hiatus hernia is an uncommon entity and results from a break in the phrenoesophageal membrane. Since the gastroesophageal junction is fixed to the preaortic fascia and the median arcuate ligament, the gastroesophageal junction remains in the abdomen. As a consequence, a pouch of peritoneum containing the fundus of the stomach rolls into the chest adjacent to the esophagus. The paraesophageal hiatus hernia is therefore also known by the term *rolling hiatus hernia*, in contrast to the common sliding variety. A paraesophageal hiatus hernia is illustrated in Figure 9.29.

Owing to the fixity of the gastroesophageal junction mentioned above, the part of the stomach that has herniated into the chest can undergo torsion, resulting in a gastric volvulus. A gastric volvulus can be either organoaxial (60%) or mesenterioaxial or mesoaxial (30%). The remaining 10% are a combination of the two. The axes of the stomach along which these torsions develop are shown in Figure 9.30.

A gastric volvulus may give rise to distension in the epigastrium and the patient makes unproductive efforts at vomiting. There can be a great deal of chest or upper abdominal discomfort. When an effort is made to pass a nasogastric tube, this is not possible. It can also be suspected at endoscopy. The endoscopist is unable to locate the pylorus and easily forms loops within the stomach. A gastric volvulus may perforate.

Case history 13

A 57-year-old man with a history of hypercholesterolemia, hypertension and tobacco use presented to the Emergency Department at night with severe lower abdominal pain. Earlier that morning he had told his family he had lower abdominal pain, but he went to work nevertheless. Upon arrival in the Emergency Department he was seen to be hypotensive. He had symmetric pulses in all four extremities. The abdomen was not distended, nor did he have guarding or tenderness. Prominent aortic pulsations were present. He was resuscitated with a bolus of normal saline. The clinical impression of the Emergency Department physicians who saw him was an intra-abdominal catastrophe, perhaps a leaking aneurysm based on the finding of prominent abdominal aortic pulsations. He was transported to the CT scanner where he underwent a contrast-enhanced abdominal and pelvic CT scan, which revealed a ruptured abdominal aortic aneurysm (Figure 9.31).

The patient was taken immediately to the operating room. Just prior to surgery he developed sudden abdominal distension and was noted at surgery to have had intra-abdominal bleeding. He developed cardiac arrest on the operating table and could not be resuscitated.

Rupture of abdominal aortic aneurysm

The location of most abdominal aortic aneurysms is from that portion of the aorta that lies between the branching off of the renal arteries and of the inferior mesenteric artery. Around 5% involve either the renal arteries or the visceral arteries. Most of them are fusiform rather than saccular in shape and are atherosclerotic in etiology. However, the pathogenesis of the so-called atherosclerotic aneurysm involves much more than atherosclerosis. Atherosclerosis probably facilitates the development of an aneurysm when the local conditions are appropriate. Such local conditions include the availability of enzymes that act on elastin and collagen and are derived from the plasma but more so from endothelial, smooth muscle and inflammatory cells in the aortic wall. Examples are plasmin, urokinase (tissue derived from prourokinase by the action of plasmin), matrix metalloproteinases 1 and 3 and cathepsins S and K, and probably cytokines (especially interleukin (IL)-6) also. Smoking and male gender are major risk factors in the development of atherosclerotic aneurysms.

Clinical aspects

Aneurysms are diagnosed when a follow-up ultrasound examination is requested following the detection of a suspicious aortic pulsation during a routine abdominal examination. Others are found serendipitously when ultrasound examinations, CT scans or magnetic resonance imaging (MRI) scans of the abdomen are ordered for other reasons. Symptoms may first arise as a consequence of so-called impending rupture. Very often such situations represent a slow leak that has occurred but has been walled off by the posterior parietal peritoneum. At other times a rapid expansion of an aneurysm may be the cause. The features associated with impending rupture are pain, which may be located in the midline of the abdomen or in the back, and tenderness over the aneurysm. Once aneurysmal rupture occurs, the patient experiences throbbing pain in the midline of the abdomen, often in the hypogastrium and/or in the lower back. The pain may be radiated to the testis, scrotum or anal region. Shock and collapse often follow. On palpation a pulsatile mass is appreciated, usually just above the umbilicus. However, one or more masses may be palpated at almost any location after a major leak, the masses representing hematomas. Contrary to popular myth, the peripheral pulses are normal and may even be bounding early on, and later may become thready as a consequence of the shock state. Patients do not always succumb immediately after a leak. The leak is often confined by the posterior parietal peritoneum and patients respond to vigorous resuscitation, allowing for the opportunity for surgical intervention. Complications include rupture into the intestinal tract, the patient presenting with hematemesis and bright red blood per rectum and aortocaval fistula with severe congestive failure.

Case history 14

A 40-year-old man with known Crohn's disease for many years presented with severe pain in the left side of his chest and in the left upper quadrant. The Crohn's disease had been relatively quiescent for a while, and the patient, on average, had two to three bowel movements a day. On occasion he might experience a little lower abdominal crampy pain that would most often be relieved by a bowel movement. There had been no change in his bowel habits of late and he had not recently experienced any lower abdominal pain. The chest and left upper quadrant pain had been continuous since its rather sudden onset a day earlier. The pain radiated to the tip of the left shoulder. He did not have fever. There was guarding in the left upper quadrant and he did not allow palpation in that area. There was no distension or any tenderness present elsewhere in the abdomen. No pulsations were noted in the abdomen. The bowel sounds were normal. The cardiovascular examination was normal. The examination of the lungs appeared normal, but because he was splinting the left side of his chest, one could not be certain of the chest examination over the left lower lobe region. However, the chest X-ray was completely normal. Since his symptoms were not typical for an exacerbation of his Crohn's disease and the pain with its radiation to the tip of the left shoulder was concerning, he underwent a CT scan with both oral and intravenous contrast to rule out a fluid collection or abscess below the left diaphragm. The CT scan revealed a splenic infarction (Figure 9.32). This was presumably due to the hypercoagulable state associated with his inflammatory bowel disease. In retrospect, it perhaps should have been thought of prior to obtaining the CT scan.

Table 9.9 Causes of splenic infarction

Idiopathic myelofibrosis
Chronic myelogenous leukemia
Acute myelogenous leukemia
Sickle cell disease
Hypercoagulable states (uncommon)

Splenic infarction

This patient had the characteristic symptoms and signs of a splenic infarction. Pain radiating to the shoulder tip is characteristic, though not always present. Of course, a fluid collection or abscess below the left diaphragm may also give rise to similar symptoms. The causes of splenic infarction are listed in Table 9.9. They are frequently seen in patients with myeloproliferative disorders such as myelofibrosis. In such cases the patient generally has splenomegaly. A splenic rub may on occasion be heard.

Case history 15

A 75-year-old woman was brought into the Emergency room by her daughter with a complaint of lightheadedness. She had had watery diarrhea and vomiting over the previous four days. The diarrhea and vomiting were clearly resolving on the day of admission. The diarrhea was not accompanied by abdominal pain. She had not been able to retain much by mouth. The patient had been eating in restaurants in her neighborhood quite regularly with her friends over the past 2 weeks. One of her friends had also developed a mild diarrhea. She had no history of recent travel. She was in fairly good health recently. Her hypertension, angina pectoris and atrial fibrillation were well controlled on hydrochlorothiazide and a β-blocker after an angioplasty performed 2 years previously. In the Emergency Department she was found to have postural hypotension by blood pressure and appeared to be dehydrated. The heart, lung and abdominal examinations were entirely normal except for her atrial fibrillation. She was not in pain on arrival at the Emergency Department. She was given a bolus of normal saline and then gradually hydrated. She had no further diarrhea and her blood pressure remained normal.

She was about to be discharged from the Emergency Department, with a diagnosis of an acute viral gastroenteritis (which was what she possibly had had), when she began complaining of diffuse abdominal pain. The pain was fairly constant and with time became more severe. She had no further vomiting or diarrhea. While she had very mild tenderness diffusely on deep palpation of her abdomen, she had no guarding or percussion tenderness. The abdomen was not distended and the bowel sounds were normal. A plain radiograph of the abdomen was normal. She was maintained on intravenous fluids. The differential diagnosis included small intestinal ischemia possibly from embolism from an atrial clot, since she was known to have atrial fibrillation. The intensity of the pain increased considerably over the next few hours and small intestinal ischemia, possibly due to embolism from an atrial thrombus, was the leading contender in the differential diagnosis, since she had atrial fibrillation. However, it was important to rule out slightly atypical presentations of appendicitis, diverticulitis or biliary colic among other considerations. The WBC count, serum amylase and lipase were normal, as was the urinalysis. A serum lactic acid level was obtained and that too was within normal limits. A CT scan of the abdomen was performed with oral and intravenous contrast, and no significant abnormalities were detected, except for a few dilated loops of small bowel. Thus, in summary, the case was one of an elderly woman with chronic atrial fibrillation, who had just recovered from what was felt to have been a viral gastroenteritis and resulting hypotension and dehydration. She had then acutely developed severe abdominal pain with a paucity of findings on both physical examination and radiological tests. An angiogram was requested (Figure 9.33).

The angiogram did not show evidence of thrombosis or embolism. What it did show was narrowing of multiple arteries from their origins in the superior mesenteric artery. Beading was evident, the intestinal arcades were very constricted and not clearly evident and the intramural arterioles were not well visualized (Figure 9.33a). Furthermore, in the venous phase of the angiogram, some pooling of blood was still evident (not shown). A diagnosis of non-occlusive ischemia in the superior mesenteric territory due to a low flow state was made. The arteriogram's intravenous catheter was maintained and papaverine was infused (50 mg/h) directly into the superior mesenteric circulation. The patient was monitored carefully. Within a short time the patient's condition improved and in a few hours the abdominal pain had almost completely resolved. The abdomen remained soft and no guarding, rigidity or percussion tenderness developed. Bowel sounds continued to be normal. The papaverine infusion rate was gradually decreased and, in a few more hours, it was stopped.

Table 9.10 The features of ischemia in the superior mesenteric artery territory early in its course

Abdominal pain out of proportion to physical findings
Abdominal pain out of proportion to radiographic findings
Paucity of helpful findings on routine laboratory tests
The following laboratory tests might provide more
   confidence with regard to a diagnosis of ischemia:
    early elevation is serum lactic acid level – not always present
    early hyperphosphatemia in a patient with acute abdominal
     and pain and normal renal function. Not always present
     and requires a foot (30 cm) of intestine to become
     ischemic
   serum amylase may be elevated 2–3 times normal. This
    may lead to an erroneous diagnosis of acute pancreatitis

A few hours thereafter, an angiogram was repeated. The arterial branches of the superior mesenteric artery were now much more evident and the arcades were clearly visualized, as were the intramural vessels (Figure 9.33b). No contrast was seen in intramural veins (not shown). The patient was discharged 2 days later.

Why was the diagnosis of intestinal ischemia in the superior mesenteric artery territory thought of so early in the presentation?

(1)   Characteristics of the patient:

    (a)   Elderly,

    (b)   Atherosclerotic disease (ischemic heart disease and hypertension) elsewhere,

    (c)   Atrial fibrillation, which could lead embolism to a branch of the superior mesenteric artery,

    (d)   Recent history of severe hypotension following dehydration from an attack of acute diarrhea, which could lead to ischemia from low flow to the mesenteric circulation;

(2)   The clinical presentation (see Table 9.10):

    (a)   Severe abdominal pain in the absence of striking physical findings on abdominal examination,

    (b)   Severe abdominal pain in the absence of striking findings on plain radiographs of the abdomen.

It is often said that an elevation in serum lactic acid occurs early in intestinal ischemia and is often of a higher degree than what might be expected from hypoperfusion of other viscera. That is true and may provide support for the clinical diagnosis. However, the finding of a normal serum lactic acid level should not dissuade one from making a diagnosis of intestinal ischemia. This patient had been hypotensive and one might have expected an elevated lactate level.

How does one explain a delay in the onset of the severe abdominal pain? There was no pain at the time the patient was dehydrated and hypotensive, but pain began after her blood pressure had returned to normal and she was adequately rehydrated.

To answer the above question one needs to consider two scenarios, the first of which represents more severe and prolonged ischemia.

(1) Hypotension low-flow state $\rightarrow$ ischemia of bowel $\rightarrow$ prolonged ischemia without reversal $\rightarrow$ infarction of bowel $\rightarrow$ severe pain and shock;

(2) Hypoperfusion $\rightarrow$ low-flow state $\rightarrow$ ischemia of bowel $\rightarrow$ initiation condition corrected and patient rehydrated $\rightarrow$ ischemia reversed and patient becomes normotensive $\rightarrow$ metabolites generated in the ischemic segment of bowel result in reperfusion injury $\rightarrow$ local ischemia $\rightarrow$ pain $\rightarrow$ if reversed patient recovers, if not bowel infarction will develop.

The patient described in Case history 15 probably belonged to the second category. She had recovered from the initiating event, the acute diarrheal illness that had since resolved. She was rehydrated and at this time reperfusion injury developed. Reperfusion injury can occur both after non-occlusive (i.e. low flow) ischemia as well as after occlusive (i.e. thrombosis or embolism) ischemia.

Case history 16

An 86-year-old woman with ischemic heart disease and previous peptic ulcer disease was admitted with severe epigastric pain that was continuous. The pain had begun a few hours earlier. The abdomen was soft, there was no guarding and there was mild to moderate tenderness on palpation all over the abdomen. Bowel sounds were normal. Examinations of the heart and lungs were normal. Her blood counts, serum electrolytes, BUN, serum creatinine, liver function test profile and serum lipase were normal. The serum amylase was twice normal, however. Plain radiographs of the abdomen (including a left lateral decubitus film) showed no free air under the diaphragm, no dilated loops of bowel and no air–fluid levels.

The pain was very severe and was fairly sudden in onset thus it's unlikely to be due to an exacerbation of peptic ulcer disease unless the ulcer had perforated. With perforation the pain is very dramatic in onset, but this patient had no evidence of peritoneal signs (guarding, rigidity, percussion tenderness) and the plain radiograph did not show air under the diaphragm. Diverticulitis was a possibility, but less so without tenderness in the left lower quadrant, although as mentioned earlier the acute abdomen in the elderly is often a bag of surprises and nothing has the propensity to surprise the clinician more than diverticulitis in the elderly. Could this be acute cholecystitis or choledocholithiasis? The pain of biliary colic is often in the epigastrium and the liver function tests may be entirely normal in patients with cholecystitis. Elevations in serum amylase may suggest acute pancreatitis, although a normal serum lipase makes this less likely but not impossible. In an elderly person, particularly with known cardiac or vascular disease, ischemia in the superior mesenteric territory is a distinct possibility and must always be seriously considered. Ischemia became higher in the differential diagnosis in this woman, since her presentation met the criteria mentioned earlier (Table 9.10):

(1) Abdominal pain out of proportion to signs on physical examination of the abdomen;

(2) Abdominal pain out of proportion to findings on the plain radiograph of the abdomen;

(3) Elevated serum amylase, in the absence of an elevated serum lipase.

Since conditions other than ischemia mentioned above required to be excluded, it was decided to order a CT scan rather than to proceed to angiography directly. It must be pointed out that the pretest probability of acute cholecystitis was not considered to be very high, and hence an abdominal ultrasound examination that would have been the best test to exclude it was not ordered. The patient's renal function was good, so it was decided to carry out an abdominal CT scan with both oral and intravenous contrast (Figure 9.34).

The gallbladder and pancreas were normal. As mentioned in the legend to Figure 9.34, in this patient a clot was demonstrated in the proximal superior mesenteric artery. It was evident that she had superior mesenteric artery thrombosis. Because the clot was clearly demonstrated, there was no reason to perform an angiogram. The patient underwent a laparotomy, which showed thrombosis of the superior mesenteric artery, severe atherosclerosis and three areas of bowel that were infarcted. She underwent a resection of 70 cm of proximal jejunum, 36 cm of distal jejunum and 15 cm of mid-ileum. Histology revealed ischemic enteritis with transmural infarction. She had to be reoperated on 4 days later. At this time, a further 29 cm of bowel were resected and included a side-to-side anastomosis constructed at the previous surgery.

Frequently, at surgery, if there is even the remotest doubt of the viability of the unresected bowel, then a definitive decision needs to be made to offer the patient a 'second look' operation to determine whether the bowel continues to be viable. This is the preferred route in such patients and is preferable to an attempt to follow the patient clinically, since clinical signs in the immediate postoperative period are very unreliable.

Pneumatosis intestinalis and portal venous air may also be seen as a result of bowel ischemia that is advanced. An example is shown in Figure 9.35 in the case of a patient who developed ischemia to the bowel following volvulus of the small bowel resulting from adhesions.

Case history 17

A 30-year-old man presented to a community hospital with diffuse abdominal pain of several days' duration. By the time he sought help at that hospital, the pain was severe and had localized to the right lower quadrant with considerable tenderness in the area. Clinically he was thought to have appendicitis and was operated on. At surgery he was found to have a perforated and ischemic cecum and small bowel. He underwent a right hemicolectomy and also resection of a foot (30 cm) of jejunum. The patient had no family history to suggest a familial coagulopathy. Initially no effort was made to investigate the cause of his ischemia. He was placed on heparin and later switched to warfarin. He did reasonably well postoperatively, but a few days later developed severe, diffuse, continuous abdominal pain again and developed a fever. He was then transferred to a tertiary care hospital where he underwent a CT scan upon arrival. The CT scan, with intravenous but not oral contrast, revealed thrombosis of the superior mesenteric vein with extension into the portal vein (Figure 9.36). At surgery the mesenteric venous thrombosis was confirmed. The small intestine was very edematous, there was cloudy fluid in the peritoneal cavity and a contained leak was identified, necessitating resection of the previous anastomosis.

Intestinal ischemia

The case histories presented above and the discussions that follow allow the following general conclusions to be drawn:

(1) Damage to the gut from ischemia can result from lesions in either the arterial or the venous sides of the mesenteric circulation.

(2) Ischemic injury can develop following either occlusive (thrombotic or embolic) or non-occlusive (low flow) events;

(3) In the case of non-occlusive arterial ischemia or low-flow states, ischemic injury may be permanent if not rapidly reversed. However, reperfusion injury may be seen even after reversal of the initiating event (e.g. correction of hypotension and hypoperfusion);

(4) The presence of certain symptoms, signs and laboratory tests should make the clinician strongly consider the possibility of gut ischemia (Table 9.10). However, it is important to reiterate that severe intestinal ischemia may be present in the absence of abnormal laboratory test results.

A clinically useful classification of the causes of ischemic bowel disease is presented in Figure 9.37. It is important to distinguish bowel ischemia that arises as a consequence of lesions, anatomic or physiological, in the arterial side of the mesenteric circulation from those in the venous side of the circulation.

For the clinician it is best to consider arterial ischemia as occurring in either the superior mesenteric artery or the inferior mesenteric artery territory. The clinical presentations, course and prognosis of ischemia occurring in these two arterial territories differ considerably. The syndromes may be acute or chronic in each territory.

Acute ischemia in the superior mesenteric artery territory

The causes giving rise to acute ischemia in the superior mesenteric artery territory are presented in Table 9.11. The vast majority is due to thrombosis, embolism or a low-flow state.

The clinical presentation is with severe abdominal pain that develops rather insiduously and may be accompanied by nausea and on occasion vomiting. The patient may pass a few loose bowel movements, which usually test positive for occult blood. The other clinical features are outlined in Table 9.10.

Table 9.11 Acute mesenteric ischemia in the superior mesenteric artery territory

Occlusive
Thrombosis
  atherosclerosis
Embolism – (arrythmias, especially atrial fibrillation)
  mural thrombus due to a myocardial infarction
  vegetations on valves: rheumatic, bacterial endocarditis,
    prosthetic
  paradoxical
  tumor embolism: atrial myxoma, lung cancer
  atheroembolism
Vasculitis
  systemic lupus erythematosus
  polyarteritis nodosa
Strangulation
  volvulus
  intussusception
  hernia
Non-occlusive or low-flow state
Hypotension→ hypoperfusion of the gut
Drugs
  digoxin
  vasopressin
  noradrenaline (norepinephrine)
  propranolol

Table 9.12 Role of computed tomography scans in acute ischemia in the superior mesenteric artery territory

In the postoperative period when other diagnoses need
  to be excluded
Whenever the clinical setting requires another cause for
  acute abdomen to be excluded
When perforation of an abdominal viscus needs to
  be excluded
When intra-abdominal abscess needs to be excluded

The dagnosis needs to be established early on in the course if the patient is to be salvaged. A high degree of clinical suspicion based on host factors is essential. Mesenteric thrombosis must be considered in the differential diagnosis of diffuse acute abdominal pain, especially in elderly patients with atherosclerotic disease elsewhere in the body (heart, peripheral vascular disease, brain, renal arteries, etc.). Patients with atrial fibrillation and valvular disease, and those in the post-myocardial infarction stage (Table 9.11) are especially prone to develop embolism to the superior mesenteric artery. Superior mesenteric ischemia due to a low-flow state (non-occlusive ischemia) must be suspected in patients who develop abdominal pain either during a prolonged period of hypotension (and consequent hypoperfusion of the gut) or shortly after recovery from such an episode. Digoxin, especially in the setting of congestive heart failure and diuretic treatment, acts as a splanchnic vasoconstrictor and can cause low-flow ischemia.

Once the diagnosis is suspected, it must be established without delay. Unless there are specific contraindications, (Table 9.12) an angiogram should be recommended to the patient and not a CT scan. CT scans obtained early in the course of the disease may be normal. Even with intravenous contrast injection, a thrombus or embolus in a branch of the superior mesenteric artery may not be detected. Certainly in the case of non-occlusive ischemia, no specific features are known on CT scanning for making the diagnosis. However, it is important to remember that, when non-occlusive ischemia is suspected, the patient should initially be resuscitated and should not be on a noradrenaline (norepinephrine) drip at the time of angiography. Severe vasoconstriction, either from hypotension or from pressors, may make the interpretation of an angiogram very difficult for making a diagnosis of low-flow ischemia.

Once the diagnosis of ischemia in the superior mesenteric territory is made, the treatment depends on whether the ischemia is occlusive or non-occlusive (Figure 9.38). Whenever bowel surgery is performed it is important to assess the viability of the bowel that is not resected. If any doubt remains of the long-term viability of the intestine that is not resected, second-look surgery within the first 2 days should be planned at the completion of the initial surgery.

Chronic ischemia in the superior mesenteric artery territory

Chronic ischemia gives rise to intestinal angina and has been described in Chapter 5.

Superior mesenteric venous thrombosis

The causes of thrombosis of the superior mesenteric vein fall into two major groups, as shown in Table 13. Even though the risks of venous thrombosis are higher with antithrombin III deficiency and protein C and S deficiencies, factor V Leiden, prothrombin mutation G20210A and hyperhomocysteinemia are more frequent causes of venous thrombosis, because they occur more frequently.

The clinical features are often different from those of superior mesenteric artery thrombosis, in that the onset is often much more insidious. The patient not infrequently presents with vague abdominal pain with or without distension, diarrhea or constipation and loss of

Table 9.13   Superior mesenteric venous thrombosis

Intra-abdominal causes
Intra-abdominal inflammation
   intra-abdominal sepsis
   acute pancreatitis
   carcinoma of the pancreas
Portal hypertension
   presinusoidal
   intrahepatic
   postsinusoidal
   (hepatofugal flow favors occurrence)
Postsplenectomy

Hypercoagulable states particularly at risk for venous thrombosis
Antithrombin III deficiency (high risk)
Protein C deficiency (high risk)
Protein S deficiency (high risk)
Resistance to activated protein C or factor V Leiden
   (moderate risk)
Prothrombin mutation G20210A (moderate risk)
Hyperhomocysteinemia (moderate risk)
Oral contraceptives (low risk)

appetite. Symptoms progress to a mid-abdominal pain, sometimes a colicky pain. Vomiting then generally develops. The diagnosis is frequently missed preoperatively. If suspected, the diagnosis is often best established by a spiral CT scan done with intravenous but not oral contrast.

The patient presented in Case history 17 probably had an underlying hypercoagulable state that resulted in the superior mesenteric vein thrombosis that was missed at the time of the first surgery, his condition being interpreted as thrombosis in branches of the superior mesenteric artery. The second surgery was probably necessitated by the anastomotic leak that resulted from continuing ischemia to the small intestine from the superior mesenteric vein thrombosis. Another factor in the perpetuation or extension of the superior mesenteric vein thrombosis was the intra-abdominal sepsis.

Whenever a superior mesenteric vein thrombosis is diagnosed, and if a clear-cut intra-abdominal cause is not detected (Table 9.13), then a work-up for a hypercoagulable state must be initiated.

Ischemic colitis

Ischemic colitis is described in Chapter 7.

Case history 18

A young Caucasian woman aged 24 years had recently been diagnosed with cystitis and had been prescribed double-strength trimethoprim/sulfamethoxazole. That night she developed severe generalized abdominal pain that was colicky and accompanied by vomiting. She did not have diarrhea. She did not complain of feeling either warm or chilled. Earlier that evening she had gone to a restaurant with some friends and had eaten a salad and a filet mignon. With her meal she had had a glass of wine and with her friends had had a couple of glasses of beer and some hors d'oeuvres at the bar prior to dinner. She had called her friends before coming to the hospital, and none of them were ill. She reported that she had a steady monogamous relationship with her boyfriend who had accompanied her to the hospital. She was on no other medications other than that prescribed for her urinary tract infection and birth control pills, which she had been taking for quite some time. She mentioned that she had experienced two similar, though much less severe, episodes of vomiting and abdominal pain over the past year. On one of those occasions she remembered having been out with friends and having drunk socially. She had not had diarrhea with either episode. On one of these occasions she had been admitted to a community hospital in a small town 200 miles away where she had been visiting her grandmother. She was discharged after a few days without a definitive diagnosis. She had not had abdominal surgery previously.

On examination she was afebrile, her heart rate was 110 beats/min and her blood pressure 160/90 mmHg. She had no known history of hypertension. Her abdomen was not distended; it was soft and not really tender. No hernias were detected. Bowel sounds were present, perhaps somewhat sluggish. The rectal examination was normal with no tenderness. There was no vaginal discharge. The rest of the physical examination was normal. She was admitted with a diagnosis of a small intestinal obstruction of unknown etiology. Plain films of the abdomen were obtained and were normal. Her blood counts were normal, including the WBC count, as were the serum electrolytes, blood glucose, liver function tests and serum amylase and lipase. She was maintained on nasogastric suction and intravenous fluids.

The abdominal pain continued to be severe and required narcotics for control. Her physical examination had not altered other than the fact that the bowel sounds, although still present, were definitely more sluggish than on admission. This was interpreted as being a reflection of her being on narcotics. Another set of plain films of the abdomen taken several hours later revealed a few loops of bowel containing some air, but overall there was no marked distension to suggest an intestinal obstruction. A diagnosis of ischemic bowel was not entertained at the onset because of the patient's young age and no previous history to suggest a systemic vasculitis. A CT scan with both oral and intravenous contrast was ordered and did not reveal any abnormal findings. Despite the patient being on birth control pills, the diagnosis of ischemia was not considered probable. Blood was sent off for antinuclear antibodies. A pregnancy test was negative. On the second day the patient became a little disoriented and by the evening was hallucinating. Her friends mentioned that they had never seen her behave in this fashion. The cerebrospinal fluid was examined and was normal. A CT scan of the head was also obtained and was normal.

The psychiatrist, consulted for what was considered to be a delirium, was impressed by the following:

(1) The acute onset of the severe abdominal pain and vomiting with a paucity of physical and radiological signs in a young Caucasian woman;

(2) The association of the abdominal pain and vomiting with acute mental status changes in the absence of a clear etiology;

(3) Persistent sinus tachycardia despite adequate hydration and a somewhat elevated blood pressure in a person with no history of hypertension;

(4) The onset of symptoms in association with alcohol consumption now on at least two occasions;

(5) The onset of symptoms on this occasion after being on a sulfa drug for a day.

The psychiatrist considered the possibility of a diagnosis of porphyria. A 24-h urine collection was obtained through an indwelling urinary catheter and the patient was empirically begun on intravenous glucose. The 24-h urine aminolevulenic acid (ALA) was 350 μmol/24 h (normal < 55 μmol/24 h) and the porphobilinogen excretion was > 500 μmol/24 h (normal < 20 μmol/24 h), whereas the urinary coproporphyrin was not elevated. A diagnosis of acute intermittent porphyria was thus established. Once the diagnosis was established, the patient was started on an infusion of heme (given as hematin). After a few days she responded well. Later, when asked, she mentioned that a cousin of hers had been diagnosed with 'porphyria' earlier.

Table 9.14 Types of hepatic porphyria that give rise to abdominal symptoms

Aminolevulenic acid-dehydratase deficiency porphyria
Acute intermittent porphyria
Hereditary coproporphyria
Variegate porphyria

Porphyria

To summarize briefly, abdominal symptoms are seen only with the hepatic porphyrias and not with erythropoietic porphyrias. The commonest hepatic porphyria is porphyria cutanea tarda, which does not have abdominal manifestations.

The porphyrias that give rise to acute episodes of abdominal pain with or without mental changes and with or without evidence of a motor proximal peripheral neuropathy are shown in Table 9.14. Figure 9.39 outlines the pathway of heme synthesis and the enzyme defects that give rise to the four hepatic porphyrias.

Aminolevulinic acid-dehydratase deficiency porphyria

This is the most rare of the hepatic porphyrias. It is an autosomal recessive condition. As expected from Figure 9.39, there is an elevation of δ-ALA levels in the urine but no porphobilinogen, thus distinguishing this rare condition from acute intermittent porphyria. As expected, δ-ALA-dehydratase in erythrocytes is < 5% of normal. Clinical features include abdominal pain and peripheral neuropathy, resembling acute intermittent porphyria.

Acute intermittent porphyria

This is an autosomal dominant condition. It is most commonly seen in Caucasians, especially those of Scandinavian ancestry. As expected from Figure 9.39, there is an elevation of both δ-ALA and porphobilinogen levels, but often only during acute attacks. The majority of heterozygotes remain asymptomatic, although symptoms may be induced by triggers. Triggers that induce symptoms are alcohol consumption and a variety of drugs that induce cytochrome P450. Examples are sulfonamides, barbiturates, dilantin, carbamazepine, valproic acid, mephenytoin, synthetic estrogen and progestogens. Clinical features including neurological symptoms are as follows:

(1) *Abdominal pain* Usually colicky but may be constant. Pain is often diffuse but may be in the lower abdomen or periumbilical region. The pain may

be moderate or very severe. Constipation may be present.

(2) *Peripheral neuropathy* Almost always motor. Upper limbs > lower limbs. Proximal > distal. Cranial nerves may be involved.

(3) *Psychiatric* Depression, delirium, confusion, hallucination, paranoia.

(4) *Autonomic* Elevated blood pressure, tachycardia, sweating.

(5) Inappropriate antidiuretic hormone secretion resulting in hyponatremia. Hyponatremia may be a cause of mental status changes in addition to the effects of the elevated porphyrins. Hyponatremia may cause seizures also.

(6) Skin lesions and photosensitivity are not seen in acute intermittent porphyria.

In treatment of an acute attack, intravenous glucose infusions often provide relief. The mechanism is not well understood. Better than glucose is an infusion of heme as hematin or other heme compounds such as heme arginate.

Hereditary coproporphyria

This is an autosomal dominant condition. Women are more commonly involved, with onset after puberty. As expected from figure 9.39, elevated levels of δ-amino-levulinic acid, porphobilinogen and corproporphyrin are seen in the urine. In addition, fecal coproporphyrins but not protoporphyrins are increased. The triggers are similar to those for acute intermittent porphyria. In addition, skin photosensitivity may be seen. Clinical features are identical to those of acute intermittent porphyria.

Variegate porphyria

This is seen largely in South African Whites of Dutch descent. As would be expected from Figure 9.39, one would see elevated levels of δ-aminolevulinic acid, porphobilinogen and copro-porphyrin in the urine. In additon, fecal copropor-phyrins and protoporphyrins are increased. Clinical features include neurovisceral symptoms, similar to those of acute intermittent porphyria and hereditary coproporphyria. However, skin lesions are seen more commonly.

Table 9.15 Systemic disorders that can mimic a surgical acute abdomen

Sickle cell anemia
Vasculitis
Henoch–Schönlein purpura
systemic lupus
polyarteritis nodosa
Diabetic ketoacidosis
Hepatic porphyrias
acute intermittent porphyria
hereditary coproporphyria
variegate porphyria
Aminolevulinic acid-dehydratase deficiency porphyria
Lead poisoning
Familial Mediterranean fever

OTHER SYSTEMIC CONDITIONS THAT CAN MIMIC A SURGICAL ACUTE ABDOMEN

The clinician must always remember systemic disorders that may masquerade as a surgical acute abdomen. Table 9.15 lists some of these conditions.

Sickle cell disease

Severe acute right upper quadrant pain and tenderness accompanied by fever and leukocytosis is seen in patients with sickle cell disease. It is believed that these patients have sickle cell formation in liver sinusoids resulting in ischemic changes. Erythrophagocytosis by Kupffer cells has been noted in the liver of these patients at autopsy or on liver biopsy. Whether liver ischemia is indeed the cause of this syndrome has been debated. As in other hemolytic anemias, patients with sickle cell disease are prone to pigment gallstones. Therefore, acute cholecysti-tis must be considered in the differential diagnosis when patients with sickle cell disease present with right upper quadrant pain, tenderness, fever and leukocytosis.

Vasculitis

Any of the vasculitides mentioned in Table 9.15 may present with severe abdominal pain, most often due to bowel ischemia. On occasion pancreatitis, also on an ischemic basis, or acalculus cholecystitis may be the cause.

Henoch-Schönlein purpura

This is more common in children, but is seen in adults also. Abdominal pain, often acute and severe, sometimes colicky and at other times steady, may develop. The small vessel vasculitis with resulting ischemia is generally the cause of the pain. The pain may be accompanied by vomiting or gastrointestinal hemorrhage. An erosive duodenitis has been reported and may be the cause of pain in some patients. Intramural hematoma may develop in the intestines and may cause bleeding, pain and intussusception. Acalculus cholecystitis due to vasculitis may occur as it also may in polyarteritis nodosa.

Diabetic ketoacidosis

Abdominal pain, occasionally severe, is present in some patients with deabetic ketoacidosis and as a rule is due to the ketoacidosis itself. Nausea and vomiting are more frequent. The abdominal pain has occasionally been diagnosed as an acute surgical abdomen and patients are taken to surgery. An important differentiation from most causes of an acute abdomen is the fact that anorexia, nausea and vomiting precede the abdominal pain, usually by quite a substantial time. An elevated WBC count is not infrequently seen in diabetic ketoacidosis and sometimes reaches leukemoid proportions, up to 40 000–50 000/mm³. Elevations in serum amylase and lipase occur in diabetic ketoacidosis even without pancreatitis. The elevated amylase is proportional to both the severity of the acidosis and the serum osmolality, whereas the elevated lipase is related only to the elevation in the serum osmolality. In one study, the majority of the amylase elevation could be attributed to an elevation in the salivary isoenzyme. True acute pancreatitis may also occur and may be related to an associated hypertriglyceridemia.

Lead poisoning

As a rule the presentation is more insidious with colicky abdominal pain, constipation, anemia with basophilic stippling and neuropsychiatric manifestations. However, on occasion severe colicky pain may develop rather acutely and can mimic an intestinal obstruction. Lead can inhibit the enzyme ALA-dehydratase resulting in an increase of δ-aminolevulinic acid. Thus, the pain in lead poisoning may be due to the same cause as the pain in porphyrias, i.e. neurovisceral.

Familial Mediterranean fever

This is more often seen in Sephardic Jews, Arabs and Armenians. It has also been described in Europeans. It is an autosomal recessive condition, with the defect arising from a mutation in the MEFV gene located on the short arm of chromosome 16. The age of presentation is generally between 5 and 15 years, but is very variable. There is no specific pathology characteristic of the disease. During an acute attack of pain, inflammation of the peritoneum is seen, with a polymorphonuclear leukocyte response. Pleurisy and joint inflammation are also noted.

Clinical features include the following:

(1) Fever is present in almost all attacks.

(2) Abdominal pain is invariably present during attacks. This begins in any one quadrant and then may spread to involve the entire abdomen. It may radiate to the back and chest. Elevation in the WBC count and erythrocyte sedimentation rate is frequently present.

(3) Nausea and vomiting may be present.

(4) Chest pain may be referred pain from the abdomen or may be a *de novo* pleurisy.

(5) An episode of arthritis is seen in three-quarters of the patients at least once. It tends to involve larger joints and is often accompanied by an effusion. Arthralgias are more common.

(6) Secondary amyloidosis may develop.

Genetic testing for several of the mutations is available.

Section II   Gastroenterology illustrated

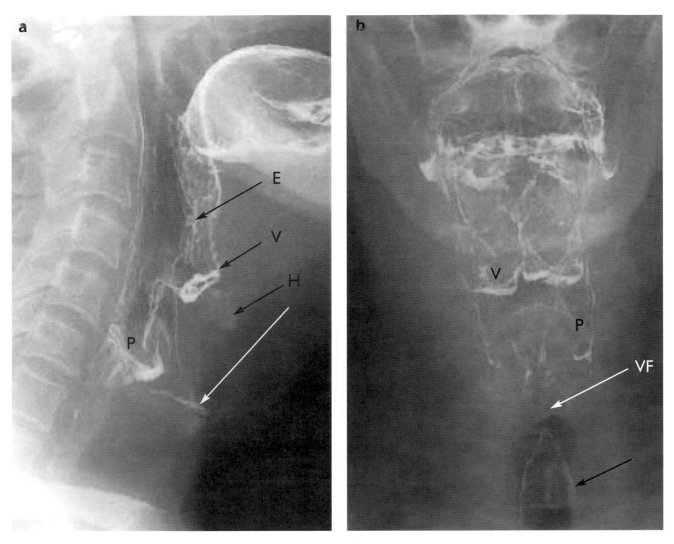

Figure 1.1 Aspiration shown during barium swallow. (a) Lateral view of oropharynx during barium swallow. Note epiglottis (E), valleculae (V), piriform sinuses (P), hyoid cartilage (H). Barium has penetrated the laryngeal inlet, and is coating the laryngeal ventricle (yellow arrow). (b) Frontal (anteroposterior) view of the oropharynx. Note the epiglottis (E), valleculae (V) and piriform sinuses (P). Vocal cords are closed (white arrow, VF), but barium has penetrated into the trachea (black arrow)

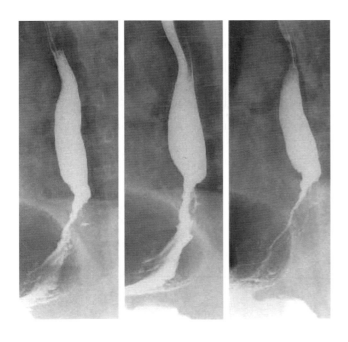

Figure 1.2 Narrowing of the lumen of the distal third of the esophagus with ulceration

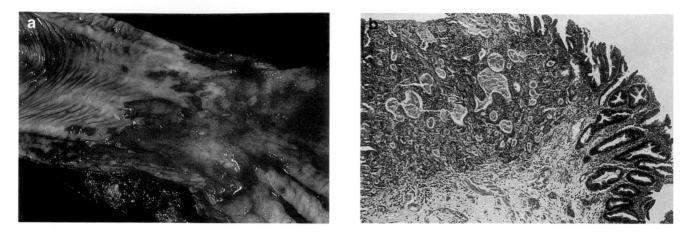

Figure 1.3 Adenocarcinoma of the esophagus. (a) Esophagogastrectomy specimen, demonstrating transformation of the lower esophagus to Barrett's mucosa, including some islands of red-granular mucosa in the midst of otherwise preserved squamous mucosa. In the center of the photograph is a raised plaque lesion. (b) Photomicrograph from the edge of the plaque lesion in this same specimen. High-grade surface dysplasia gives way to moderately differentiated adenocarcinoma, invasive through strands of the muscularis mucosa into the submucosa (Hematoxylin and eosin, 100 ×)

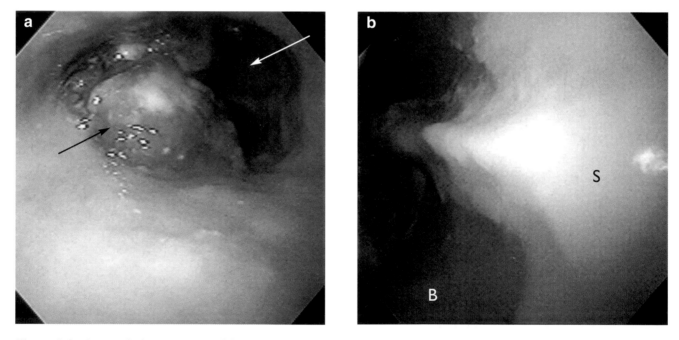

Figure 1.4 A case of adenocarcinoma of the esophagus (NB. this is not the patient described in Case history 1). (a) Large eccentric tumor (black arrow) obstructing the lumen of the distal esophagus (white arrow). Biopsy revealed it to be an adenocarcinoma. (b) Endoscopic view of the esophageal lumen proximal to the tumor seen in (a), shows pink mucosa (marked 'B' for Barrett's) quite distinct from the more proximal normal pearly squamous mucosa (S) of the esophagus

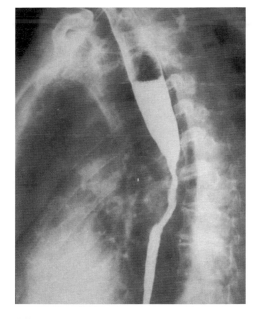

Figure 1.5 Mid-esophageal malignant stricture

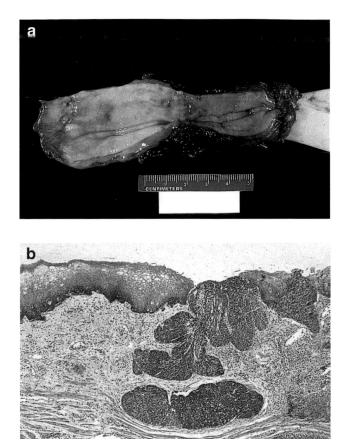

Figure 1.6 Squamous cell carcinoma of the esophagus. (a) Esophagectomy specimen, showing a stricture in the central portion and an irregular small exophytic lesion at the point of stricture. (b) Low-power photomicrograph from the edge of the lesion, demonstrating normal esophageal squamous mucosa on the left, and squamous cell carcinoma on the right, invasive into the lamina propria and pressing against the muscularis mucosa at the lower portion of the image (Hematoxylin and eosin, 40 ×)

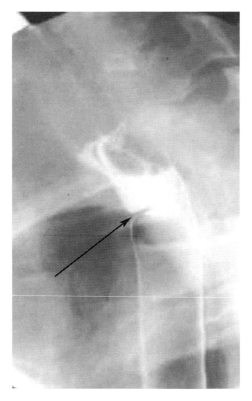

Figure 1.7 Esophageal web (arrowed)

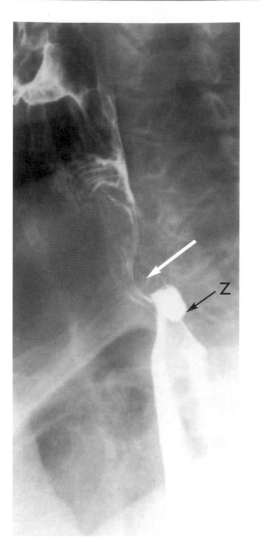

Figure 1.8 Zencker's diverticulum (Z) arising at Killian's dehiscence in an 82-year-old man. Note the prominent cricopharyngeus (arrowed)

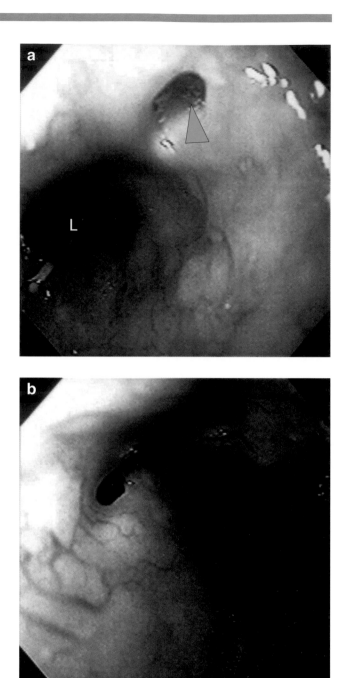

Figure 1.9 (a) A small diverticulum (arrow head) high in the esophagus incidentally noted during endoscopy (L indicates the lumen). (b) Another view looking down into the diverticulum

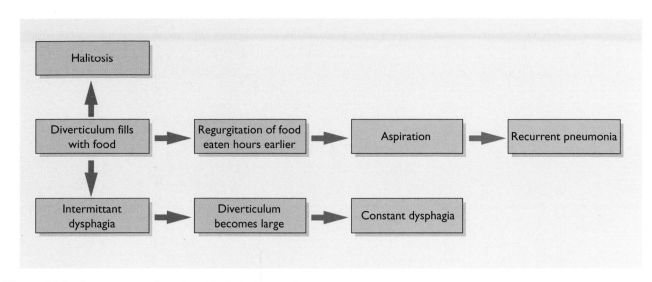

Figure 1.10   Symptoms resulting from Zenker's diverticulum

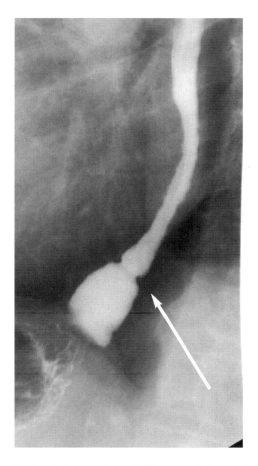

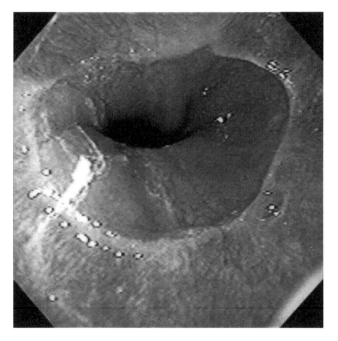

Figure 1.12   A typical Schatzki ring

Figure 1.11   A Schatski ring (white arrow) is radiologically identified as a mucosal fold at the gastroesophageal junction, associated with a hiatal hernia or proximal displacement of the gastroesophageal junction, and is usually asymptomatic. It is a relatively common finding (occurring in about 15%). The pathogenesis is unclear, but shortening of the longitudinal muscle of the esophagus has been postulated. Fibrosis can develop in a small percentage of patients, leading to thickening of the fold to 4–5 mm in width. Once the lumen becomes less than 12 mm in diameter, symptoms of dysphagia to solid food can occur

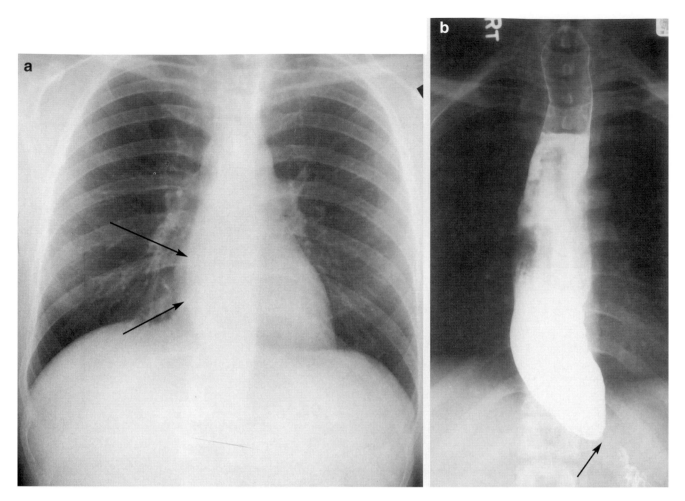

Figure 1.13 (a) Chest radiograph, showing absence of stomach bubble and bulge along azygoesophageal recess (arrowed) due to dilated, fluid-filled esophagus. (b) Beaking at the gastroesophageal junction (arrowed), and air–fluid level in the mid-esophagus

Innervation the lower two-thirds of the body of the esophagus and of the lower esophageal sphincter (LES):

Inflammatory degeneration of intrinsic neurons:
Myenteric plexus: diminished to absent neurons (ganglion cells) in circular and longitudinal muscle layers: diminished number of neurons.
Lymphocytes and a few eosinophils surround the neurons that remain. **Degeneration is mostly of the NO (nitric oxide) – containing inhibitory neurons***
Most of the excitatory cholinergic neurons are preserved

Extrinsic nerve supply of the esophagus:
Most of the vagal nerve supply is preserved. There may be some Wallerian degeneration of these nerves and some degeneration seen in the dorsal motor nucleus of the vagus.
Neuropeptide-Y perivascular neurons preserved in the myenteric plexus, suggesting an intact extrinsic nerve supply

Impaired peristalsis in the lower two-thirds of the esophagus

Impaired LES relaxation with swallowing

*NO synthase-containing neurons can be detected by histochemical methods that use nicotinamide adenine dinucleotide phosphate (NADPH) diaphorase

Figure 1.14   Achalasia – pathology and pathophysiology

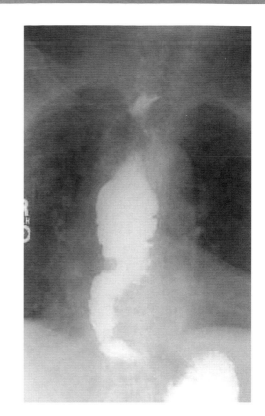

Figure 1.15   An esophagram in a 77-year-old woman with dysphagia, showing beaking and also marked dysmotility with tertiary contractions, consistent with vigorous achalasia. This patient presented on numerous occasions with esophageal food impaction requiring endoscopic intervention

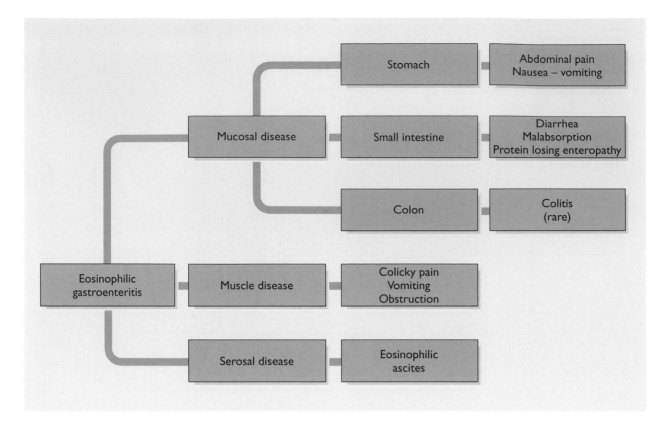

Figure 1.16   Eosinophilic gastroenteritis – the spectrum

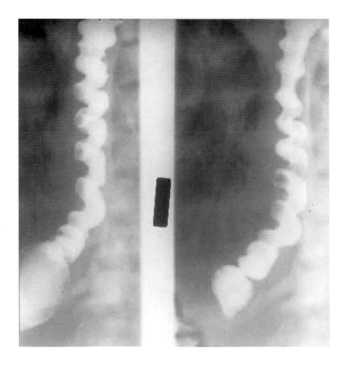

Figure 1.17   In diffuse esophageal spasm, barium swallow showed the classic appearance of 'corkscrew' esophagus

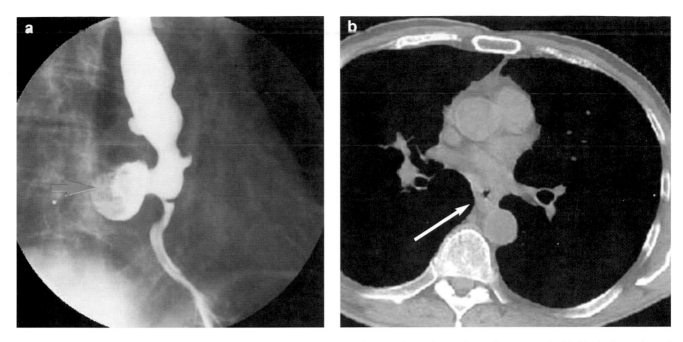

Figure 1.18 (a) Epiphrenic diverticulum (green arrow) demonstrated in distal esophagus during barium study. (b) Marked esophageal wall thickening (arrowed) confirmed on computerized tomography in same 64-year-old patient with a long history of dysphagia to liquids and solids, with a 30 lb weight loss. Endoscopy confirmed the presence of a diverticulum, and the patient underwent a laparoscopic cricomyotomy with relief of symptoms

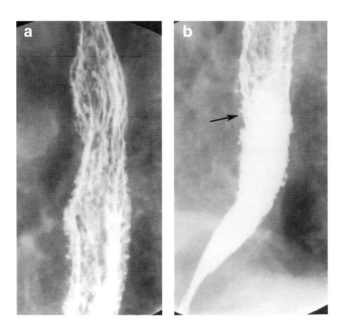

Figure 1.19 Chronic candida esophagitis with pseudo-diverticulosis in a 64-year-old man with odynophagia and insulin-dependent diabetes mellitus. The esophagus had markedly reduced peristalsis, and contained innumerable pseudo-diverticula extending beyond the lumen into the submucosal region (arrowed). (a) Barium esophogram of mid-esophagus; (b) barium esophogram of distal esophagus

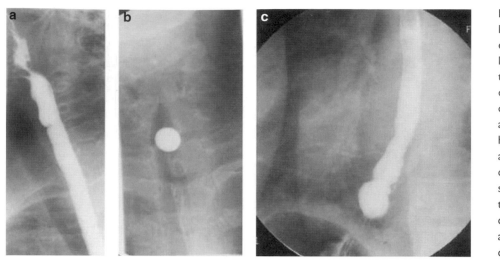

Figure 1.20 (a) Barium swallow demonstrates upper cervical esophageal web as anterior linear incomplete thin band at the level of C5. (b) Transient delay was noted to passage of barium pill at the same level as the esophageal web. (c) A hiatal hernia is present, and additionally, submucosal pinpoint collections of barium and linear submucosal tracking parallel to the esophageal lumen are indicative of pseudo-diverticulosis associated with esophageal candidiasis

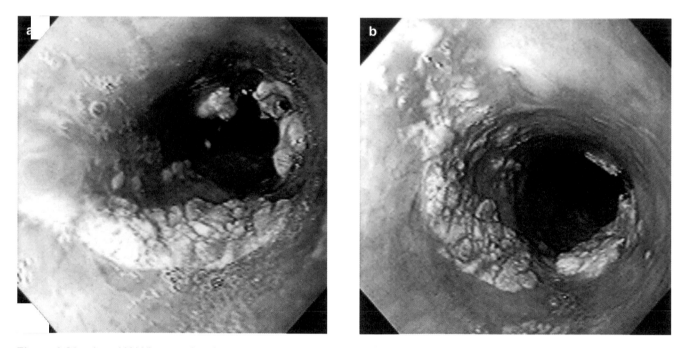

Figure 1.21 (a and b) White exudate firmly adherent to underlying mucosa, typical for esophageal candidiasis

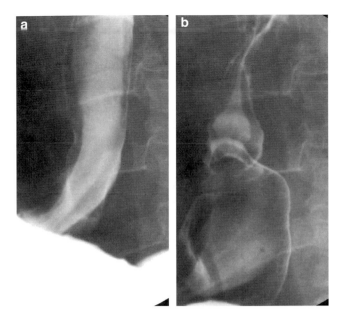

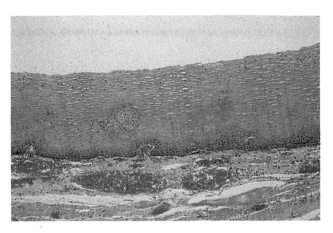

Figure 2.2 Normal esophageal mucosa. (Hematoxylin and eosin, 100 ×)

Figure 2.1 Type III hiatal hernia demonstrated during double-contrast barium esophagram. (a) Distal esophagus is incompletely distended with barium; gastric folds are identified within non-distended hiatal hernia. (b) Air-filled view of distended esophagus shows Schatski ring proximal to hernia sac

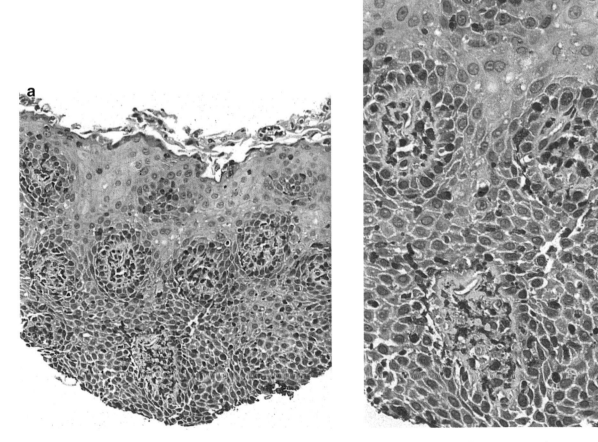

Figure 2.3 Reflux esophagitis. (a) Mucosal biopsy showing expansion of the basal proliferative zone, elongation of rete papillae, and superficial inflammatory exudate. (Hematoxylin and eosin, 200 ×). (b) Higher power photomicrograph demonstrating intramucosal infiltrate of eosinophils. (H & E, 1000 ×)

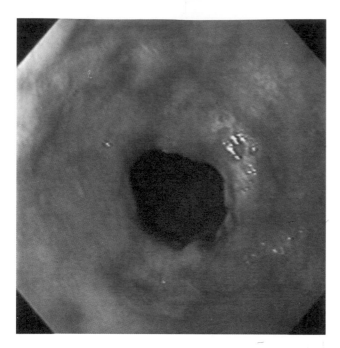

Figure 2.4 Benign esophageal stricture. Markedly erythematous esophageal mucosa with narrowing of the lumen

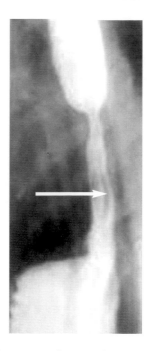

Figure 2.5 Barium esophogram demonstrates a long stricture involving the distal esophagus due to reflux esophagitis

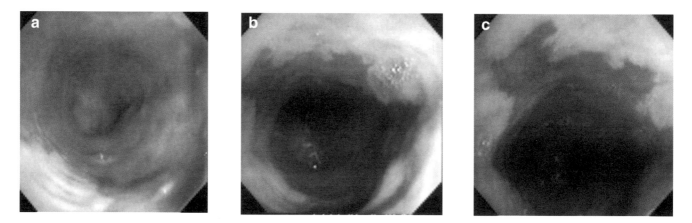

Figure 2.6 Barrett's esophagus. A patient with long segment Barrett's esophagus. Contrast the pink metaplastic (Barrett's) mucosa with the adjacent, proximal pearly white squamous mucosa

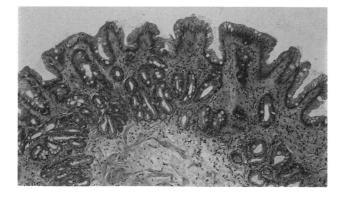

Figure 2.7 Barrett's esophagus. Normally this should be a stratified non-keratinizing squamous mucosa. Shown is the abnormal villiform columnar mucosa of Barrett's esophagus, with a mixture of columnar absorptive and columnar mucin-secreting goblet cells. (Hematoxylin & eosin stain, × 40). Figure courtesy of Dr Melissa Li, University of Florida

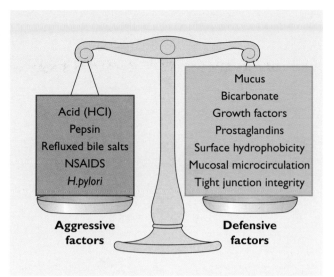

Figure 3.1 Maintenance of mucosal integrity. Aggressive vs. defensive factors

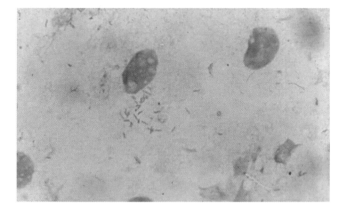

Figure 3.2 *H. pylori* cultured from an antral mucosal biopsy obtained from a patient with duodenal ulcer (Gram stain)

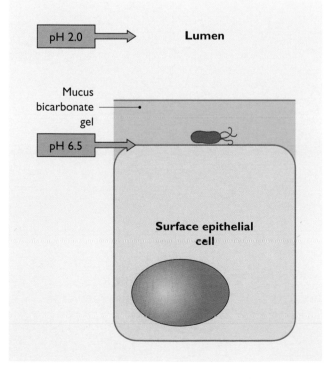

Figure 3.3 The surface epithelial cell with the mucus–bicarbonate gel at its surface. *H. pylori* (red rod) is adherent to the surface where the pH is around 6.5, whereas in the lumen the pH could be as low as 2.0

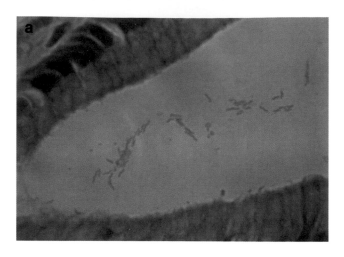

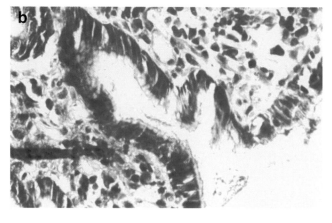

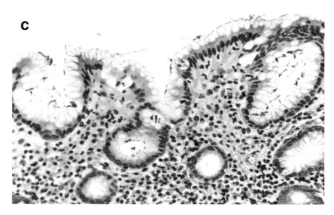

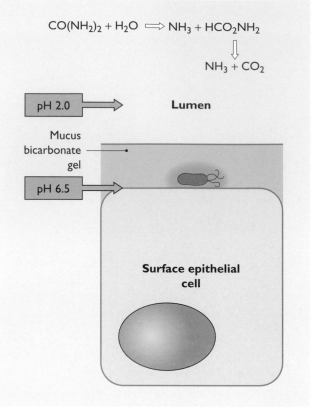

$$CO(NH_2)_2 + H_2O \implies NH_3 + HCO_2NH_2$$

$$\Downarrow$$

$$NH_3 + CO_2$$

pH 2.0 → **Lumen**

Mucus bicarbonate gel

pH 6.5 →

Surface epithelial cell

Figure 3.5 *H. pylori* surrounded by a cloud of ammonia. *H. pylori* represented by the red rod, adherent to the surface of the S E cell within the mucus–bicarbonate gel, protected in part by the cloud of ammonia (green) generated by its urease activity

Figure 3.4 *H. pylori* in its 'natural environment', adjacent to surface epithelium within the mucus layer. (a) Hematoxylin and eosin stain; (b) Giemsa stain; (c) silver stain, microorganisms stain black

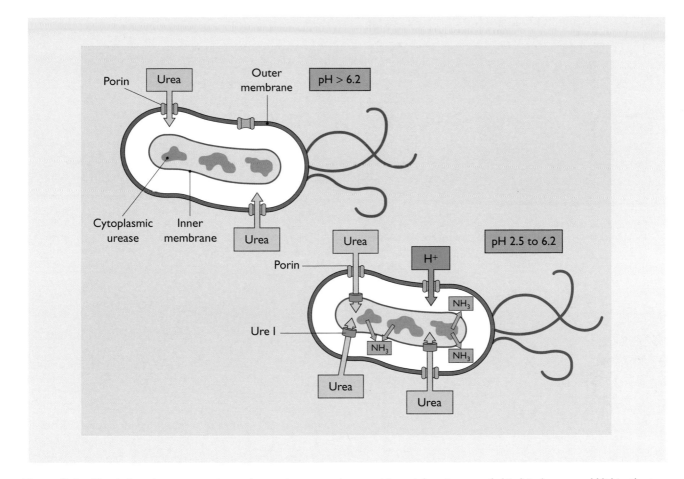

Figure 3.6 *H. pylori*: red outer membrane, brown inner membrane with periplasmic space (white) in between. Within the inner membrane is the cytoplasm, which contains cytoplasmic urease (orange). Left panel: the *H. pylori* in stomach at near neutral pH. Urea can enter via porins in the outer membrane, but does not have access to the cytoplasm, where urease is located. Right panel: when the pH drops below 6.2, H^+ ions enter via porins on the outer membrane. Ure I proton-gated urea channels (green pores on the inner membrane) are opened and urea transport is accelerated into the cytoplasm. This provides for abundant substrate for the cytoplasmic urease, which is then activated. The activity of cytoplasmic urease results in NH_3 generation and diffusion (green arrows) into the periplasmic space. The periplasmic pH is thus maintained at physiological levels. A cloud of ammonia is also generated at the surface of the organism

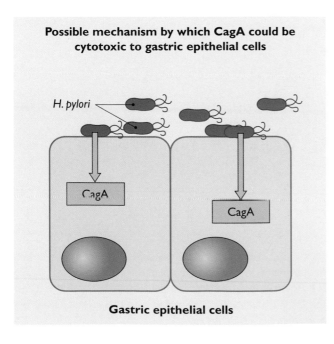

Figure 3.7 CagA-positive *H. pylori* in tissue culture with gastric epithelial cells. *H. pylori* adhere to the surface and translocate the CagA protein into cells in culture. The CagA protein is then tyrosine phosphorylated within the gastric epithelial cells

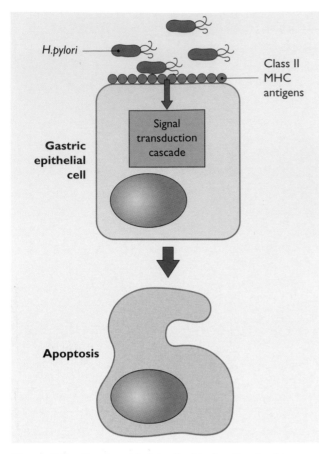

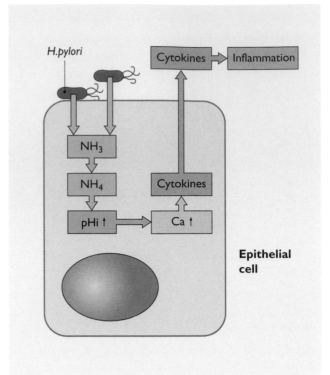

Figure 3.8 Gastric epithelial cell with class II major histocompatibility complex (MHC) antigen on surface. When *H. pylori* attaches to the class II MHC complex it initiates a signal transduction cascade using the Fas ligand/antigen pathway leading to apoptosis

Figure 3.9 NH_3 generated by cytoplasmic urease from *H. pylori* on the surface of epithelial cells diffuses out of the organism and into the cell. Inside the cell it becomes protonated to NH_4 and thus trapped within the cell. The intracellular pH (pHi) rises, resulting in an increase in intracellular calcium. This could give rise to the generation and secretion of cytokines such as interleukin 8 and others, and to the initiation of inflammation

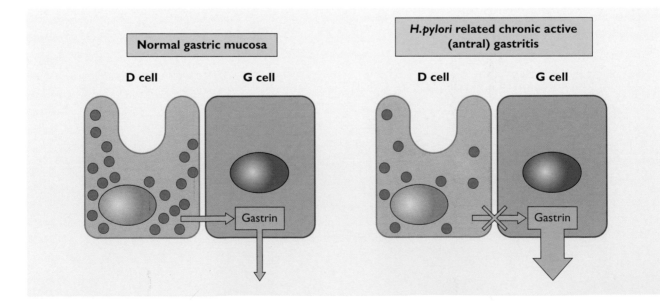

Figure 3.10 Left panel: In normal antral mucosa, the paracrine release of somatostatin from the D cell inhibits the endocrine release of gastrin from the adjacent G cell. Gastrin release is thus regulated by somatostatin. Right panel: As a consequence of *H. pylori* infection and the resulting chronic active gastritis, somatostatin release from antral D cells is inhibited. Thus, more gastrin is released from the G cell. Experimental data suggest that the defect in the D cell is at the transcriptional level

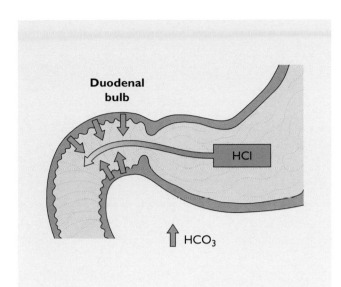

Figure 3.11   Neutralization of HCl reaching the duodenal bulb from the stomach by HCO_3 secreted by the surface epithelial cells of the duodenum

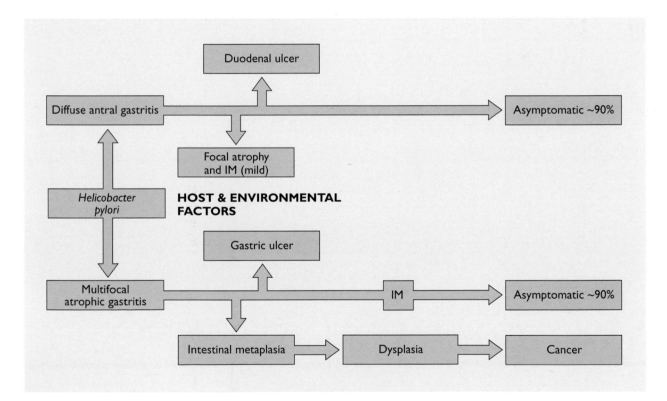

Figure 3.12   The spectrum of *H. pylori* related gastritis. IM, intestinal metaplasia

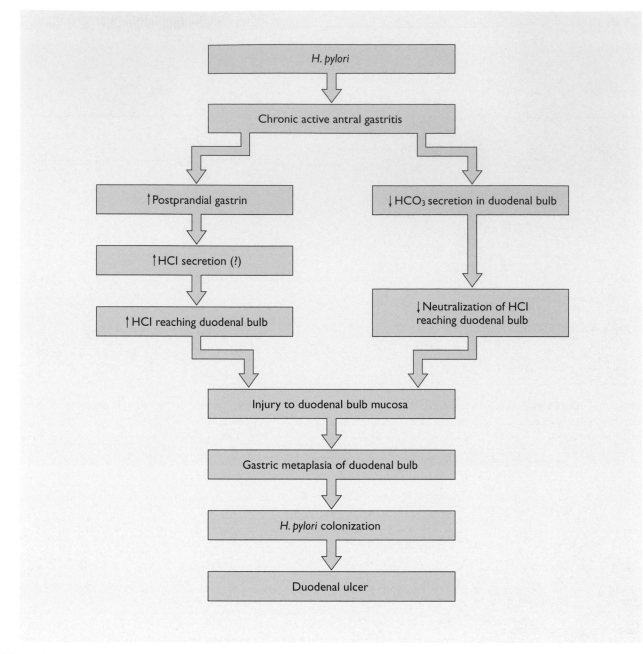

Figure 3.13 Development of a duodenal ulcer

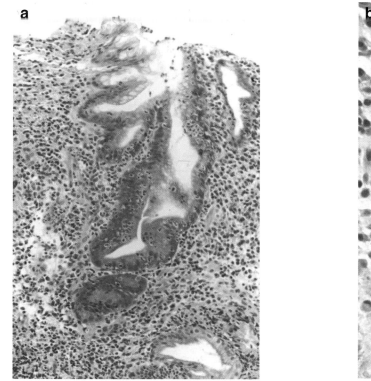

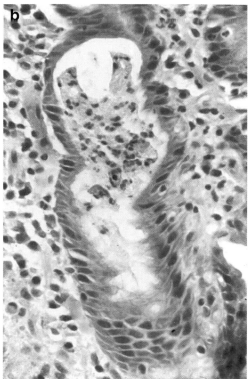

Figure 3.14 Chronic active (superficial) gastritis of the antrum, the typical lesion of *H. pylori*. Note the marked infiltration of the lamina propria with lymphocytes and plasma cells and also polymorphonuclear leukocytes. 'Active' is an old term used by pathologies to imply the presence of polymorphonuclear leukocytes. This lesion is superficial and there is no mucosal atrophy. (a) Lower power view; (b) higher power view, showing infiltration of a single antral gland

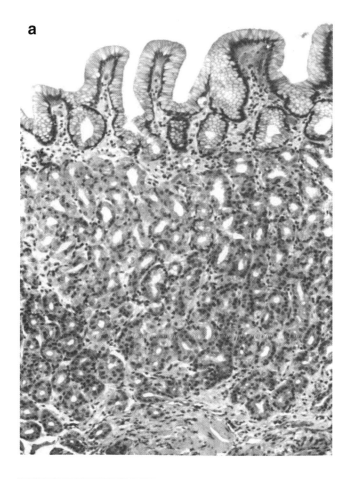

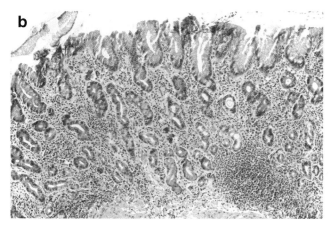

Figure 3.15 (a) Normal gastric mucosa from the body (corpus) of the stomach. Note the presence of the specialized long glands containing the parietal and chief cells. (b) Atrophic gastritis of the body of the stomach. Note the replacement of the specialized corpus glands by mucous cells

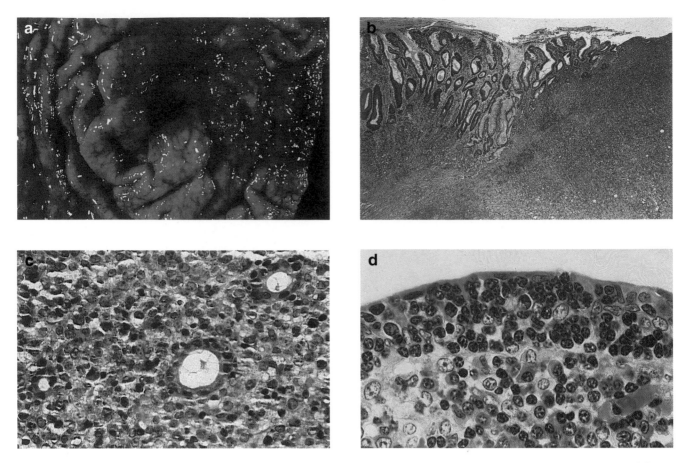

Figure 3.16 MALT lymphoma of stomach. (a) Mucosa of the greater curvature of the stomach in resected specimen, exhibiting cerebreform mucosal folds, marked vascular congestion and a central depression resulting from local ulceration. (b) Low-power photomicrograph demonstrating replacement of mucosa and submucosa by a dense cellular infiltrate; the residual gastric mucosa exhibits chronic atrophic gastritis. (Hematoxylin and eosin, 20 ×) (c) High-power photomicrograph of mucosa, showing separation of gastric glands by a dense lymphomatous infiltrate; some lymphocytes are present in the epithelial layer of the glands (hematoxylin and eosin, 400 ×). (d) High-power photomicrograph of mucosal surface, showing 'lymphoepithelial lesion' of lymphocytes heavily populating the surface epithelial layer (H & E, 1000 ×)

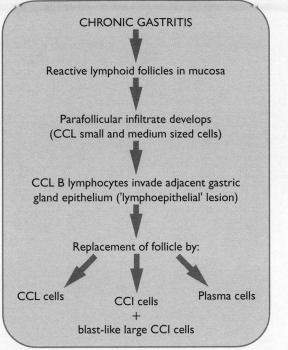

CCL, centrocyte-like. Plasma cells are differentiated from CCL cells

Figure 3.17   Development of low-grade MALT lymphoma

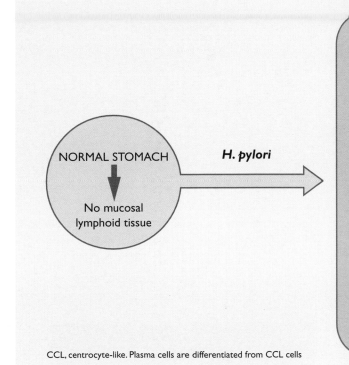

Figure 3.18   The stomach and duodenum, showing sites at which peptic ulcers commonly occur

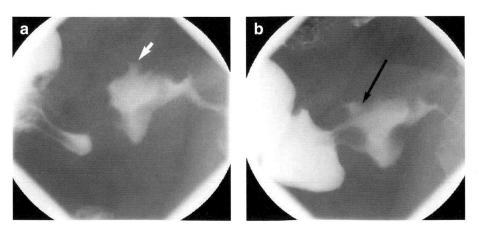

Figure 3.19   Duodenal ulcer. Abdominal pain persisted while patient was using H₂ blockers. Duodenal bulb shows ulcer crater (arrowed) in profile (a) and *en face* (b) with zone of edema around crater

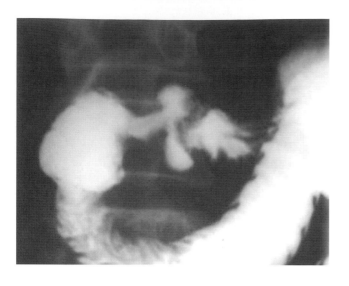

Figure 3.20 A 2-cm duodenal ulcer with cloverleaf deformity (73-year-old died of other cause, confirmed at autopsy)

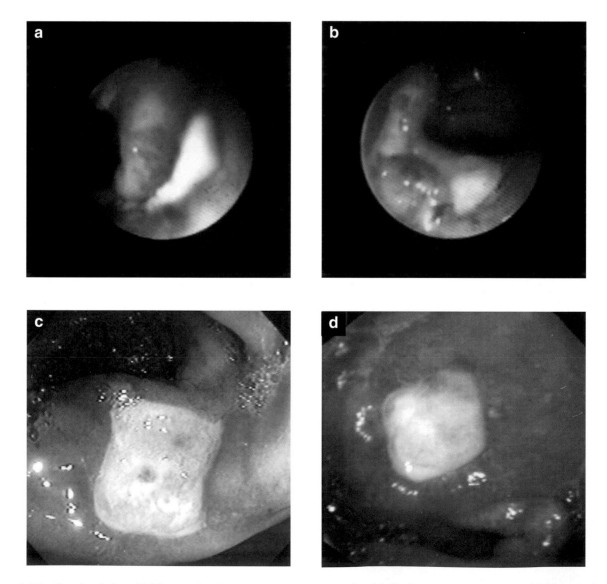

Figure 3.21 Duodenal ulcer. (a) Ulcer in the duodenal bulb; (b) two duodenal bulb ulcers on opposite walls; (c) Ulcer in duodenal bulb; (d) Ulcer in duodenal bulb

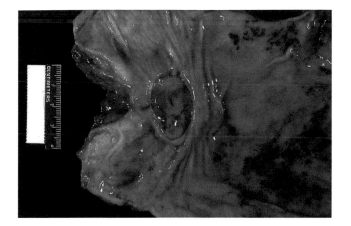

Figure 3.22 Duodenal ulcer. Healed peptic ulcer in the antral channel, leaving a residual crater; the mucosa of the adjacent stomach body exhibits moderate acute hemorrhagic gastritis

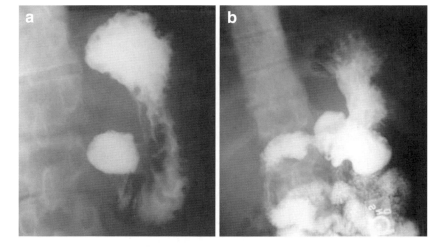

Figure 3.23 A 34-year-old male with a 2-week history of abdominal pain and vomiting with occasional hematemesis. He regularly used alcohol. Stool examination was Guiac-positive. A large penetrating gastric ulcer is shown on the lesser curve of the stomach (confirmed on endoscopy), in this upper gastrointestinal series

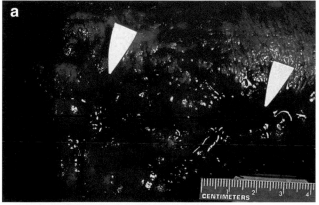

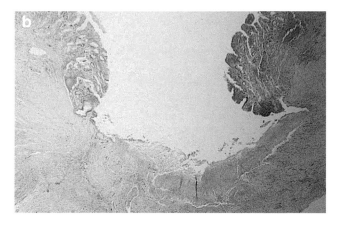

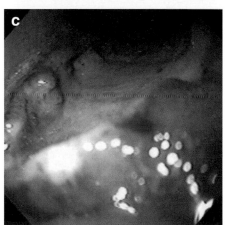

Figure 3.24 Gastric ulcer. (a) Acute peptic ulceration, with two hemorrhagic ulcers necessitating a partial gastric resection. (b) Low power photomicrograph showing reactive gastric mucosa at the edges, and a central crater at the depth of the muscularis propria. (Hematoxylin and eosin, 20 ×). (c) Large antral ulcer

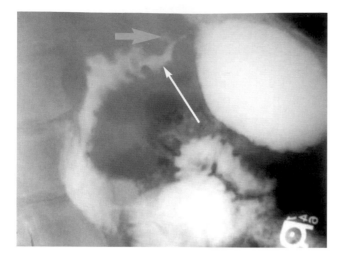

Figure 3.25 Zollinger–Ellison syndrome. A young male had H$_2$ blocker treatment after complaining of epigastric pain, with little relief of symptoms. This radiograph, performed during an upper gastrointestinal series to evaluate melena, showed a pyloric channel ulcer (not shown), duodenal ulcer (green arrow) and post-bulbar deformity (white arrow)

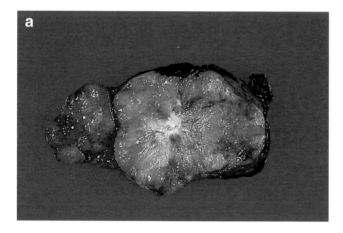

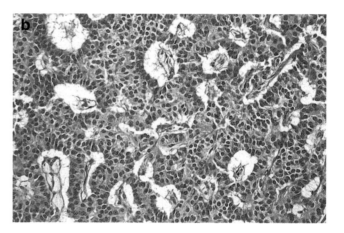

Figure 3.26 Gastrinoma. (a) Pancreatic islet cell tumor, 3.5 cm maximum dimension, in a patient with Zollinger–Ellison syndrome. (b) Photomicrograph demonstrating characteristic pattern of uniform tumor cells with palisading around vascular stromal stalks ('insular' pattern). (Hematoxylin and eosin, 400 ×)

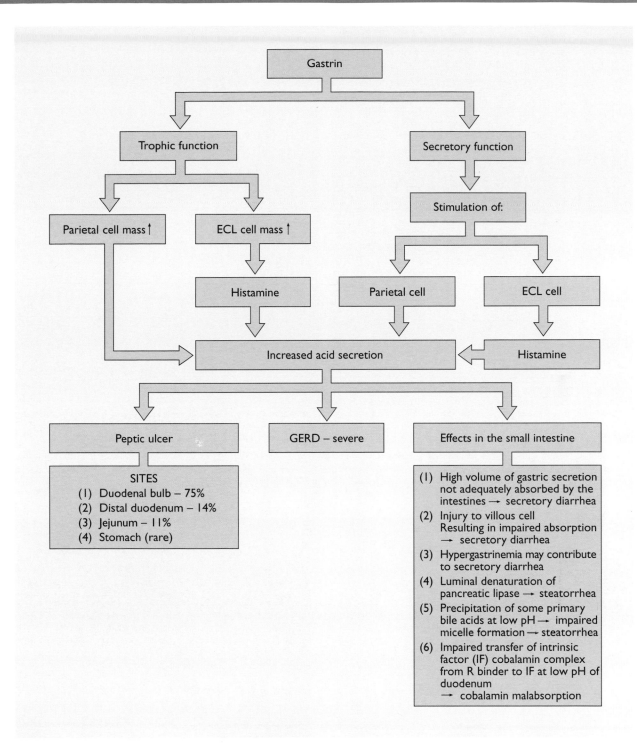

Figure 3.27 Zollinger–Ellison syndrome – pathophysiology

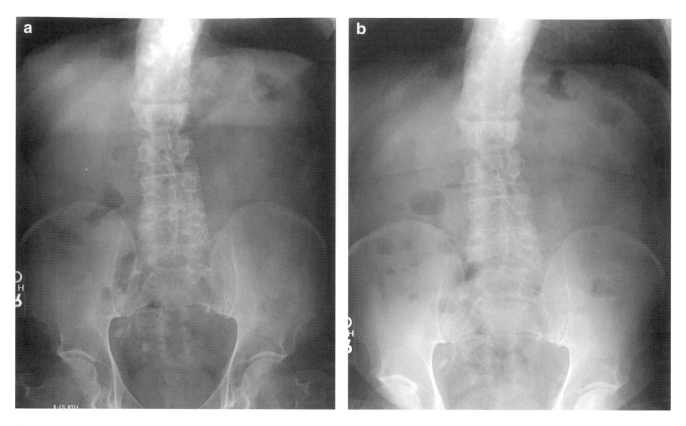

Figure 3.28 A 70-year-old man presented to the primary care urgent visit clinic with several hours of acute epigastric pain and symptoms of reflux. He also complained of increasing lower abdominal pain and constipation. He denied fever, chills, nausea or vomiting. He received two Fleet enemas in the clinic with little result. Plain radiographs of the abdomen were unremarkable. Supine (a) and upright (b) radiographs show no evidence of free air. A few air–fluid levels are present in non-distended small bowel (see Figure 3.29)

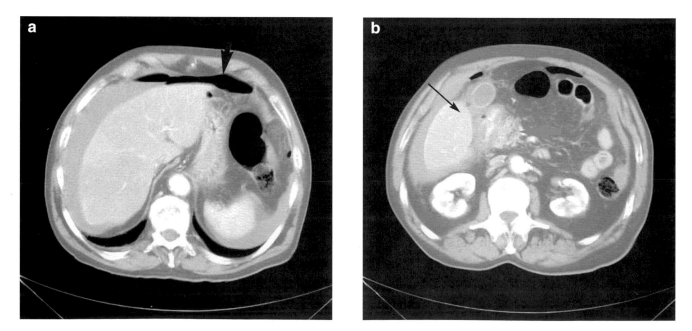

Figure 3.29 Duodenal perforation. The patient (as described in Figure 3.28) was referred for an emergency computerized tomography (CT) scan of the abdomen, which was performed after administration of intravenous and oral contrast. (a) CT scan of the upper abdomen shows free air (arrowed) and ascites around the liver. (b) Scan through the second part of the duodenum shows duodenal wall thickening. A small amount of air is seen just lateral to the duodenum (black arrow). Fluid tracks into Morison's pouch. The pancreatic head is indicated (green arrow). These findings were interpreted as an upper gastrointestinal tract perforation, most likely of duodenal origin, given the distribution of free air adjacent to the duodenum and upper abdomen and the duodenal thickening and paraduodenal fluid. The patient developed peritoneal signs with percussion tenderness and rigidity. He was taken for emergency surgery, where a perforated duodenal ulcer was repaired

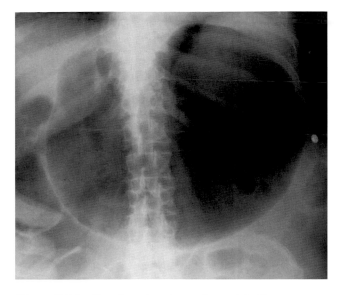

Figure 3.30 Gastric outlet obstruction - plain X-ray

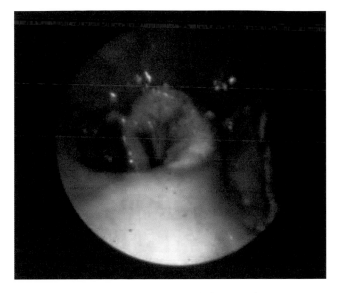

Figure 3.31 Large pyloric channel ulcer resulting in gastric outlet obstruction. 'Channel ulcers' tend to behave more like duodenal ulcers, with higher amounts of acid secretion, than like typical more proximal antral ulcers

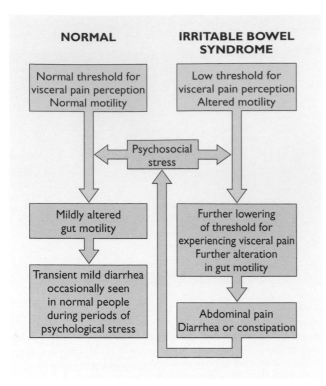

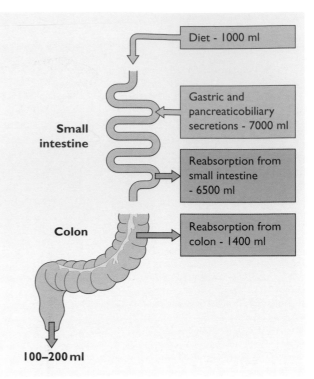

Figure 4.1 Working hypothesis for the pathogenesis of irritable bowel syndrome

Figure 4.2 Colonic salvage of fluid

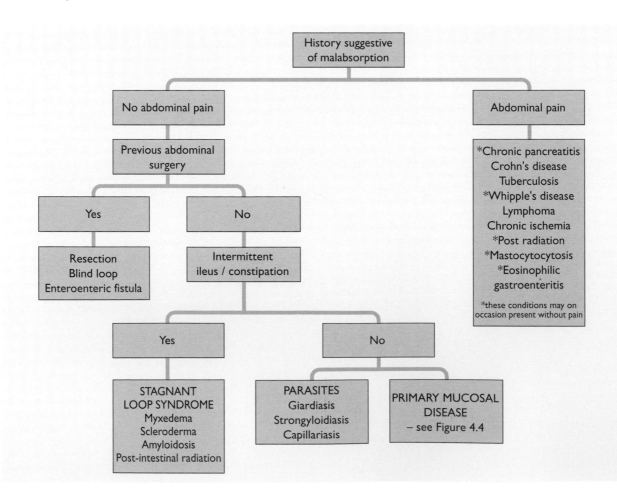

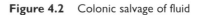

Figure 4.3 An approach to the elucidation of the etiology of intestinal malabsorption

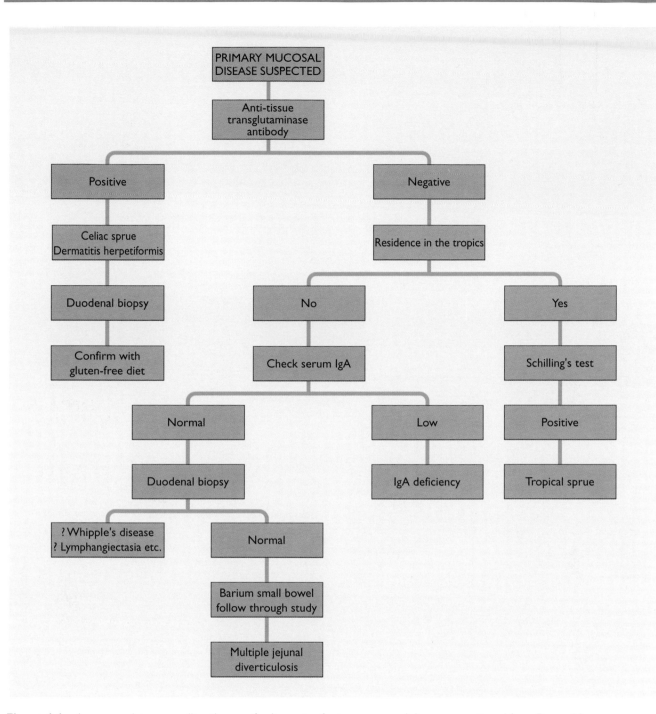

Figure 4.4 An approach to unravelling the specific diagnosis of primary mucosal disease – continued from Figure 4.3

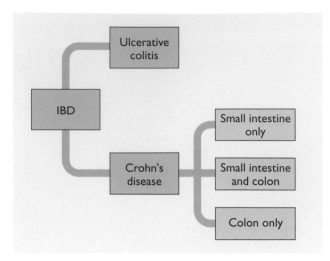

Figure 4.5   The spectrum of inflammatory bowel disease (IBD). Note: rarely, Crohn's disease may involve the esophagus and stomach

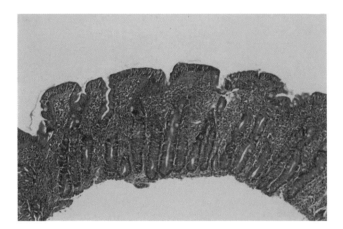

Figure 4.6   Celiac sprue. Normally the small intestinal mucosa should exhibit tall narrow villi and short crypts. In this specimen, the villiform architecture is essentially gone, with subtotal villous blunting, expansion of the lumina propria by a dense lymphoplas-macytic inflammatory infiltrate, and expansion of the crypt zone as the result of regenerative activity. (Hematoxylin & eosin stain, 40 ×). Figure courtesy of Dr Melissa Li, University of Florida

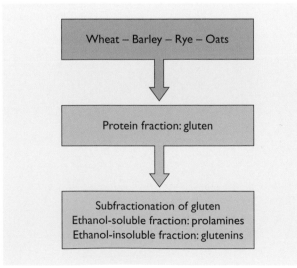

Figure 4.7   The protein fractions of cereals

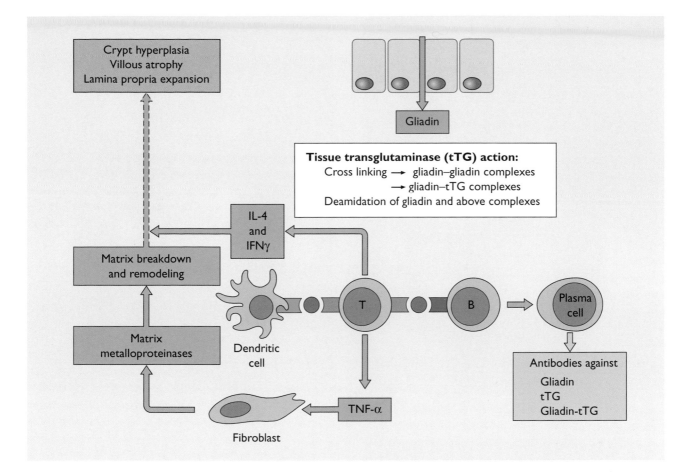

Figure 4.8 A tiny amount of gliadin enters between surface epithelial cells of the mucosa. In the lamina propria gliadin is acted on by tissue tranglutaminase (tTG), forming deamidated gliadin, and a variety of complexes between proteins rich in glutamine. The deamidated gliadin or the complexes (●) are captured, processed and presented on the surfaces of antigen-presenting cells (dendritic cells) along with class II MHC molecules, in most cases HLA-DQ2 (▨), to the surface receptors (▨) on both CD4 Th1 and Th2 cells (marked T). Cytokines generated from these T cell subtypes are believed to contribute to the lesion in celiac sprue. A mechanism for the generation of antibodies to gliadin and tTG is also illustrated in the Figure. B cell is marked B. TNF, tumor necrosis factor; IL, interleukin; IFN, interferon

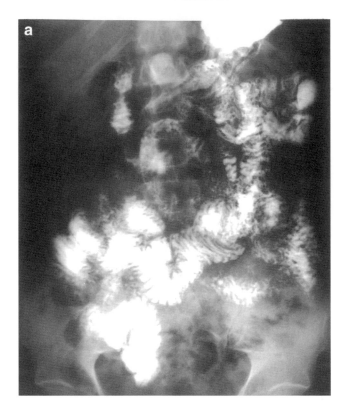

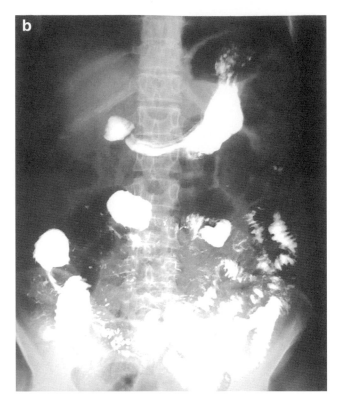

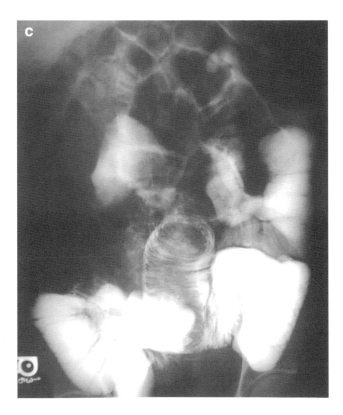

Figure 4.9 (a) Non-tropical (celiac) sprue is radiographically demonstrated as small intestinal dilatation, and evidence of hypersecretion. In this example, a 58-year-old man with a 2-month history of diarrhea and 10lb (4.5 kg) weight loss had a small bowel study showing dilatation of the small bowel, with normal thickness folds. Hypoproteinemia is often associated with fold thickening. The duodenal folds are somewhat thickened. Transit time is often somewhat increased (in the 3–5-h range), but occasionally can be reduced or markedly increased. (b) A 48-year-old woman presented with tetany due to hypocalcemia, steatorrhea and osteopenia. Radiograph from a barium study shows flocculation of barium within the small bowel, with segmentation due to pooling of barium in regions containing extensive secretions. The areas of narrower bowel opacified with barium are described as a 'moulage' or cast-like pattern. (c) Intussusception can occur in sprue. It is usually transient, and usually does not cause obstruction. The intussuscepted portion of bowel is seen in the mid-abdomen with a typical 'coiled spring' appearance

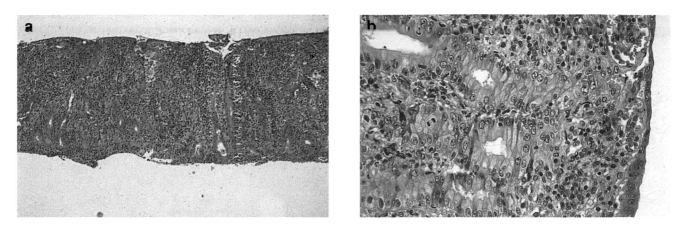

Figure 4.10 Tropical sprue. (a) Low-power photomicrograph of small intestinal mucosa, demonstrating complete absence of villi. The mucosal thickness is normal, however, owing to marked expansion of the crypt proliferative zone. (Hematoxylin and eosin, 100 ×). (b) Higher-power photomicrograph of superficial mucosa, showing attenuated superficial epithelium and dense mononuclear inflammatory infiltrate of the lamina propria. Intraepithelial lymphocytes and surface enterocyte vacuolization are not as evident in this specimen; otherwise the features are similar to those of celiac sprue. (Hematoxylin and eosin, 1000 ×)

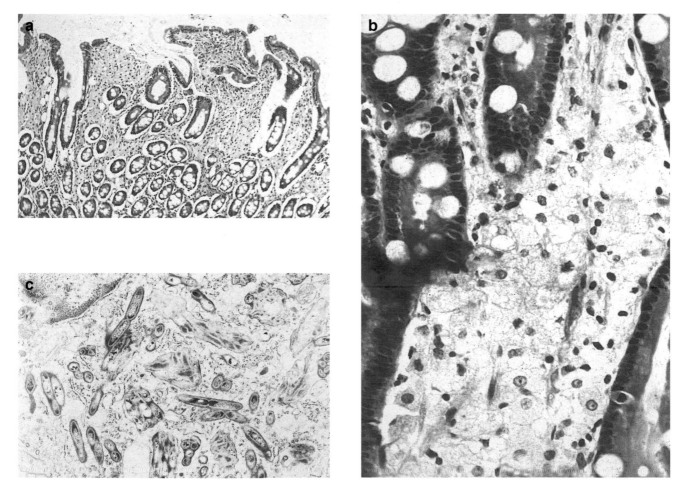

Figure 4.11 Whipple's disease (a) Low-power photomicrograph of small intestinal mucosa, demonstrating blunting of villi and expansion of the lamina propria by an inflammatory infiltrate. (Hematoxylin and eosin, 100 ×). (b) Higher-power photomicrograph demonstrating that the lamina propria is filled with foamy macrophages. (H & E, 400 ×). (c) Electron micrograph demonstrating intact and fragmented bacilli within lamina propria macrophages (5000 ×). Figure courtesy of Dr Jerry Trier, Brigham and Women's Hospital, Boston, MA

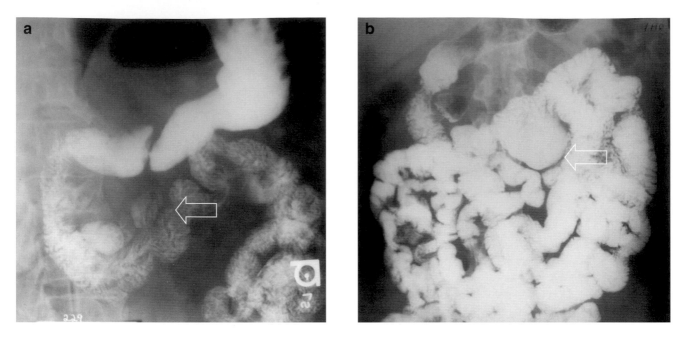

Figure 4.12 Multiple jejunal diverticula may also host bacterial flora. This 42-year-old man presented with diarrhea and was found to have multiple jejunal diverticula. Figure courtesy of Dr M. Burrell, MD, Yale University School of Medicine, CT

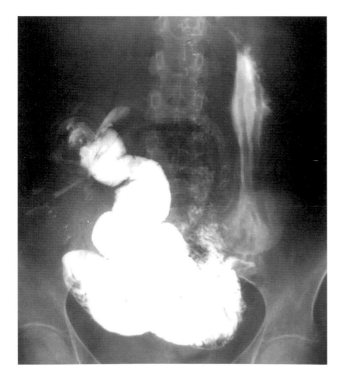

Figure 4.13 A patient with long-standing Crohn's disease and multiple surgical procedures has only 35 cm of bowel remaining. A barium gastrointestinal study demonstrates barium within somewhat dilated but non-obstructed small bowel proximal to the ileocolic anastomosis in the right upper quadrant

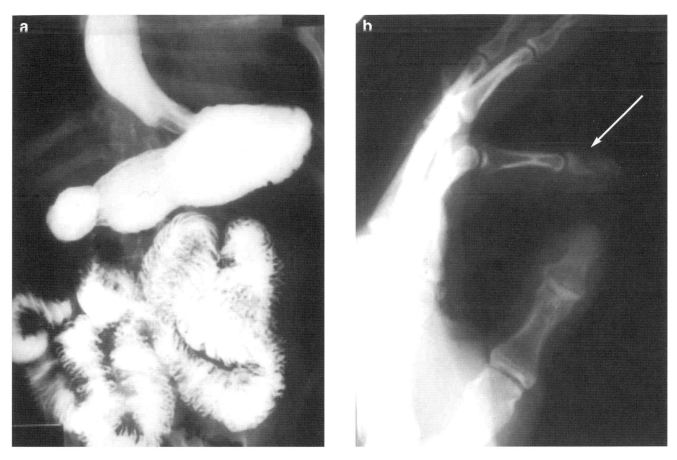

Figure 4.14 (a) Scleroderma is a systemic disease that may be associated with malabsorption, as in this young woman with weight loss and Reynaud's phenomenon. Note free reflux of barium into a patulous, immotile esophagus, and a dilated small bowel with generalized hypomotility and slightly thickened valvuli conniventes and 'concertina' folds. Other radiological manifestations (b): note acro-osteolysis (arrowed) affecting the terminal phalanx of the index finger

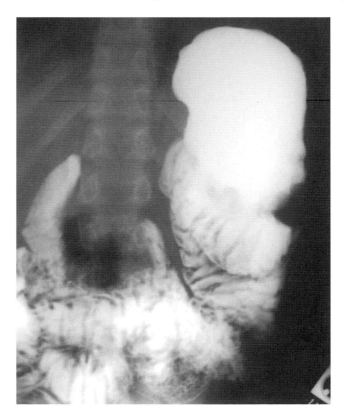

Figure 4.15 Occasionally bacterial overgrowth can create malabsorption, as in this case of an unfortunate 15-year-old male who had undergone a Bilroth II procedure for duodenal ulcer disease prior to an understanding of the pathogenetic role of *Helicobacter pylori*. He developed bacterial overgrowth in the 'blind loop', causing growth retardation. He improved after the anastomoses were revised to a Billroth I configuration

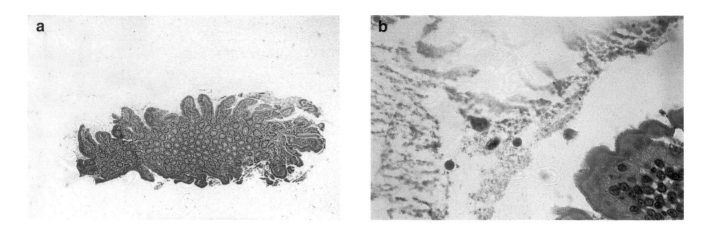

Figure 4.16 Giardiasis. (a) Small-bowel biopsy, demonstrating only minimal blunting of villi; adherent mucus is present (hematoxylin and eosin, 100 ×). (b) High-power photomicrograph of superficial mucus, showing a tear-drop-shaped *Giardia* organism *en face*, with its two nuclei evident. (Hematoxylin and eosin, 1000 ×)

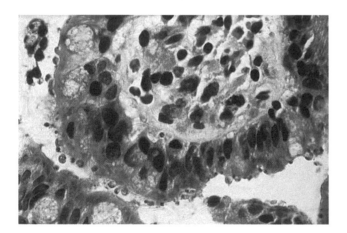

Figure 4.17 Cryptosporidia. Superficial small intestinal mucosa, showing damaged enterocytes with loss of microvillus brush border, and abundant cryptosporidia organisms adherent to the apical surfaces of enterocytes. (Hematoxylin and eosin, 1000 ×)

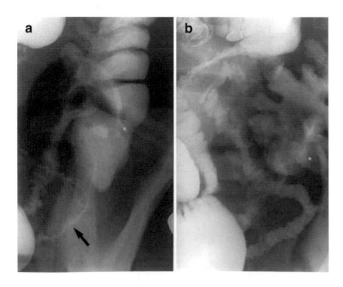

Figure 4.18 (a) Spot film obtained during a small-bowel follow-through shows barium in the terminal ileum, ileocecal valve and cecum. There is narrowing of the terminal ileum and loss of normal mucosal contours. Overlying the terminal ileum is a second loop of markedly narrowed and strictured small bowel (arrowed) – the 'string sign' described in Crohn's disease which correlates with strictures in rigid, fibrotic loops of ileum. (b) Spot film of terminal ileum and right lower quadrant shows better filling of the distal small bowel loop, but it is still stenotic with loss of normal folds and shows an irregular nodular contour. The patient is in a prone position

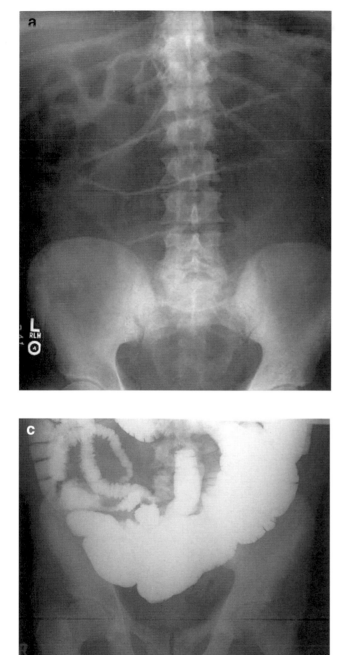

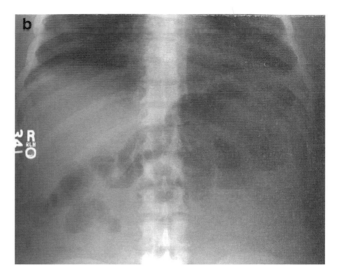

Figure 4.19 The same patient as in Figure 4.18 presented with nausea, abdominal pain and distension. A supine abdominal radiograph (a) demonstrates multiple loops of dilated small bowel, and minimal air within transverse colon, suggesting a partial small bowel obstruction. Upright film (b) shows multiple air–fluid levels in dilated small bowel. (c) Small-bowel follow-through series showing partial obstruction of small bowel due to strictures within distal small bowel loops and terminal ileum

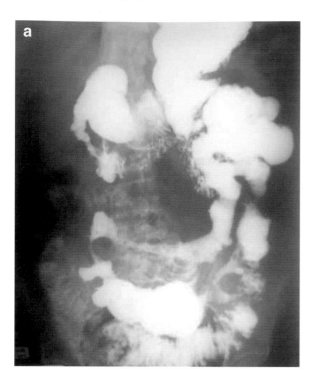

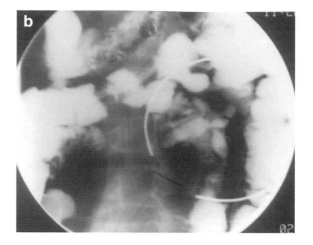

Figure 4.20 A 35-year-old woman with a history of diarrhea. (a) An upper gastrointestinal series with small-bowel follow-through shows involvement of the duodenum, which is narrowed, with loss of a normal mucosal pattern. Multiple segments of stricture formation are present in the jejunum, with focal dilatation and loss of normal mucosal detail. (b) Ulceration and fistula formation

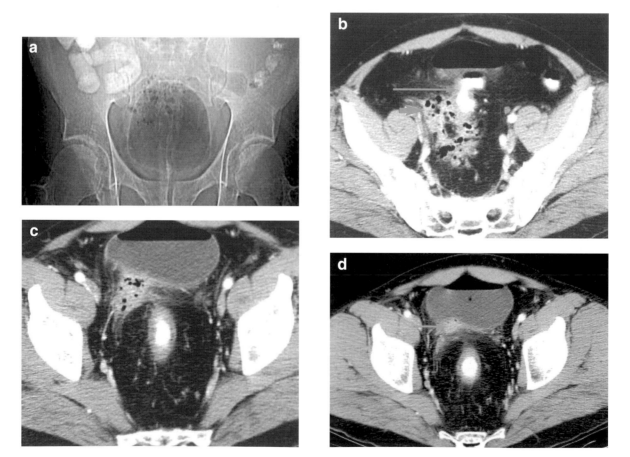

Figure 4.21 A 36-year-old with history of Crohn's colitis treated with 6-mercaptopurine and steroids presented with fever and urinary frequency with pneumaturia. (a) Digital scout radiograph from CT scan shows air within the bladder and abnormal mottled lucencies superimposed, suspicious for abscess. (b) Scan though the pelvis of the same patient following administration of intravenous and oral contrast shows mottled air collection (short arrow) adjacent to and to the right of the sigmoid colon (long arrow), with air–fluid level in the bladder. (c) CT scan at a lower level in the pelvis shows that the mottled region of air is adjacent to the posterior right wall of the bladder. Note the thickening of the rectosigmoid colon. (d) Colovesical fistula extends toward the bladder base. Note enhancement adjacent to air collection extending into posterior right bladder wall (arrowed)

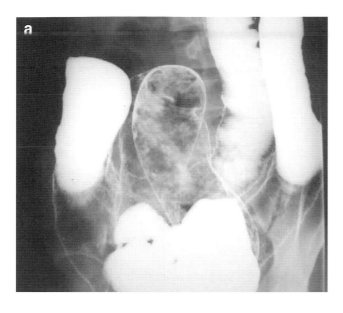

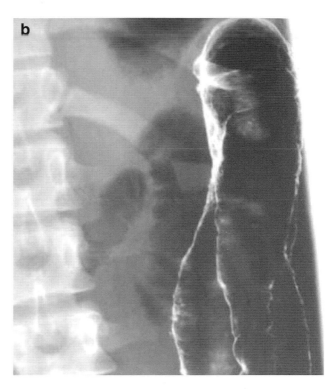

Figure 4.22 An 18-year-old woman with active ulcerative colitis (a) Barium enema showing ulceration in the sigmoid colon; (b) spot film showing ulceration at the splenic flexure

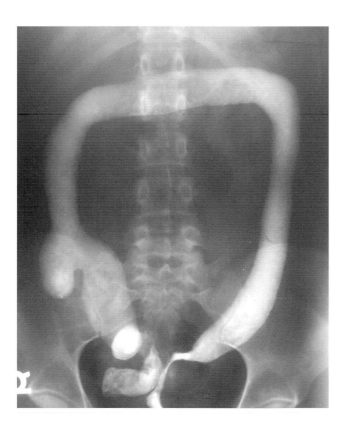

Figure 4.23 The terminal ileum is abnormal in up to 20% of cases of ulcerative colitis, with a phenomenon described as 'backwash ileitis' where the valve is open and incompetent, the terminal ileum is dilated, occasionally with granularity (but not ulceration). Malignant transformation is the most serious complication

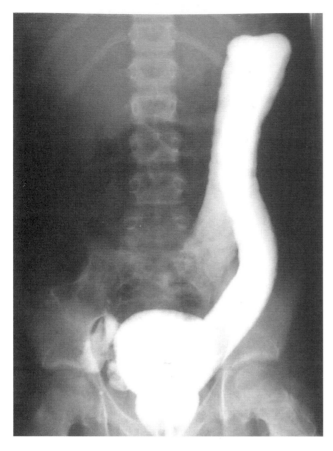

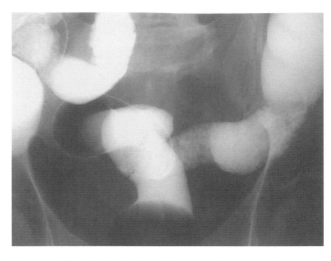

Figure 4.25 Crohn's colitis. Disease is limited to the sigmoid colon. The nodularity correlated grossly with nodularity seen on endoscopy

Figure 4.24 Advanced disease is associated with fibrosis, shortening of the colon and stricture formation. The haustral markings are lost, as in this case of an 11-year-old girl with chronic ulcerative colitis. Figure courtesy of Dr M. Burrell, MD, Yale University School of Medicine, CT

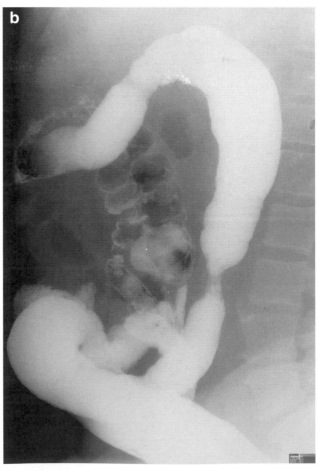

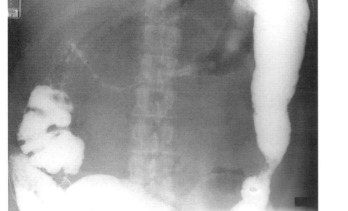

Figure 4.26 (a) Colonic stricture (descending colon) secondary to long-standing Crohn's disease. (b) Benign strcture in Crohn's disease. Lateral view of colon during barium enema shows the stricture in the descending colon, with smooth margins

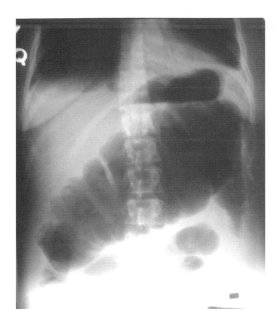

Figure 4.27 Complications in ulcerative colitis. A young female with a several-year history of ulcerative colitis presented with abdominal pain, distension and fever. Radiographs of the abdomen showed marked dilatation of the colon consistent with the clinical suspicion of toxic megacolon

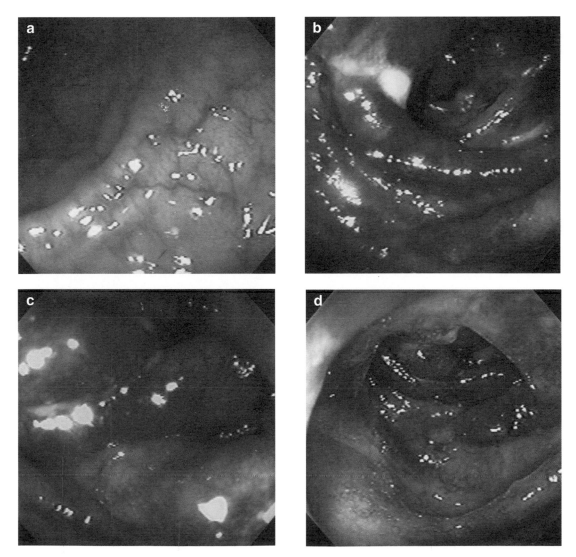

Figure 4.28 Crohn's colitis. (a) Normal appearing mucosa of the rectum and recto-sigmoid area ('rectal sparing'). (b–d) Rest of the sigmoid and descending colon show very marked erythema, exudate and edema. Colon beyond the splenic flexure was also spared. This case demonstrates the rectal sparing and skip areas so characteristic of Crohn's colitis

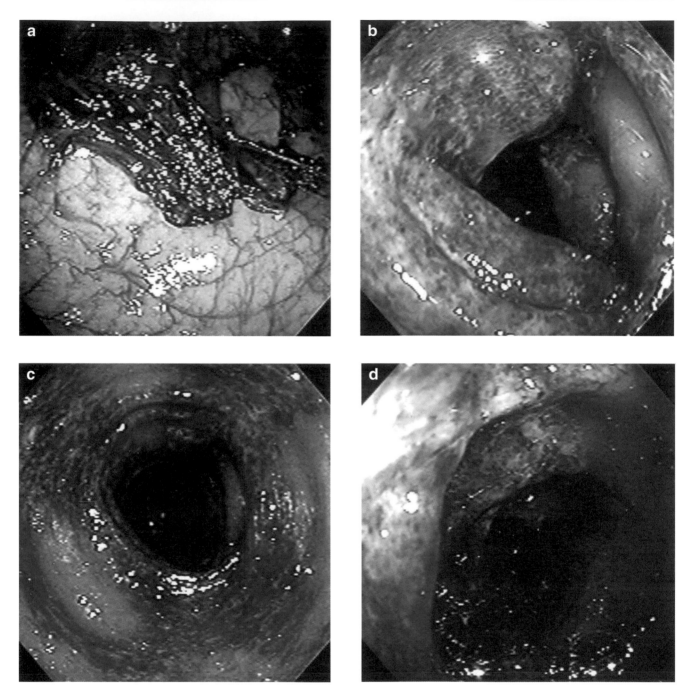

Figure 4.29 Crohn's colitis. (a) Normal appearing mucosa seen in the entire sigmoid colon and most of the descending colon of this patient. (b–d) The splenic flexure and the transverse colon were markedly involved with erythema, edema tiny ulcerations and exudate

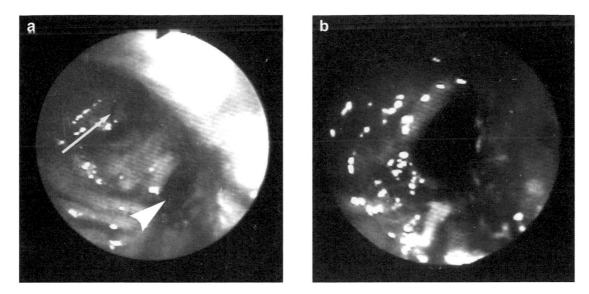

Figure 4.30 (a) Patient with Crohn's colitis. Within the lumen of the colon two openings were seen. The one marked by the yellow arrow represents the true colonic lumen, whereas the white arrowhead depicts the opening of an enterocolic fistula. (b) Close-up view of the mouth of the fistula

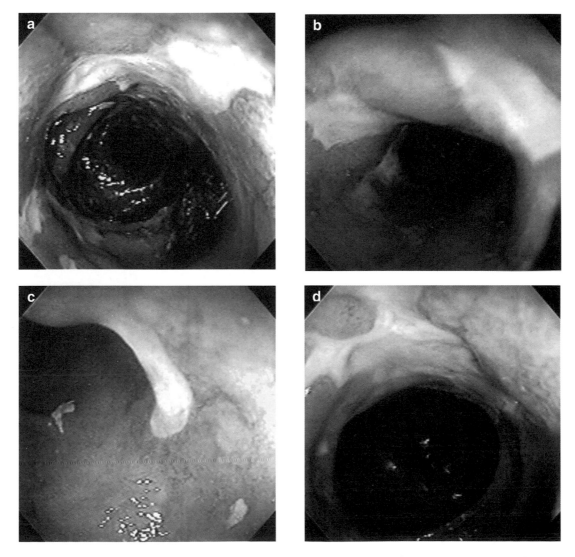

Figure 4.31 Terminal ileum visualized at colonoscopy in a patient with Crohn's disease. Several ileal ulcers, some fairly deep, are seen with distinct margins and necrotic bases

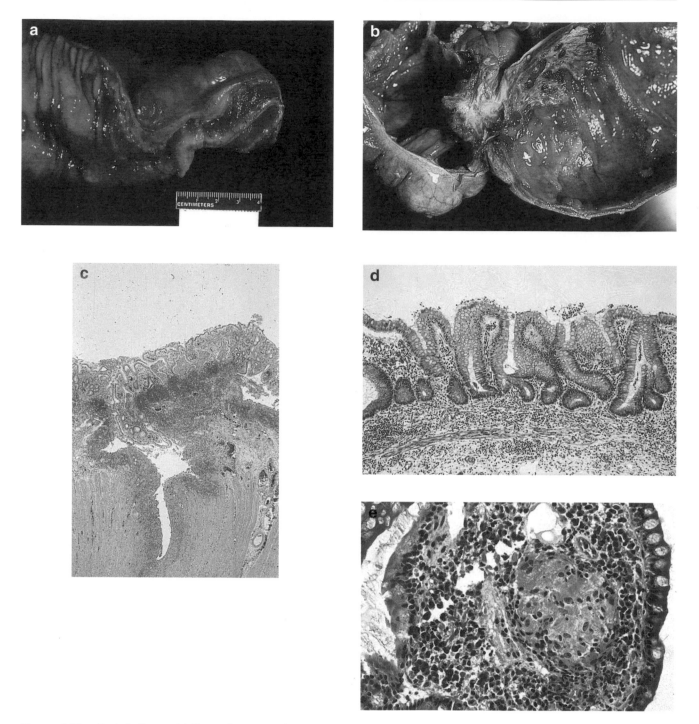

Figure 4.32 Crohn's disease. (a) Opened portion of ileum, demonstrating an extensive stricture ('string sign' by radiographic barium examination) with a longitudinal ulcer also extending into the more preserved portion of the small intestinal segment. (b) Sigmoid colon, opened after formalin fixation, demonstrating focal stricture, dilatation of adjacent colonic segments and additional ulceration of colonic mucosa in dilated colonic segment. (c) Low-power photomicrograph of colonic Crohn's disease, showing superficial mucosa with sub-mucosal lymphoid aggregates (blue-stained), and a deep fissure into the muscularis propria. (Hematoxylin and eosin, 40 ×). (d) Colonic mucosa in patient with Crohn's disease, exhibiting chronic colitis with architectural distortion but no ulceration. (H & E, 200 ×). (e) Ileal mucosa in patient with Crohn's disease, showing non-caseating granuloma in lamina propria. (H & E, 1000 ×)

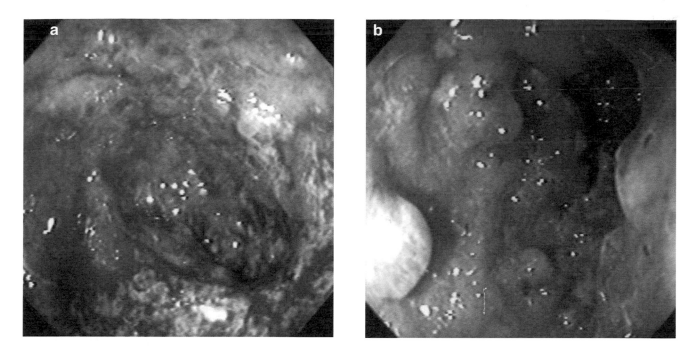

Figure 4.33 Colon in ulcerative colitis. (a) Mucosa uniformly erythematous with exudate and shallow ulcerations. (b) Colon with pseudopolyps. Pseudopolyps may be seen in Crohn's colitis also

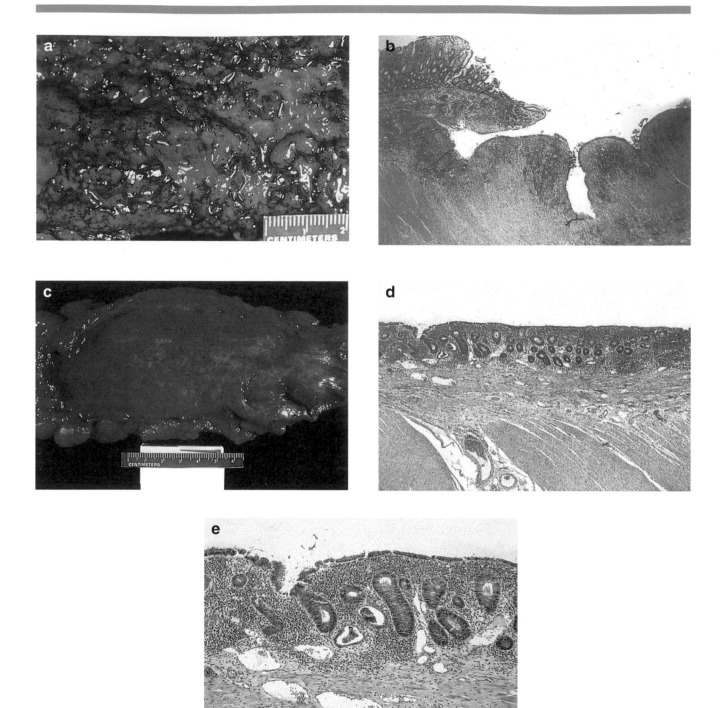

Figure 4.34 Ulcerative colitis. (a) Severe acute phase of ulcerative colitis, showing abundant pseudopolyps of residual inflamed mucosa, with extensive ulceration of remainder of mucosa. The pale pink areas of the image are exposed muscularis propria. The entire colon exhibited this severe degree of ulceration. (b) Low-power photomicrograph from the same case as (a), showing that, in the most severe cases of ulcerative colitis, the ulcer bed can rest on the muscularis propria, with focal compromise to the integrity of even the muscularis propria, thereby raising the risk of perforation. Residual inflamed but preserved mucosa is present at the edge of the photomicrograph. (Hematoxylin and eosin, 40 ×). (c) Atrophic stage of ulcerative colitis. All mucosal features have been obliterated by the atrophy of the mucosa. (d) Low-power photomicrograph of (c), showing extensive atrophy of colonic mucosal crypts, dense lamina propria inflammatory infiltrate, and absence of ulceration. (H & E, 100 ×). (e) Higher-power photomicrograph of (d), showing crypt abscesses (neutrophils within the crypt lumina) in center of image. Adjacent crypts exhibit hyperchromasia, attributable to regenerative changes of crypt epithelium (enlarged nuclei and mucin depletion), and there is extensive architectural distortion of crypts. (H & E, 200 ×)

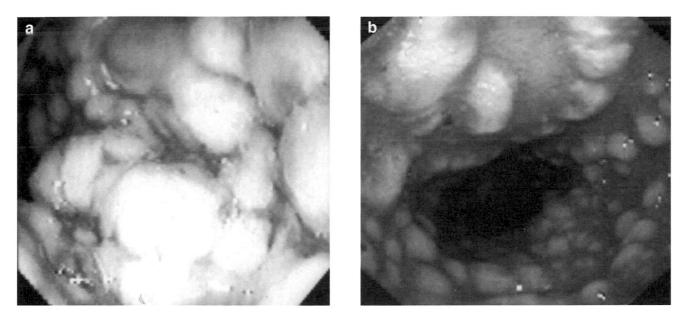

Figure 4.35 (a and b) Typical fluffy, firmly adherent pseudomembranes covering erythematous mucosa, almost obscuring it

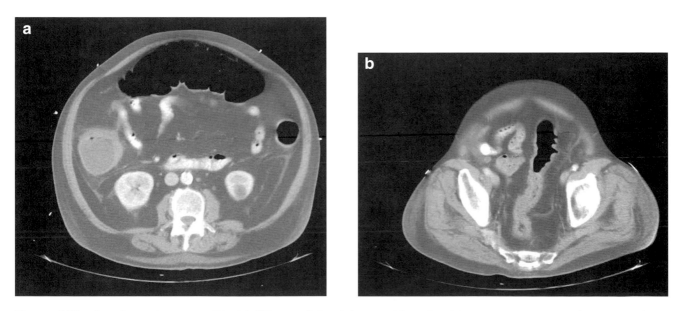

Figure 4.36 Pseudomembranous colitis. (a) CT scan of the abdomen with oral and intravenous contrast enhancement shows thickening of the ascending colon. (b) The sigmoid colon is also involved, showing transmural thickening and no pericolic inflammatory changes

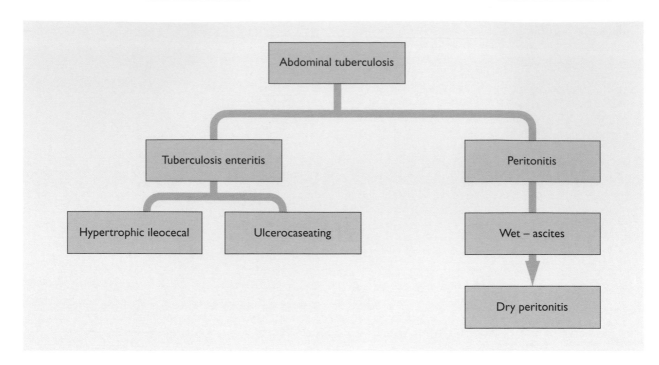

Figure 5.1   Classification of abdominal tuberculosis

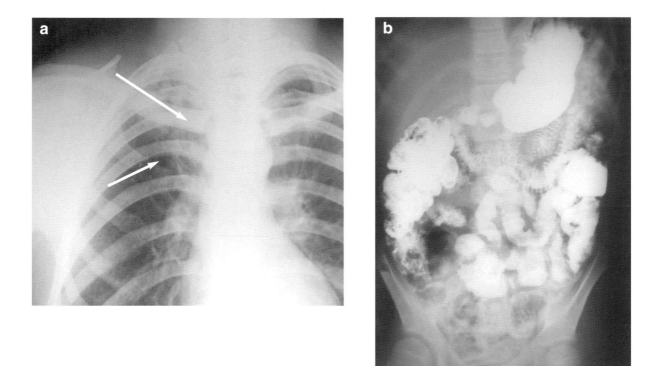

Figure 5.2   A 25-year-old male presented with cough, abdominal pain and weight loss. (a) The chest radiograph showed an ill-defined opacity in the right upper lobe, with no evidence of hilar adenopathy, calcifications, or pleural effusion. This close up view of right apex demonstrates the right upper lobe opacity (arrowed). (b) It is unusual to see primary tuberculosis targeting the GI tract in the general US population, although with the emergence of resistant strains this may again become more common. Infection can occur from ingestion of infected milk (now of course rare due to universal pasteurization) through ingestion of infected sputum, or from hematogenous dissemination of pulmonary infection. Barium study of the small intestine shows abnormal loops of ileum, with loss of normal mucosal pattern, with angulated loops and several focally dilated segments. This represents underlying fibrotic change and stricture formation. No active ulcers are seen. Although the terminal ileum was not involved in this case, such involvement may be difficult to differentiate radiographically from Crohn's disease.

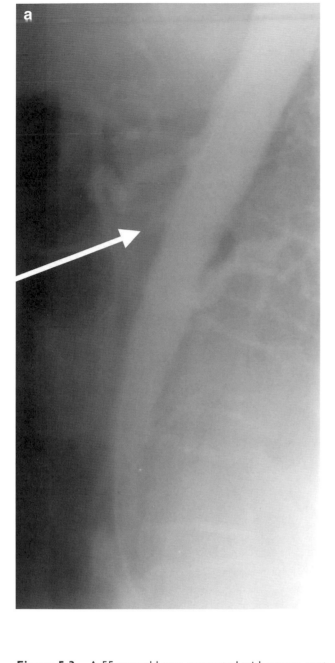

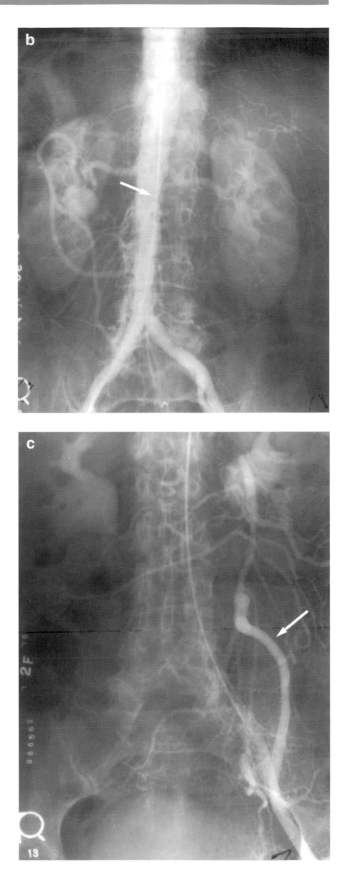

Figure 5.3 A 55-year-old man presented with severe post-prandial abdominal pain occurring 30 min after a meal, accompanied by significant weight loss over several months. An aortogram was performed because of a suspicion of intestinal angina. (a) A lateral aortogram reveals the origin of the celiac and superior mesenteric arteries, which are poorly opacified. Only the origin of the superior mesenteric artery is visualized (arrow). (b) Aortogram (frontal projection) shows a patent and enlarged inferior mesenteric artery which fills the middle colic artery in a retrograde fashion and reconstitutes the superior mesenteric artery near its origin. (c) The patient had an end-to-side saphenous vein graft (arrowed) placed from the left common iliac artery to the superior mesenteric artery, with resolution of his symptoms. Figure courtesy of Dr M. Glickman, MD, Yale University School of Medicine, CT

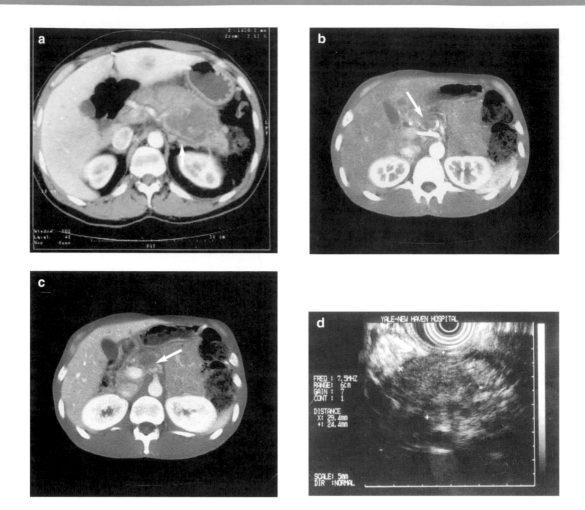

Figure 5.4 (a) A 45-year-old male presented with weight loss and mid-epigastric abdominal pain, and was referred for contrast enhanced CT of the abdomen because of concern for underlying malignancy. Scans through the body of the pancreas show a focal hypoattentuating mass within the tail, with evidence for encasement and narrowing of the splenic vein (white arrow). Several hypoattenuating lesions of the liver were also present (yellow arrow), consistent with metastatic disease. The patient underwent a biopsy of a liver mass that was positive only for inflammatory cells, and a biopsy of the tail of the pancreas subsequently showed anaplastic carcinoma. (b) A 48-year-old male presented with weight loss and abdominal pain. An abdominal CT scan was performed. An arterial phase CT through the pancreas showed a 1.4 × 2.6 cm hypodense mass. The remainder of the body and tail of the pancreas (not shown) was atrophic, with a dilated distal pancreatic duct. (c) Same patient as in (b), portal venous phase CT shows a low attenuation lesion within the body of the pancreas, and soft tissue infiltration posteriorly adjacent to the splenic vein. (d) Image obtained at endoscopic ultrasound evaluation shows a 2.9 × 2.4 cm hypoechoic mass with an irregular border, in the body of the pancreas, delineated by cursors. There was loss of tissue plane over a 9.7 mm segment between the mass and the splenic vein, suggestive of invasion. Adjacent lymph nodes adjacent to the duodenal wall and within the celiac axis were present (not shown). A biopsy of the lesion was performed at the time of the EUS

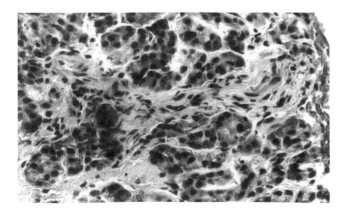

Figure 5.5 Biopsy specimen from tail of pancreas (high magnification), from patient in Figure 5.4a, shows in addition to necrosis, pleomorphic tumor cells, some tumor giant cells and inflammation at the periphery of the specimen consistent with an anaplastic carcinoma of the pancreas

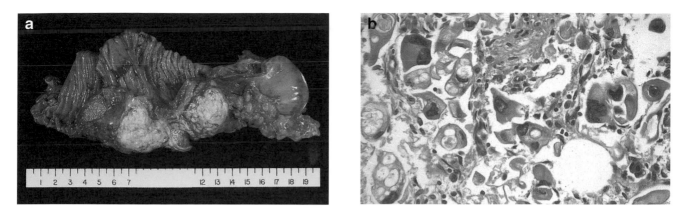

Figure 5.6 Pancreatic cancer. (a) Pancreatoduodenectomy (Whipple) specimen, with pancreas bisected to demonstrate 3-cm solid tumor mass of pancreas (Figure courtesy of Dr Melissa Li, University of Florida). (b) High-power photomicrograph demonstrating poorly differentiated mucin-containing malignant cells within the pancreatic stroma

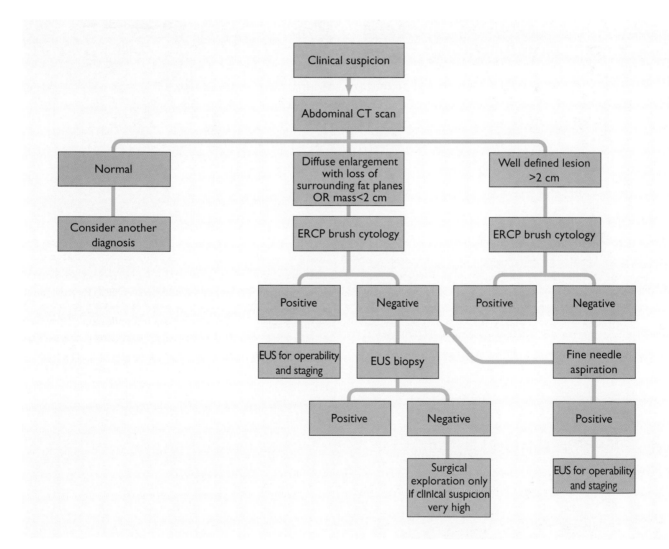

Figure 5.7 An approach to the diagnosis of pancreatic cancer. For suspicious lesions in the pancreatic head, endoscopic ultrasound scan (EUS) may be used sooner than indicated in this algorithm. CT, computerized tomography; ERCP, endoscopic retrograde cholangiopancreatogram

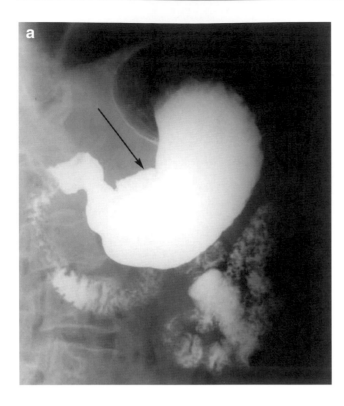

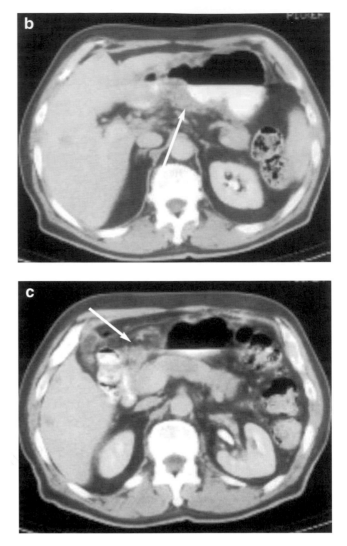

Figure 5.8 A 77-year-old male presented with a 6-month history of epigastric fullness, bloating and early satiety, unrelieved by antacids. He had lost 12 pounds in weight and his hematocrit was 33 (prior 49). Stool was Guiac positive. (a) An upper gastrointestinal series showed an antral lesion with a large ulcer in the antrum (arrowed), confirmed endoscopically as an 8-cm ulcerated mass on the lesser curvature noted approximately 2–3 cm distal to the gastroesophageal junction. (b) Staging contrast enhanced CT shows antral wall thickening posteriorly (arrowed), and a hypoattenuating lesion within the right lobe of liver suspicious for a metastasis. (c) A section inferiorly shows an enlarged peripancreatic lymph node (arrowed) and additional hepatic lesions

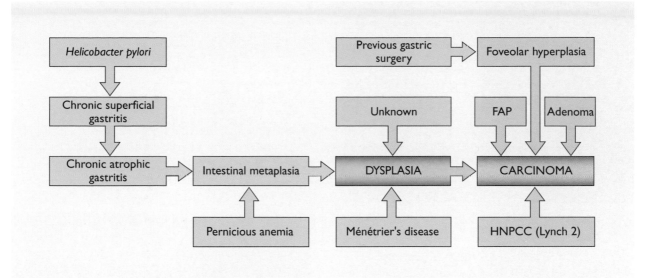

Figure 5.9 Etiopathogenesis of gastric adenocarcinoma. FAP, familial adenomatous polyposis; HNPCC, hereditary non-polyposis colorectal cancer. Refer also to Chapter 3 and Figure 3.12

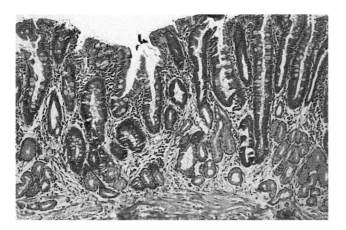

Figure 5.10 Chronic gastritis with intestinal metaplasis. Although chronic gastritis is common in the general population, this mucosal lesion is the background from which gastric carcinoma, intestinal type, arises. (Hematoxylin & eosin, 100 ×)

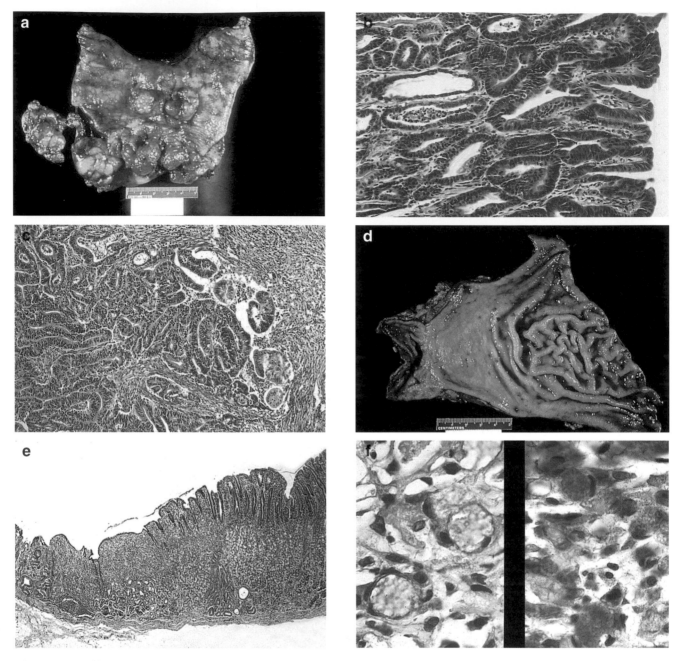

Figure 5.11 (a) Distal gastrectomy, showing an irregular polypoid mass involving much of the antral region. (b) Photomicrograph of superficial portion of polypoid mass in (a), showing extensive intraepithelial dysplasia. (Hematoxylin and eosin, 100 ×). (c) Photomicrograph of base of polypoid mass, showing moderately differentiated intestinal-type adenocarcinoma invading the submucosa. (H & E, 100 ×). (d) Distal gastrectomy, photographed after formalin fixation, showing effacement of the mucosal folds throughout the antral region. (e) Low-power photomicrograph of transition zone from preserved gastric mucosa to effaced mucosa in (d), showing attenuated thickness of mucosa and loss of mucosal glands. (H & E, 40 ×). (f) High-power photomicrographs showing hematoxylin and eosin staining (left) and mucin staining (right) of 'signet ring' cells of poorly differentiated diffusely infiltrative carcinoma, from (d) and (e) (1000 ×)

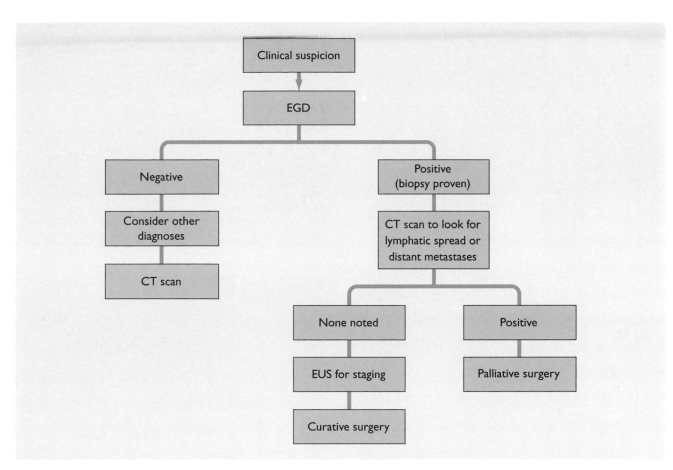

Figure 5.12   Gastric cancer – an approach to the diagnosis. EGD, esophagogastroduodenoscopy; CT, computerized tomography; EUS, endoscopic ultrasound scan

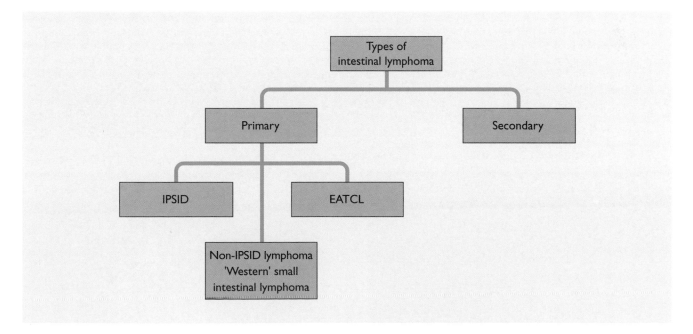

Figure 5.13   Intestinal lymphoma – a classification. IPSID, immunoproliferative small intestinal disease; EATCL, enteropathy-associated T-cell lymphoma

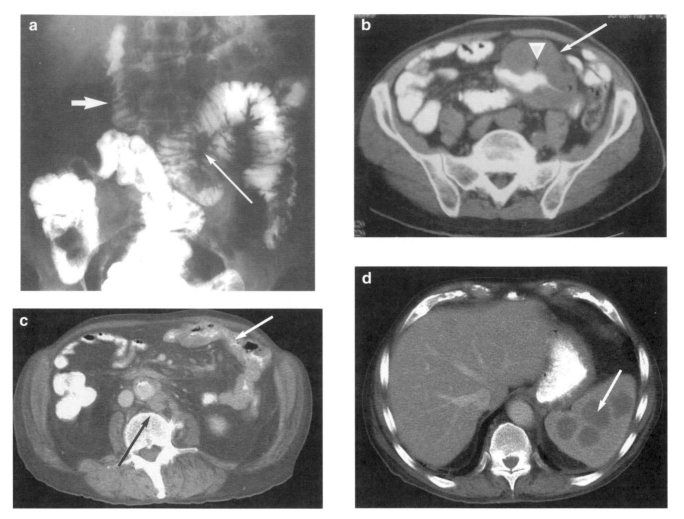

Figure 5.14 Lymphoma of small bowel. (a) Small bowel barium study demonstrates some dilatation of small bowel, with intraluminal nodules (thin arrow). Duodenal folds are thickened (large arrowhead). In more advanced cases, loss of mucosal folds occurs, with 'aneurysmal' dilatation, and ulcerations and excavations occur in larger masses, often with fistula formation. (b) Lymphoma of jejunum: CT of the mid-abdomen, following administration of oral contrast. There is an area of extensive involvement of the jejunum in this patient who presented with abdominal pain several years after a renal transplant. There is marked transmural thickening (arrowed) and loss of normal mucosal contour, with ulceration into the mass containing a small quantity of air (yellow arrowhead). (c) An 82-year-old male with non-Hodgkin's lymphoma presented with weakness and anemia. A segment of jejunum is involved, with thickening of the wall. Lymph nodes are also present in the mesentery and left para-aortic region (red arrow). A bone marrow biopsy revealed a transformation to a less well differentiated large cell lymphoma. (d) Contrast enhanced CT of the abdomen (same patient as Figure 5.14c) shows multiple hypoattenuating lesions in the spleen (arrowed)

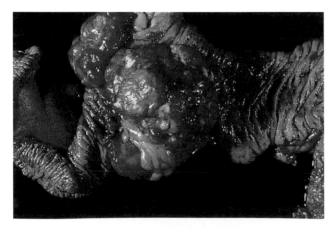

Figure 5.15 Lymphomatous mass astride the ileocecal valvular region. The small intestine is the narrower caliber segment of bowel

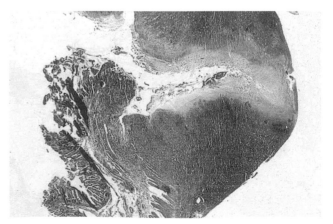

Figure 5.16 Low-power photomicrograph, demonstrating replacement of the small-intestinal segment by lymphomatous infiltrate; perforation has occurred. (H & E, 20 ×)

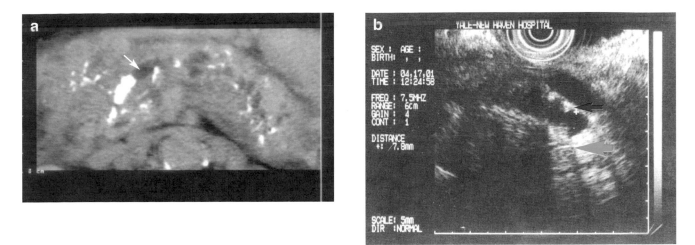

Figure 5.17 (a) Computed tomogram of the pancreas (non-contrast study) of an elderly male with chronic alcoholism demonstrates calcific pancreatitis, with irregular dilatation of the main pancreatic duct (arrowed). Numerous calcifications are present along the course of the duct. (b) Endoscopic US in a patient with chronic pancreatitis shows dilated pancreatic duct (arrowed) with intraductal concretions (red arrow) which shadow posteriorly (green arrow)

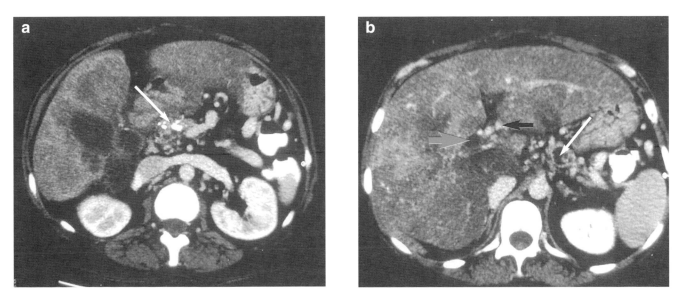

Figure 5.18 A 42-year-old female alcoholic with chronic pancreatitis presenting with abdominal pain. (a) A CT scan with contrast enhancement (portal venous phase) shows calcifications in head of pancreas (arrowed) indicating chronic calcific pancreatitis. The liver is diffusely heterogeneous due to portal vein occlusion and fatty infiltration of the liver. (b) CT scan, portal venous phase image shows atrophy of distal pancreas with dilated segment of pancreatic duct. The splenic vein is thrombosed (white arrow). There are tortuous enhancing vascular structures (red arrow) within the porta hepatis, consistent with cavernous transformation due to portal vein occlusion. Thrombus is present in the main portal vein (green arrowhead). The liver (L) is heterogeneous due to a combination of fatty infiltration and perfusion abnormalities associated with the thrombosis of the portal system

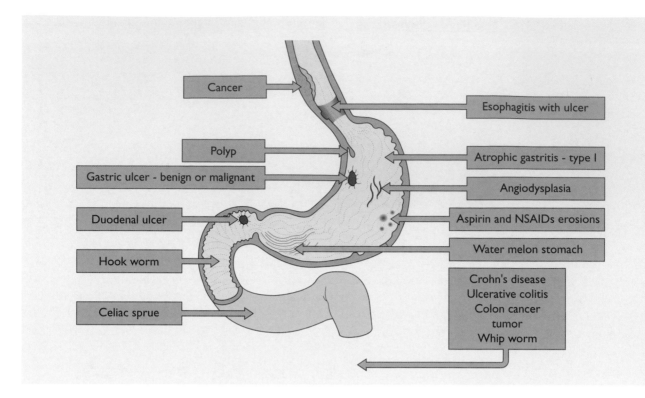

Figure 6.1 Various lesions of the gastrointestinal tract that can give rise to iron deficiency anemia

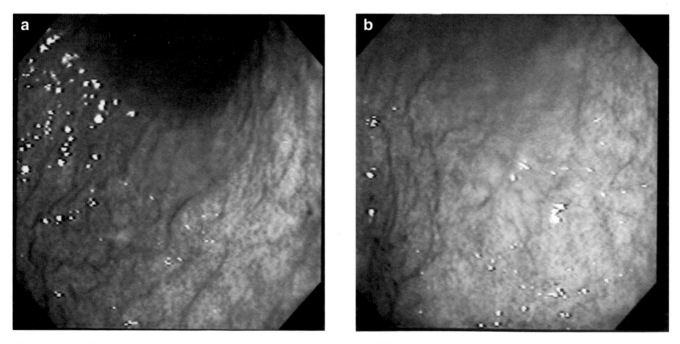

Figure 6.2 (a, b) Atrophic gastritis. The normal gastric folds are obliterated. The mucosa is thin resulting in the underlying vascular architecture (thin bluish vessels) appearing more prominent. Such a lesion may be seen in pernicious anemia (confined to the fundus and body of the stomach) and in atrophic gastritis resulting from chronic *H. pylori* colonization.

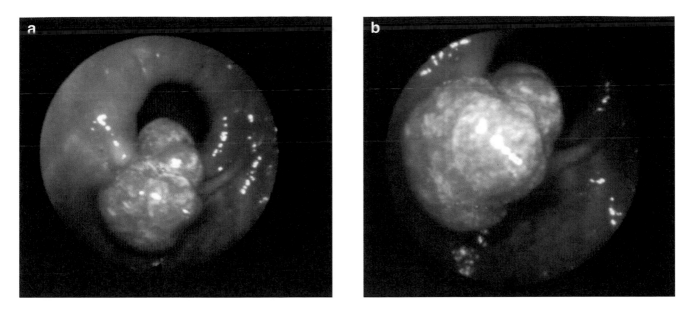

Figure 6.3 (a, b) Gastric adenomatous polyps arising from the distal stomach in a patient with atrophic gastritis. The polyps are large and multilobulated

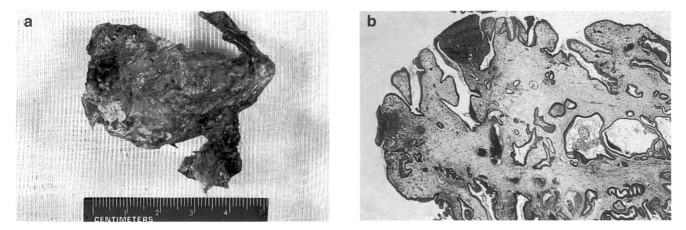

Figure 6.4 Gastric hyperplastic polyp. (a) Gross photograph of an irregular polyp retrieved from the stomach cavity; it was attached to the body mucosa by a slender stalk. (b) Photomicrograph of (a), showing edematous stroma, disorganized embedded hyperplastic glands, and superficial foci of inflammation and granulation tissue (blue-staining in this image) resulting from superficial erosion of the polyp. (Hematoxylin and eosin × 20)

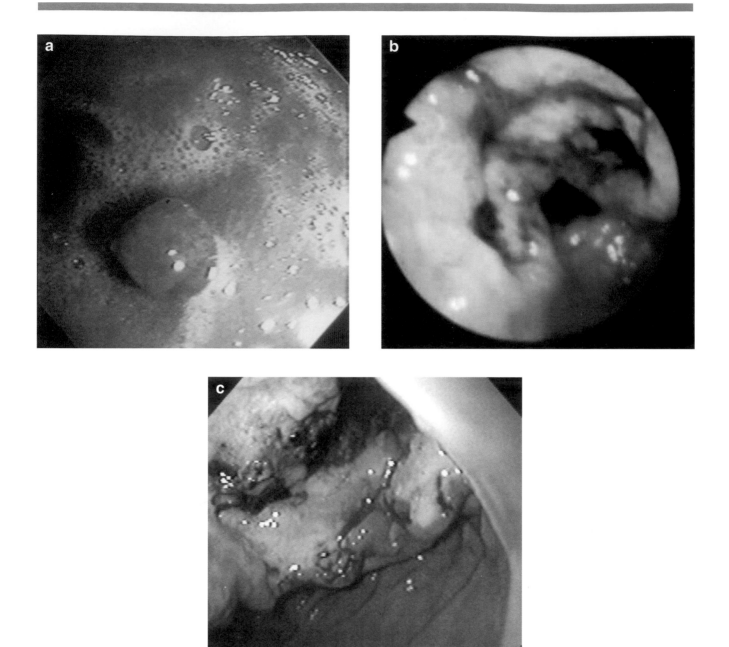

Figure 6.5 Gastric lymphoma. Endoscopic appearance of (a) gastric polyp; (b) a distal antral ulcer; and (c) a large ulcerating and fungating mass at the cardia of the stomach resembling a gastric carcinoma

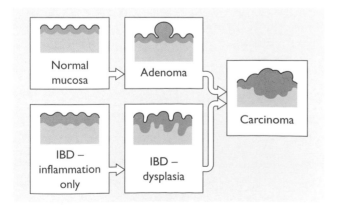

Figure 6.6 The sequence of conditions giving rise to carcinoma. IBD, inflammatory bowel disease

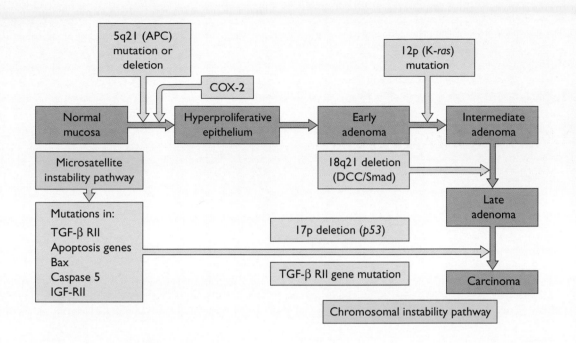

Figure 6.7 Transition from normal mucosa to carcinomia

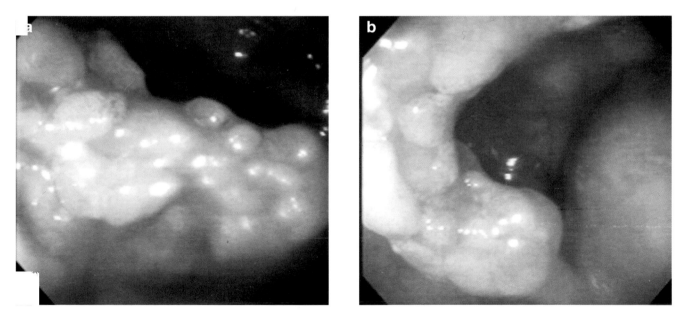

Figure 6.8 (a, b) Large rounded sessile mass occupying at least two-thirds of the lumen of the colon. Biopsy revealed it to be an adenocarcinoma

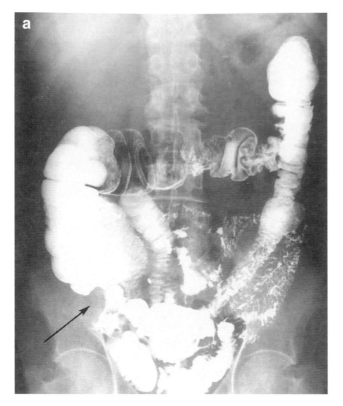

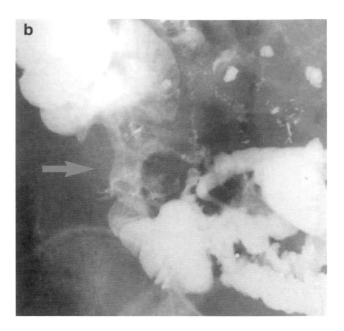

Figure 6.9   (a) Overhead AP radiograph obtained following a barium enema, with (b) spot film of cecum. There is a filling defect in the cecum due to a colonic neoplasm (arrows). Barium has refluxed into the terminal ileum

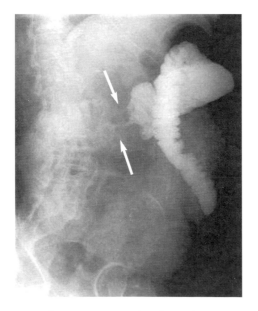

Figure 6.10   Barium enema with radiograph in lateral projection demonstrates 'cored apple' appearance of lesion in the mid-transverse colon (white arrows)

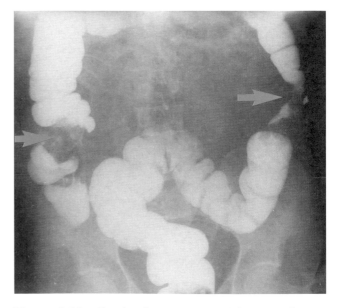

Figure 6.11   Overhead view obtained following barium enema shows synchronous lesions within ascending and descending colon (arrowed)

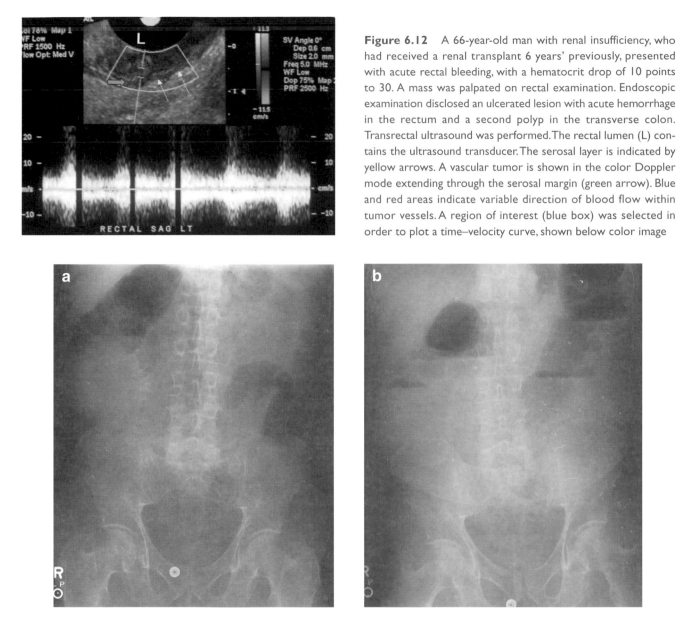

Figure 6.12 A 66-year-old man with renal insufficiency, who had received a renal transplant 6 years' previously, presented with acute rectal bleeding, with a hematocrit drop of 10 points to 30. A mass was palpated on rectal examination. Endoscopic examination disclosed an ulcerated lesion with acute hemorrhage in the rectum and a second polyp in the transverse colon. Transrectal ultrasound was performed. The rectal lumen (L) contains the ultrasound transducer. The serosal layer is indicated by yellow arrows. A vascular tumor is shown in the color Doppler mode extending through the serosal margin (green arrow). Blue and red areas indicate variable direction of blood flow within tumor vessels. A region of interest (blue box) was selected in order to plot a time–velocity curve, shown below color image

Figure 6.13 (a) Supine abdominal radiograph shows distension of colon and fluid-filled small bowel. (b) Erect abdominal radiograph shows multiple air–fluid levels in the large bowel and no air within the rectosigmoid

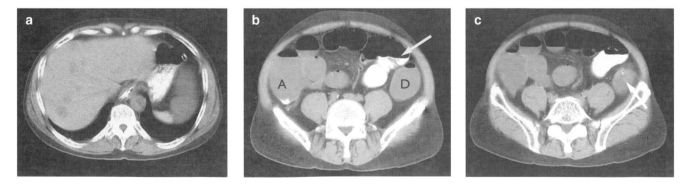

Figure 6.14 (a) Body CT scan (with oral but not intravenous contrast) demonstrates multiple focal hypoattenuating liver lesions consistent with liver metastases. (b) CT scan through mid-abdomen shows dilated loop of contrast-filled small bowel, with air–fluid level (yellow arrow). Air–fluid levels are present in fluid filled and dilated ascending (A) and descending (D) colon. (c) CT scan at more inferior level shows a soft tissue mass causing a large bowel obstruction at the junction of the descending and sigmoid colon (arrowed), with multiple air–fluid levels in distal small bowel

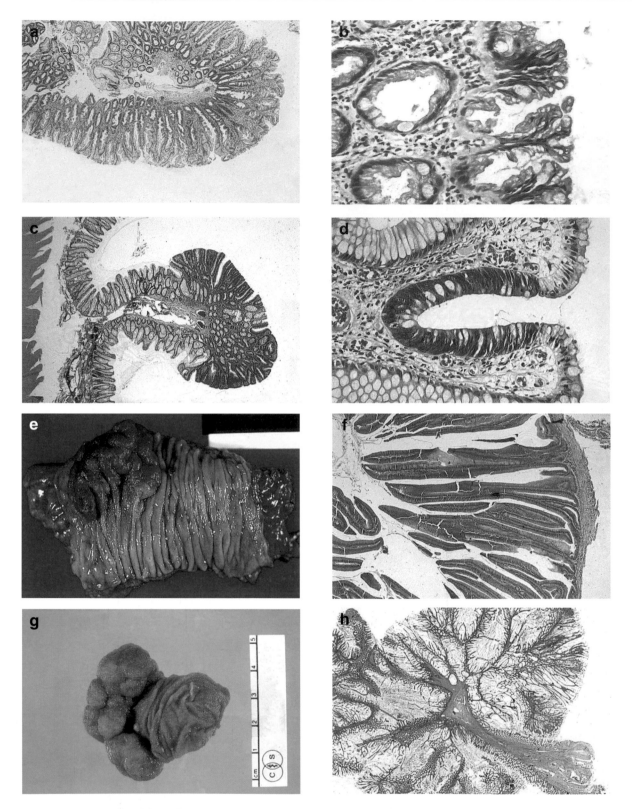

Figure 6.15 Colonic polyps. Hyperplastic polyp, (a) low-power photomicrograph showing absence of nuclear hyperchromasia, modest thickening of the mucosal layer, and a 'serrated' profile to the glandular lumens (hematoxylin and eosin, 100 ×). (b) High-power photomicrograph showing heaped up superficial colonic epithelial cells, without nuclear features of dysplasia (H & E, 400 ×). (c) Tubular adenoma, low-power photomicrograph demonstrating pedunculated (stalked) polyp with superficial tubular adenomatous features (H & E, 100 ×). (d) Focal adenomatous transformation of a colonic crypt, showing 'tubular' architecture (H & E, 100 ×). (e) Villous adenoma of cecum, sessile and 10 cm in maximum diameter. (f) Villous adenoma, medium-power photomicrograph showing frond-like villous projections of adenomatous mucosa (H & E, 40 ×). Peutz-Jegher polyp (g) gross photograph; (h) low power photomicrograph showing central muscular stalk, splayed muscle fibers into polyp head, and abundant mucinous stalk epithelial component (H & E, 40 ×)

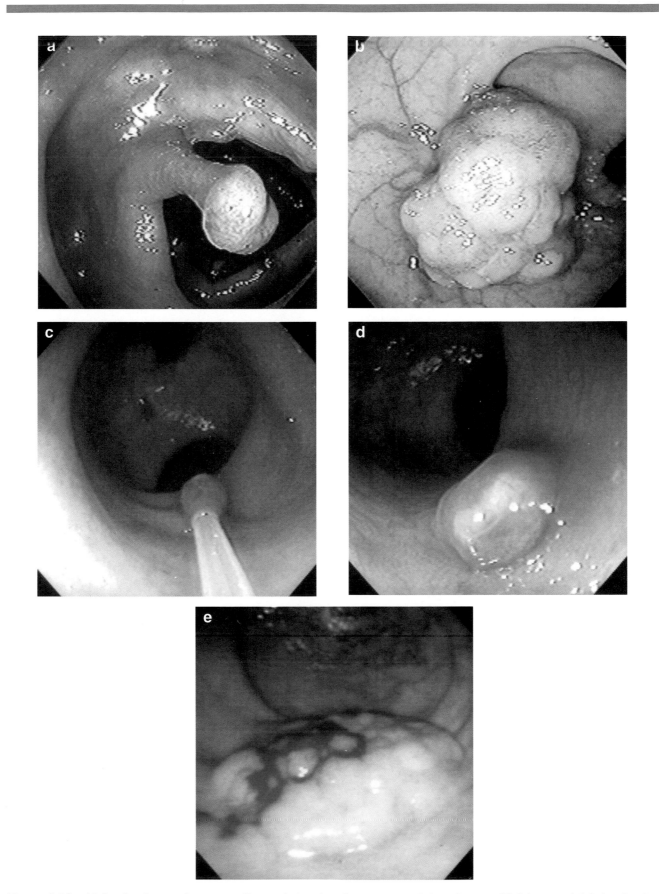

Figure 6.16 (a) Small colonic polyp on a stalk, revealed on histology to be a tubular adenoma. (b) A large multilobulated polyp, revealed on histology to be chiefly a tubular adenoma but with some villous components. (c) Small stalked polyp with snare around it prior to application of cautery. (d) Small sessile polyp tubular adenoma. (e) Flat, sessile, polyp with 'fronds' on the surface. Biopsy revealed it to be a villous adenoma. It required saline injection into the submucosa in order to remove it by snare cautery safely

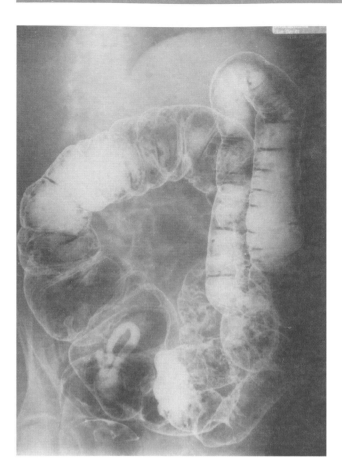

Figure 6.17 Air contrast barium enema, showing innumerable tiny polyps throughout the colon. The patient had polyposis coli

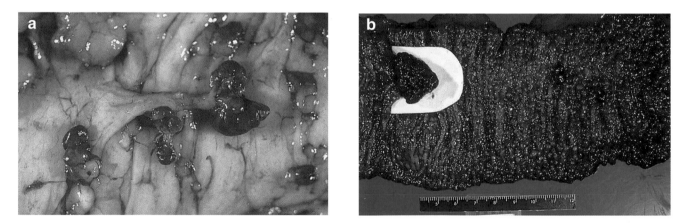

Figure 6.18 Familial adenomatous polyposis (adenomatous polyposis coli). (a) Gross photograph showing both small sessile polypoid lesions of colonic mucosa, and one pedunculated larger adenoma. (b) Gross photograph showing a colonic mucosa carpeted with small adenomatous polyps, and one large pedunculated polyp. Both patients were in their early twenties

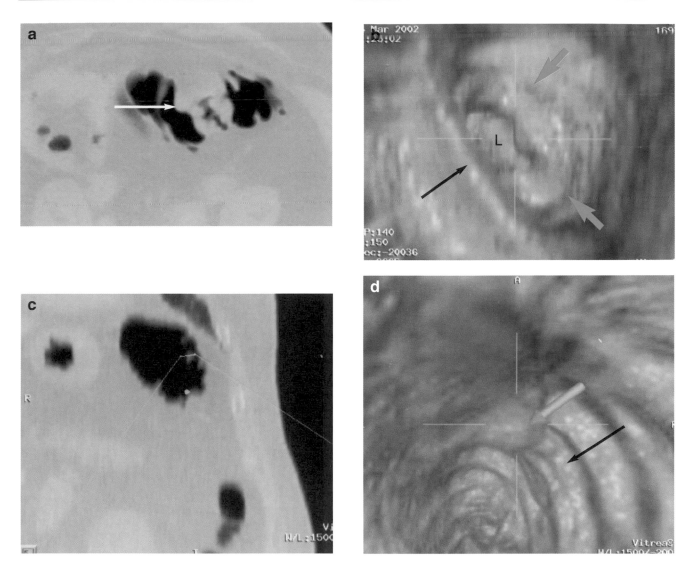

Figure 6.19 (a) CT scan of the colon obtained during CT colonography, 3 mm sections, axial projection viewed with wide windows optimizing the air–colon interface. Note 'cored apple' lesion in rectosigmoid (arrow) that could not be passed at endoscopy. (b) Same patient, demonstrating polypoid sigmoid carcinoma (green arrows) almost occluding the colonic lumen, as viewed from the rectosigmoid aspect in virtual colonoscopy (3-D color reformatted) projection. A normal colonic haustral fold (black arrow) is in the foreground. (c) Multiplanar reconstruction, coronal view of same patient proximal to the sigmoid lesion, shows the splenic flexure. A polypoid lesion of less than 1 cm diameter is tagged with a yellow mark. (d) Virtual colography reconstruction of tagged area at splenic flexure, descending colon, reveals a sessile polyp (yellow arrow) adjacent to a haustral fold (black arrow) corresponding to the coronal view. The presence of the polyp was confirmed at surgery for the sigmoid carcinoma and a left hemicolectomy was performed

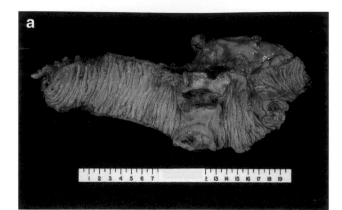

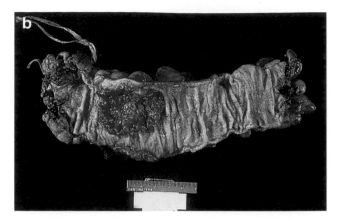

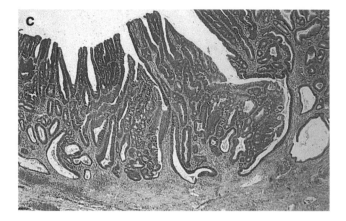

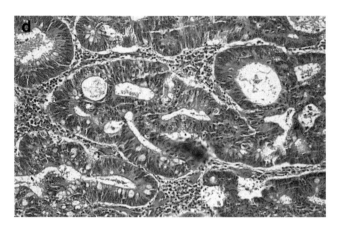

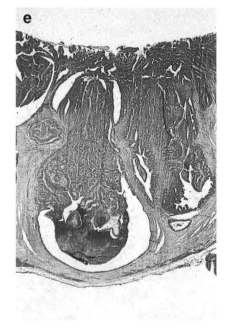

Figure 6.20 Colon carcinoma. (a) Colon adenocarcinoma of cecum in opened ileocecal resection specimen, showing near-circumferential mass with central ulceration. Figure courtesy of Melissa Li, MD, University of Florida. (b) Colon adenocarcinoma of descending colon in opened specimen, showing heaped up edges and a large central ulcerated crater. Villous adenoma low-power photomicrograph (c) with intramucosal carcinoma present in the mid-portion of the image; glandular architecture is partially obliterated. (Hematoxylin & eosin, 40 ×). (d) High-power photomicrograph showing intramucosal malignant glands with cribiform architecture (H & E, 200 ×). (e) Low power photomicrograph of colon adenocarcinoma invasive through the wall (muscularis propria) but not yet at the serosal surface (H & E, 20 ×)

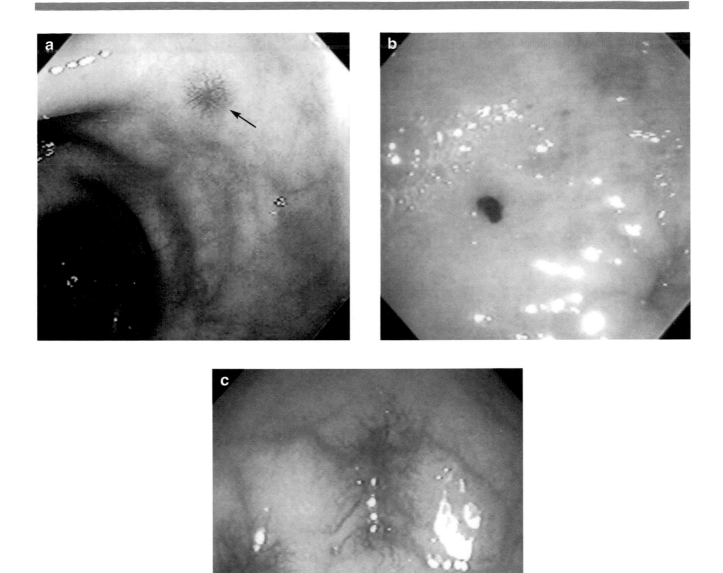

Figure 6.21 Angiodysplasias of the colon. (a) Lesion resembling a telangiectasia (arrowed). (b) 'Cherry red spot'. (c) Multiple telangiectasias in the colon of a patient with scleroderma

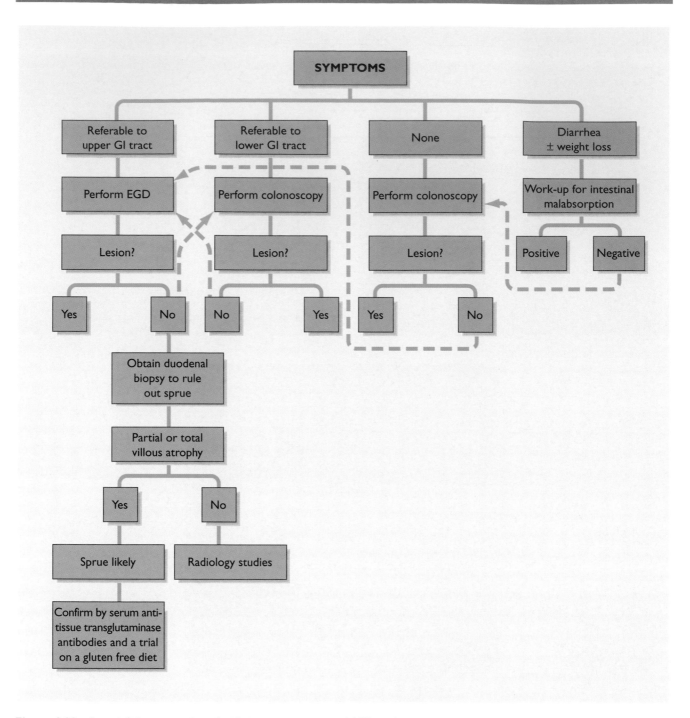

Figure 6.22 Iron deficiency anemia – elucidating a gastrointestinal (GI) etiology

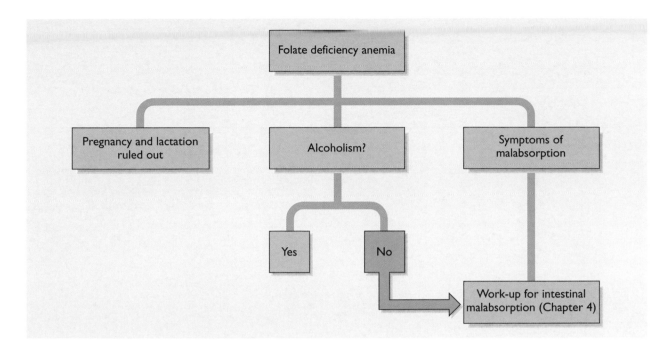

Figure 6.23 Elucidation of the etiology of folate deficiency anemia

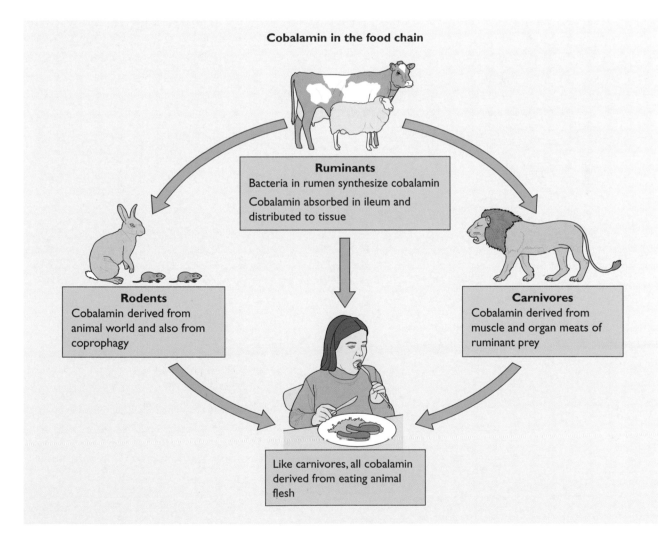

Figure 6.24 Cobalamin in the food chain

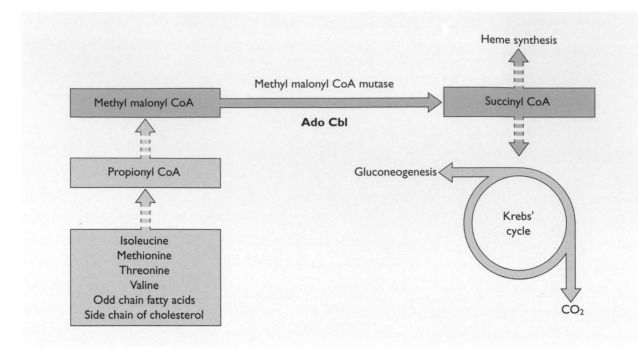

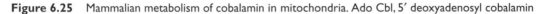

Figure 6.25 Mammalian metabolism of cobalamin in mitochondria. Ado Cbl, 5′ deoxyadenosyl cobalamin

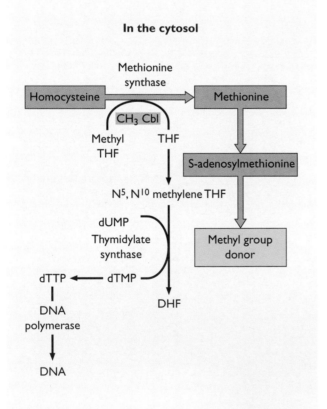

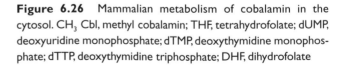

Figure 6.26 Mammalian metabolism of cobalamin in the cytosol. CH₃ Cbl, methyl cobalamin; THF, tetrahydrofolate; dUMP, deoxyuridine monophosphate; dTMP, deoxythymidine monophosphate; dTTP, deoxythymidine triphosphate; DHF, dihydrofolate

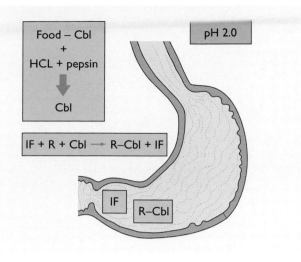

Figure 6.27 The gastric phase of cobalamin absorption. Cbl, cobalamin; R, R protein; IF, intrinsic factor; R–Cbl, R protein–cobalamin complex; IF–Cbl, intrinsic factor–cobalamin complex

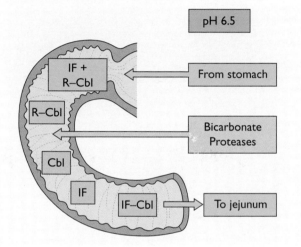

Figure 6.28 The duodenal phase of cobalamin absorption. IF, intrinsic factor; R–Cbl, R protein–cobalamin complex; IF–Cbl, intrinsic factor–cobalamin complex

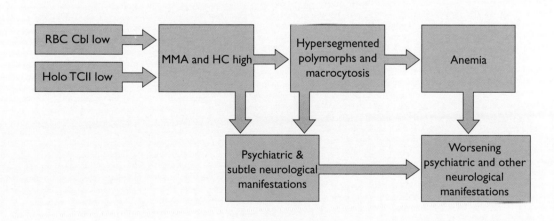

Figure 6.29 Serial progression of cobalamin deficiency. RBC, red blood cell; Cbl, cobalamin; Holo TCII, holotranscobalamin II; MMA, methylmalonic acid; HC, homocysteine

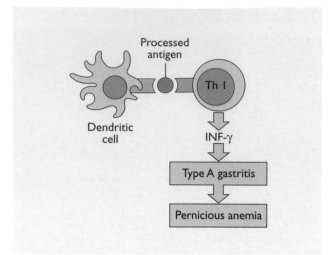

Figure 6.30 Pathogenesis of pernicious anemia – a hypothesis based on a model of murine gastric atrophy. The antigen presenting cell (dendritic cell) presents the processed antigen (β subunit of the proton pump) coupled to a MHC class two molecule to the surface receptor on CD4 Th1 cells. Th1 cytokines, especially interferon β, are secreted and are responsible, at least in part, for the development of Type A gastritis, the lesion of pernicious anemia

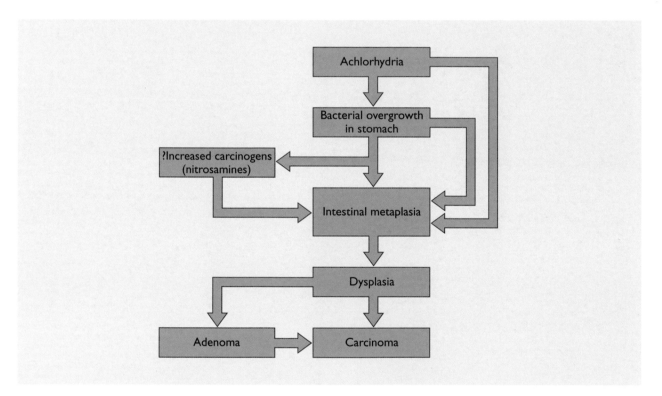

Figure 6.31   The sequence from achlorhydria to adenoma and carcinoma

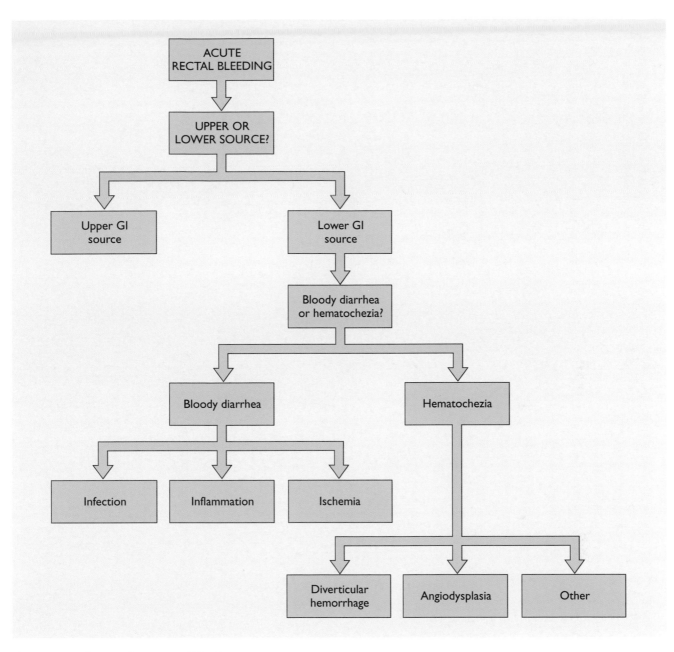

Figure 7.1   Causes of acute rectal bleeding

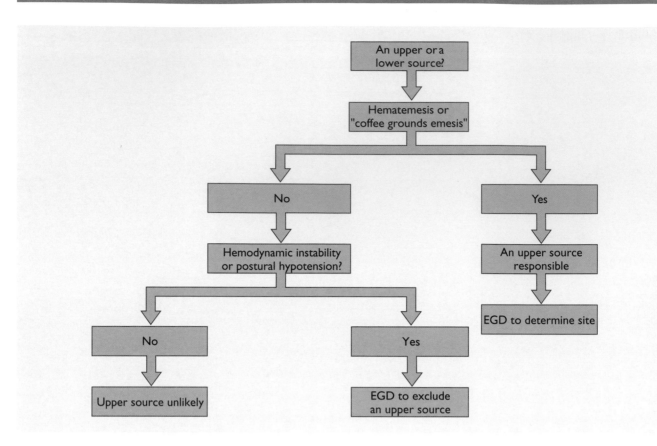

Figure 7.2 Source of acute rectal bleeding

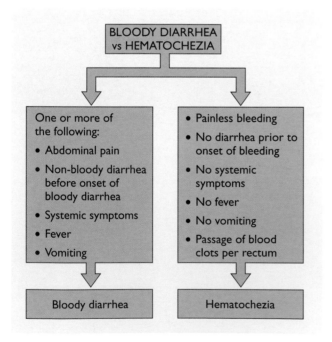

Bloody diarrhea

Hematochezia

Figure 7.3 Algorithm to distinguish between bloody diarrhea and hematochezia

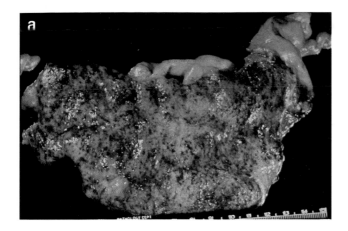

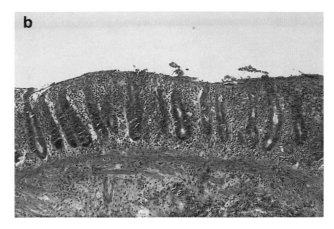

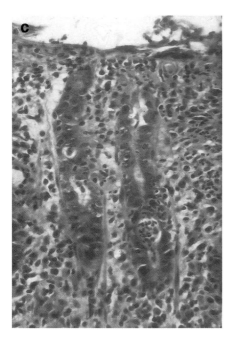

Figure 7.4 (a) Gross image of *Shigella* colitis, showing hemorrhagic mucosal surface. (b) Low-power photomicrograph of 'acute self-limited colitis', in this case from enterotoxigenic *E. coli*. Preservation of crypt vertical orientation is evident (in contradistinction to the chronic colitis of Crohn's disease or ulcerative colitis), but with separation of crypts by a lamina propria inflammatory infiltrate (hematoxylin & eosin, 100 ×). (c) High-power photomicrograph of (b), showing intraepithelial neutrophils of both surface and crypt epithelium, crypt abscesses and mixed lamina propria inflammatory infiltrate (H & E, 400 ×)

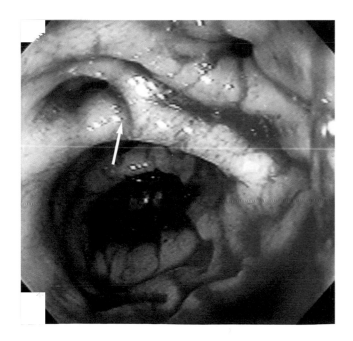

Figure 7.5 The patient had several diverticula in the left and right colon, one of which (arrow) was noted to be bleeding at the time of colonoscopy together with pooling of blood in the lumen

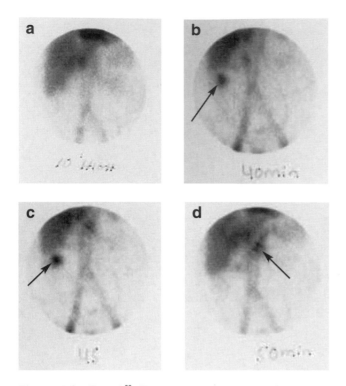

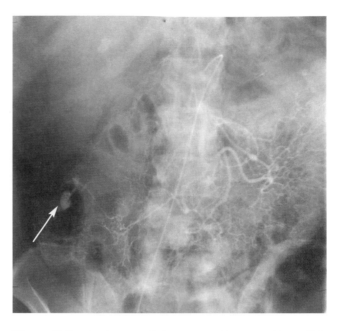

Figure 7.7 Angiogram of the same patient as in Figure 7.6. A superior mesenteric artery injection of contrast reveals extravasation of the contrast from a branch of the right colic artery (arrow)

Figure 7.6 Tagged ^{99m} Tc red-cell study imaged at (a) 10 mins demonstrates hepatic activity with no focus seen within gastrointestinal tract; imaging at (b) 40 mins, (c) 45 mins, and (d) 50 mins shows activity (black arrow) appearing in the right mid-abdomen below the liver, probably within hepatic flexure. On the later phase image (d), the activity becomes more linear as it moves into the mid-abdomen, consistent with radiolabeled tracer within blood passing through the transverse colon.

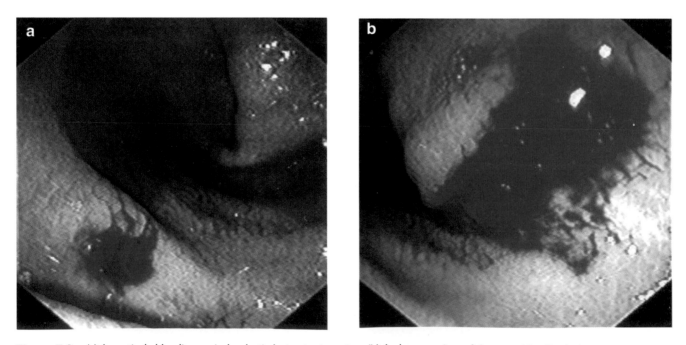

Figure 7.8 (a) An actively bleeding angiodysplastic lesion in the colon. (b) A close-up view of the same bleeding lesion

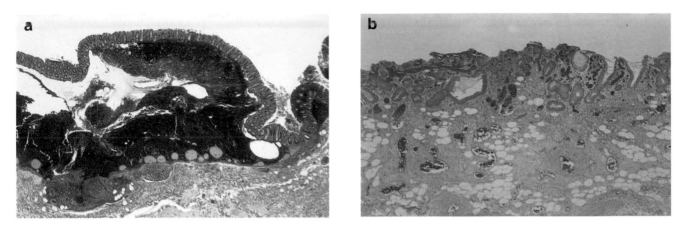

Figure 7.9 Angiodysplasia. (a) Low-power photomicrograph of cecal mucosa from resected specimen showing intramucosal hemorrhage at far right of image and extensive hemorrhage splitting the mucosal epithelial layer from the muscularis mucosa in a patient with angiodysplasia. Incidental dilated lymphatic channels resting just on top of the muscularis mucosa are evident in sharp contrast to the hemorrhagic blood (hematoxylin & eosin, 20 ×). (b) Different area of the same specimen showing prominent submucosal and mucosal vascular channels with focal intramucosal hemorrhage (H & E, 20 ×)

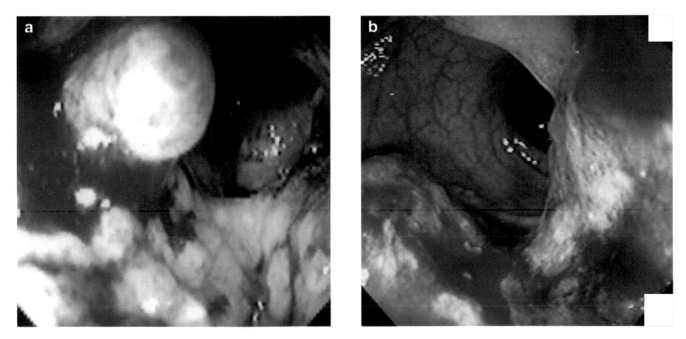

Figure 7.10 (a) A polypoid lesion, later determined to be a benign adenomatous polyp, in the sigmoid colon was bleeding at a brisk rate. The patient had been on warfarin. (b) A large, flat, concentric cancer of the sigmoid colon oozing blood

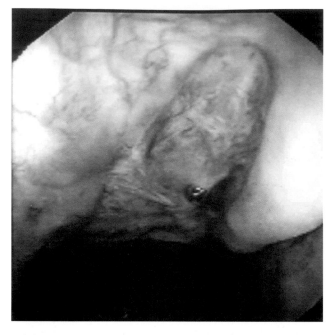

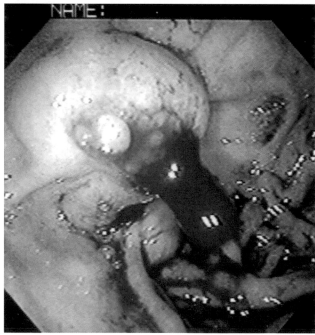

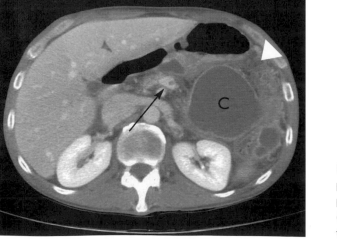

Figure 7.11 A rectal stercoral ulcer from an elderly, constipated patient who bled off and on, although never as briskly as the patient described in Case history 3. The patient was not bleeding at the time of colonoscopy

Figure 7.12 A large single gastric varix spurting blood

Figure 7.13 Contrast enhanced CT demonstrates large pseudocyst (C) arising from tail of pancreas with several smaller pseudocysts peripherally. There is a low attenuation thrombus (arrowed) within the splenic vein. A collateral vessel is also identified adjacent to stomach (arrowhead)

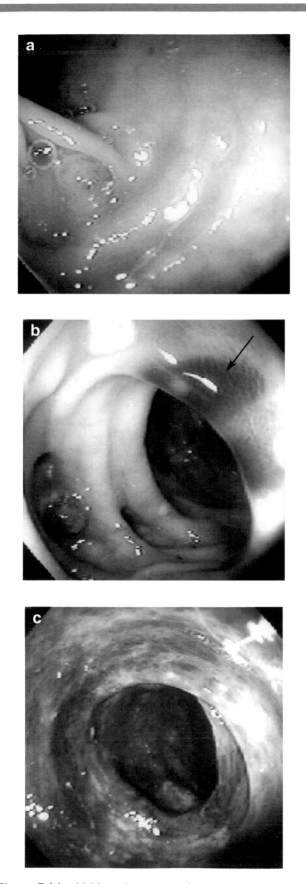

Figure 7.14 (a) Normal mucosa at the rectosigmoid junction. (b) Submucosal hemorrhages in distal sigmoid colon (arrow). (c) Erythema, mild edema and exudates in the proximal sigmoid and distal descending colon

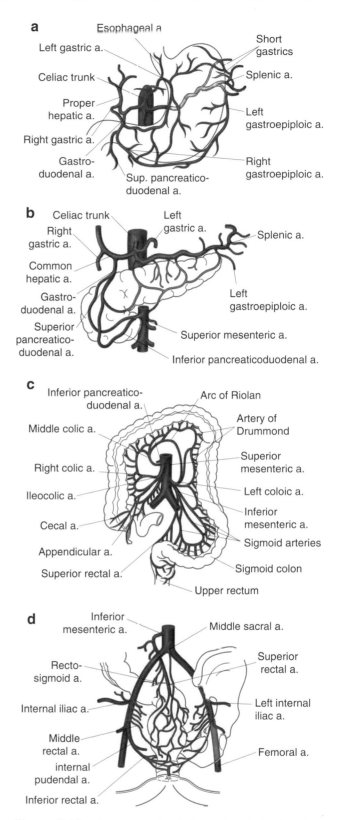

Figure 7.15 Artery supply of the gastrointestinal system: (a and b) the celiac trunk; (c) superior mesenteric artery (SMA); (d) inferior mesenteric artery

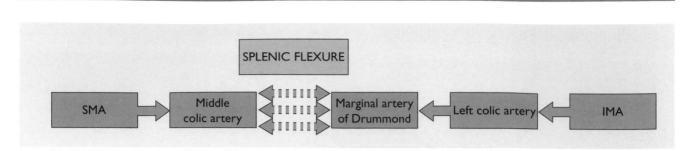

Figure 7.16   Griffith's point: anastomosis of the superior mesenteric artery (SMA) with the inferior mesenteric artery (IMA)

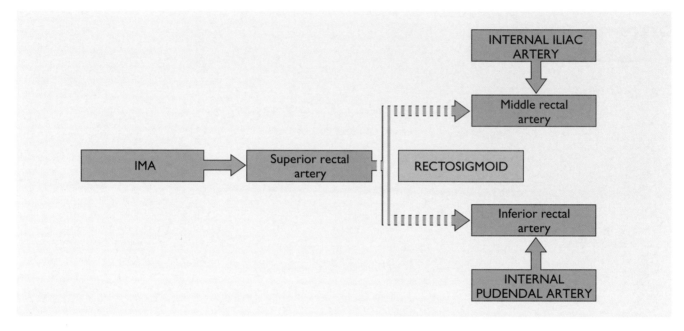

Figure 7.17   Sudeck's point: anastomosis of the inferior mesenteric artery (IMA) (splanchnic circulation) with arteries of the systemic circulation

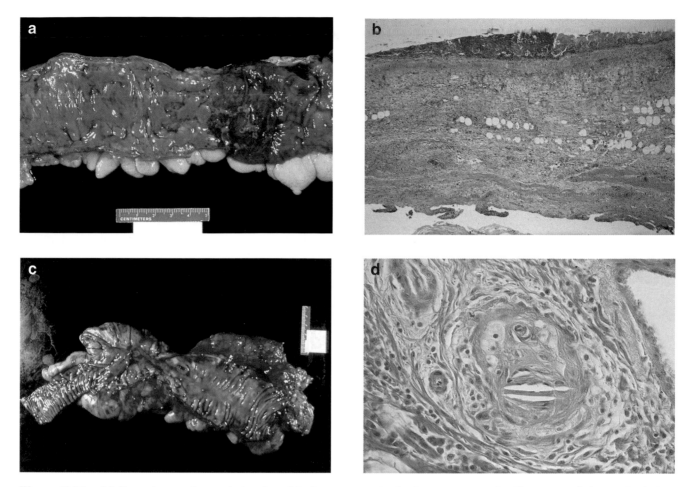

Figure 7.18 (a) Gross image of acute ischemic colitis due to systemic circulatory compromise. The mucosa is hemorrhagic in a segmental, patchy distribution. (b) Photomicrograph of (a) showing mucosal infarction and extensive edema with minimal inflammation of the submucosa and muscularis propria (hematoxylin & eosin, 40 ×). (c) Gross image of chronic ischemic colitis with focal stricture attributable to mural scarring. (d) Photomicrograph from (c), showing cholesterol crystals within mesenteric thromboembolism in region of stricture (H & E, 200 ×)

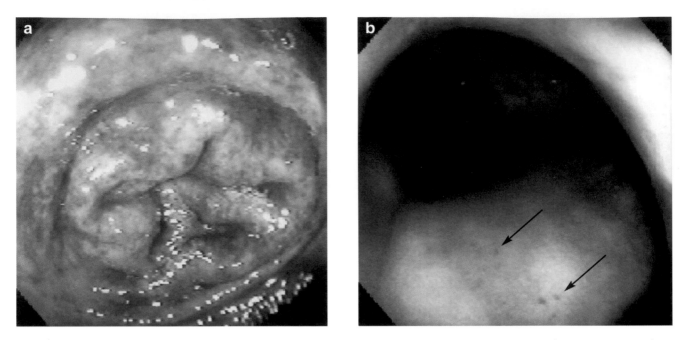

Figure 7.19 An 88-year-old woman with a history of occult blood in the stool and iron deficiency anemia for some years, resulting from previously identified angiodysplasia in the stomach and colon, presented with an episode of passing bright red blood per rectum in the absence of any abdominal pain. She fainted and on examination was hypotensive. She had a history of hypertension, degenerative joint disease and an aneurysm of the thoracic aorta. She was not on non-steroidal anti-inflammatory drugs, but was on one tablet a day of aspirin for her heart. Colonoscopy revealed normal rectal mucosa, but from the rectosigmoid junction there was marked erythema, edema, and purple 'ecchymotic spots'. These lesions, typical for ischemic colitis, were confined to the sigmoid colon. The remainder of the colon was studded with hundreds of angiodysplasias, varying in shape from cherry red spots to some with a typical fern leaf architecture. (a) Ischemia with marked edema, (b) normal mucosa with numerous little cherry red spots (arrows)

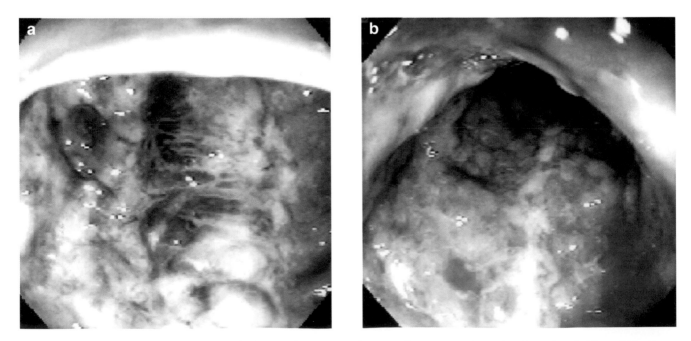

Figure 7.20 (a, b) An 87-year-old man with chronic obstructive pulmonary disease was admitted with painless bright red blood per rectum. Colonoscopy revealed patchy edematous areas of mucosa that were slightly erythematous but mostly bluish in color that extended from the sigmoid to the mid transverse colon

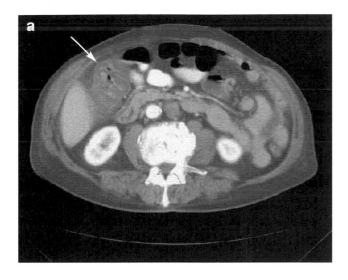

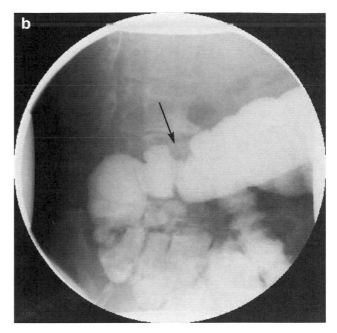

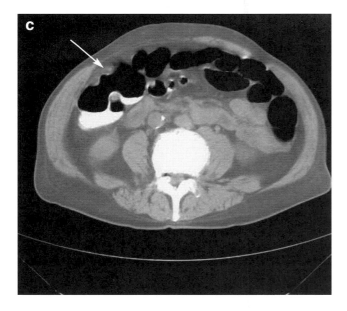

Figure 7.21 (a) Contrast enhanced CT scan though the abdomen shows thickening of the colonic wall (arrowed), which was confined to the distal ascending colon, hepatic flexure, and proximal transverse colon. These appearances could be seen in colitis, ischemia, or neoplasia, so the clinical history must be carefully integrated with these findings. (b) A hypaque enema with retrograde filling of the transverse and ascending colon shows 'thumbprinting' of the colon (arrowed) characteristic for ischemia. (c) Abdominal CT scan with oral contrast, performed several days after the initial scan, shows oral contrast in the ascending colon with resolution of the diffuse edema and wall thickening but showing the CT appearances of thumbprinting (arrowed) equivalent to those demonstrated on the hypaque enema

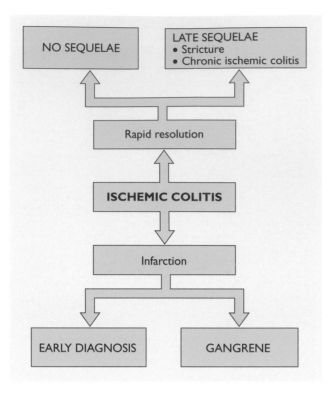

Figure 7.22   The clinical course of ischemic colitis

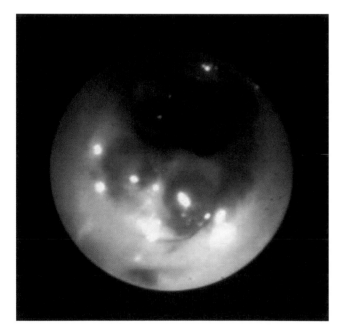

Figure 7.23   Submucosal hemorrhages in the colon of a patient with hemophilia who presented with rectal bleeding

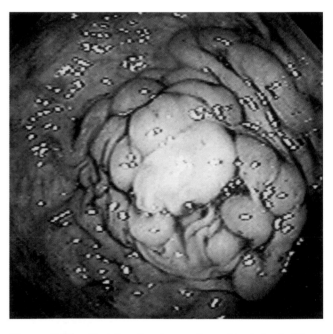

Figure 7.24   Rectal varices in a patient with cirrhosis. These may bleed giving rise to massive hemorrhage

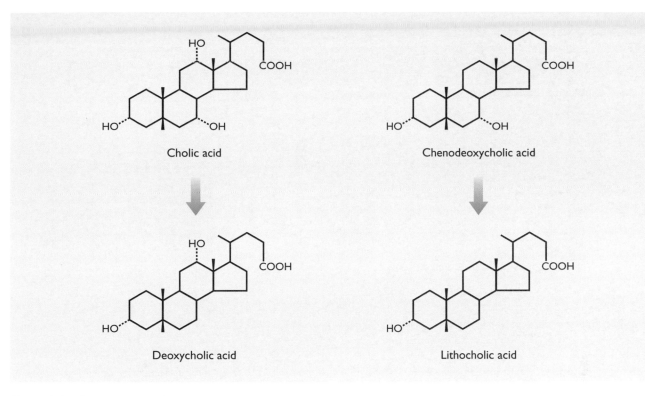

Cholic acid

Chenodeoxycholic acid

Deoxycholic acid

Lithocholic acid

Figure 8.1 The structures of bile acids

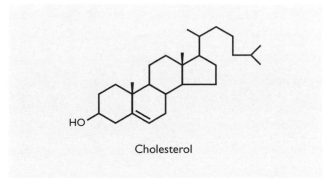

Cholesterol

Figure 8.2 The structure of cholesterol

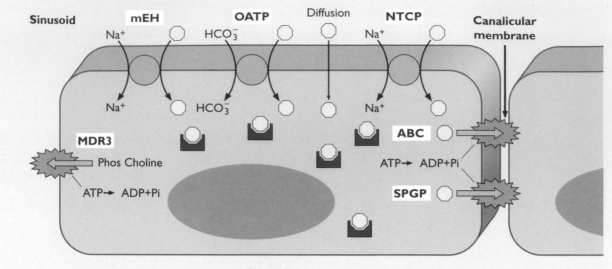

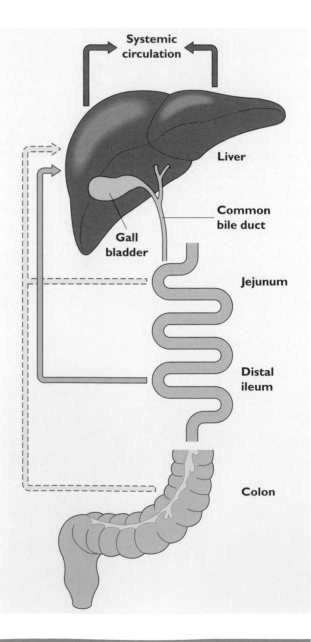

Figure 8.3 Bile acid transporters in the liver. Bile acids (○) are transported across the sinusoidal membrane into the hepatocyte both by passive diffusion and by carrier-mediated mechanisms. The carriers on the sinusoidal membrane (●) are: (1) NTCP or the Na⁺-dependent Taurocholate transporter Protein; (2) mEH or microsomal Epoxy Hydrolase, also a Na⁺-dependent transporter identified in the rat; (3) OATP or Organic Anion Transport Protein, which probably transports other organic anions such as estrone-3-sulfate and estradiol-17β-glucuronide preferentially. Within the cytosol bile acids are transported either bound to bile acid binding proteins (◖) or in intracellular vesicles. Bile acids are transported in the canaliculus by transporters located on the canalicular membrane. Energy for transport is derived from the hydrolysis of ATP into ADP + Pi. These transporters are: (1) MDR3 (Multi-Drug Resistant); (2) SPGP (Sister of P Glycoprotein); (3) probably a transporter related to the ABC transport gene family (see text)

Figure 8.4 Enterohepatic circulation of bile acids. Dashed arrows represent passive non-ionic absorption of bile acids from the jejunum and colon. Bold green arrows depict active bile acid absorption from the ileum. The red arrow shows bile acids entering the systemic circulation from the liver

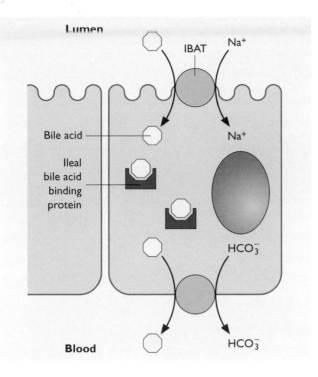

Figure 8.5 Active reabsorption of conjugated bile acids through the ileal enterocyte. Luminal bile acids (◯) are transported across the apical membrane by a Na⁺-coupled transporter (IBAT). Internalized conjugated bile acids are then transported to the basolateral membrane bound to a cytosolic ileal bile acid binding protein. A bicarbonate exchanger probably helps transport the bile acid into the portal blood

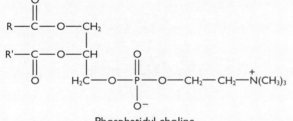

Figure 8.6 The structural formula of lecithin (phosphatidyl choline). R and R′ represent hydrophobic long-chain fatty acids. The phosphoric acid is a strong acid and the choline a strong base over most of the physiological pH range. With both hydrophobic and hydrophilic groups, lecithin is an amphipathic molecule

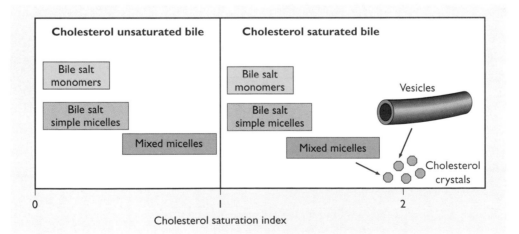

Figure 8.7 Bile salts, phospholipids (phosphatidyl choline or lecithin is the major constituent) and cholesterol constitute the biliary lipids. Beyond the critical micellar concentration (0.5–5.0 mmol/l for different bile acids), bile salt monomers form simple micelles (20–30 Å). When phospholipids and cholesterol are also present with bile acids, they interact to form a variety of lipid aggregates in bile. The nature of the aggregate formed depends on the total concentration of lipids in bile and on the concentration of each lipid type relative to the other two. At a high bile:salt phospholipid ratio, mixed micelles are formed which also incorporate cholesterol. At high total lipid concentrations, these are small and round (40–80 Å), and become larger and rod-shaped at low total lipid concentration (several hundred angstrom units). When the concentration of cholesterol is increased in mixed micelles, (at cholesterol saturation index > 1.5), unilamellar vesicles form (500–1000 Å). These can fuse and form multilamellar vesicles (1000–10 000 Å). Vesicles are thermodynamically very unstable and cholesterol crystals may precipitate out

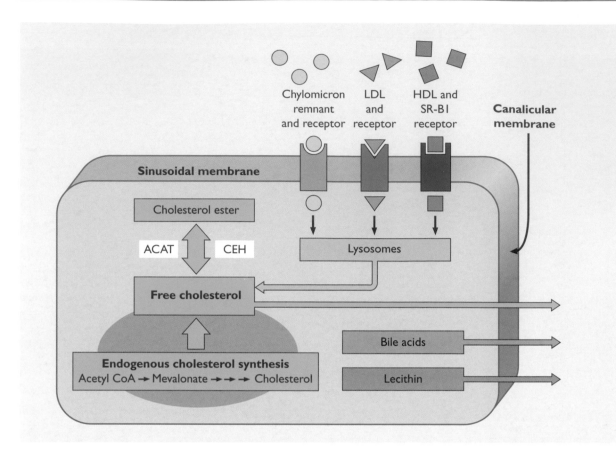

Figure 8.8 Cholesterol synthesis, uptake, secretion and metabolism

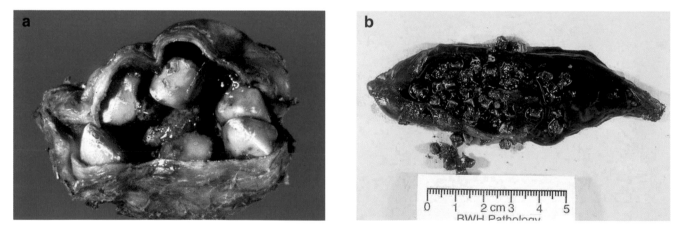

Figure 8.9 (a) Opened gallbladder specimen with several yellow, hard cholesterol gallstones. (b) Opened gallbladder specimen with numerous small, pigmented gallstones. (Photograph courtesy of Dr Martin Carey, Brigham and Women's Hospital)

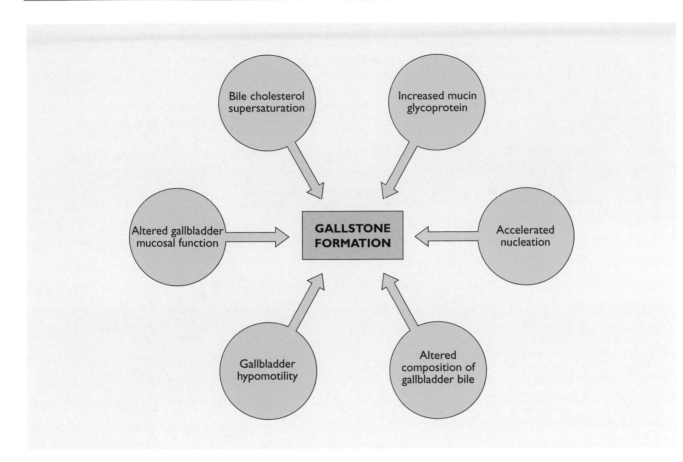

Figure 8.10 Factors responsible for gallstone formation

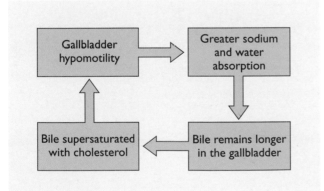

Figure 8.11 Vicious cycle of cholesterol-supersaturated bile and gallbladder hypomotility

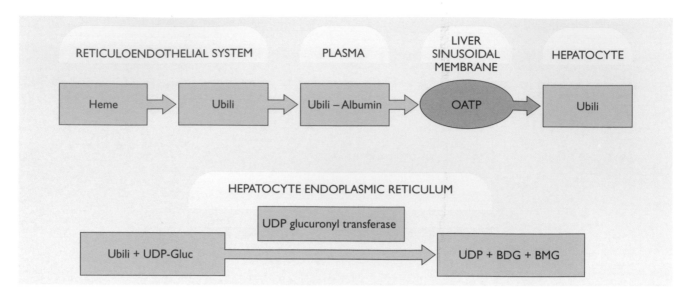

Figure 8.12   Bilirubin conjugation in the liver. Ubili, unconjugated bilirubin; BDG, bilirubin diglucuronide; BMG, bilirubin monoglucuronide; UDP-Gluc, uridine diphosphate-glucuronic acid; OATP, organic anion transport protein located on the sinusoidal membrane of hepatocytes

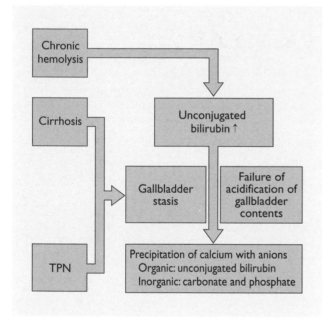

Figure 8.13   Pathogenesis of black pigment stone formation. TPN, total parenteral nutrition

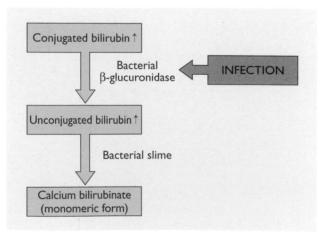

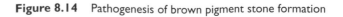

Figure 8.14   Pathogenesis of brown pigment stone formation

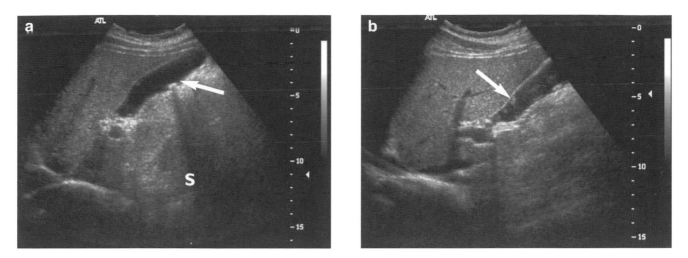

Figure 8.15 (a) Gallstones are shadowing structures within the gallbladder (arrowed), which move with position change. The shadowing effect (S) is due to mineral content of the gallstone which reflects the ultrasound beam almost totally. Polyps (see (b)) related to the gallbladder wall do not move with positional changes and will not cast a strong shadow. (b) Another patient, referred for liver ultrasound hepatitis C screen, was shown to have gallbladder polyps (arrowed, adherent to the anterior gallbladder wall)

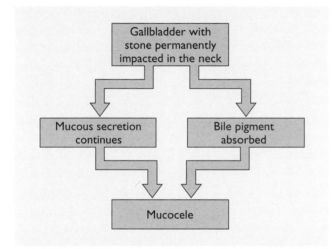

Figure 8.16 Formation of a mucocele of the gallbladder

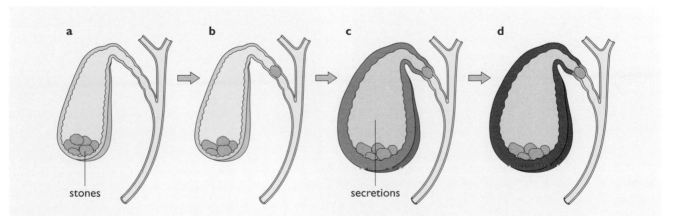

Figure 8.17 Pathogenesis of acute calculous cholecystitis. (a) Gallbladder with stones; (b) one stone obstructing the cystic duct causing biliary colic; (c) stone remains in the cystic duct hours later, leading to inflammation and thickening and edema of the gallbladder wall and pericholecystic fluid formation. The gallbladder becomes filled with secretions and is dilated. (d) The gallbladder wall becoming ischemic (maroon) and necrotic

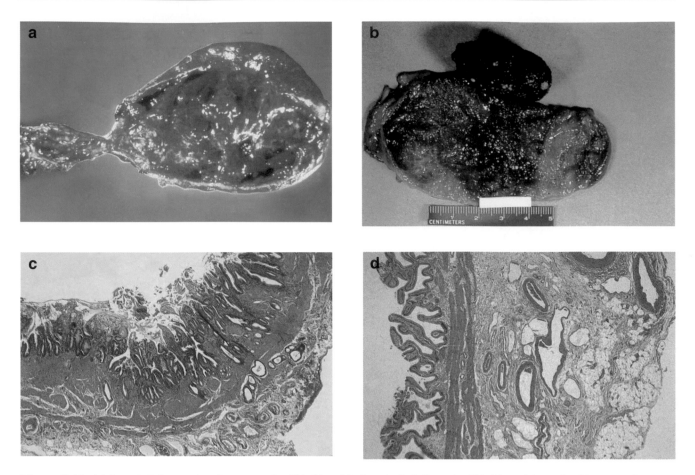

Figure 8.18 (a) Acutely inflammed and congested gallbladder; (b) chronically inflamed gallbladder with retained large single stone. This was a cholesterol stone containing trapped bile pigments; (c) low-power photomicrograph of (b) showing gallbladder wall thickened by muscular hypertrophy, mucosal inflammation and outpouchings of gallbladder mucosa termed Rochitansky–Aschoff sinuses (hematoxylin and eosin, 20 ×); (d) photomicrograph of normal gallbladder wall for comparison (H & E, 20 ×)

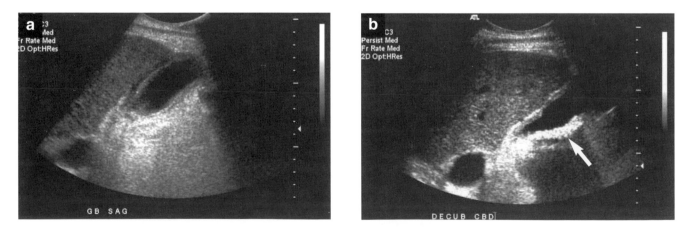

Figure 8.19 (a) A patient presenting with acute right upper quadrant pain, tenderness and fever can be rapidly evaluated by real-time ultrasound. The signs of acute cholecystitis include thickening of the gallbladder wall, pericholecystic fluid, gallstones (usually) and an ultrasonic Murphy's sign which, if elicited, can increase diagnostic confidence to almost 100%. In cases where ultrasound is equivocal, a HIDA is helpful in confirming absence of uptake in the gallbladder, indicating cystic duct obstruction. Pericholecystic fluid and edema can also occasionally be seen in cirrhosis and chronic hypoalbuminemia. (b) In the same patient, an ultrasound scan showing shadowing gallstones (arrowed), layering posteriorly

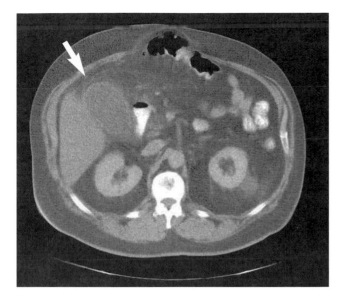

Figure 8.20 Acute cholecystitis: computed tomography scan demonstrates similar findings in a different case: there is thickening of the gallbladder wall, with edema and stranding of the pericholecystic fat (arrowed). Gallstones may not be visualized. In approximately 30% of patients, the stones consist of mixed bilirubinate salts and cholesterol which have the same attenuation as the surrounding bile, and therefore cannot be visualized

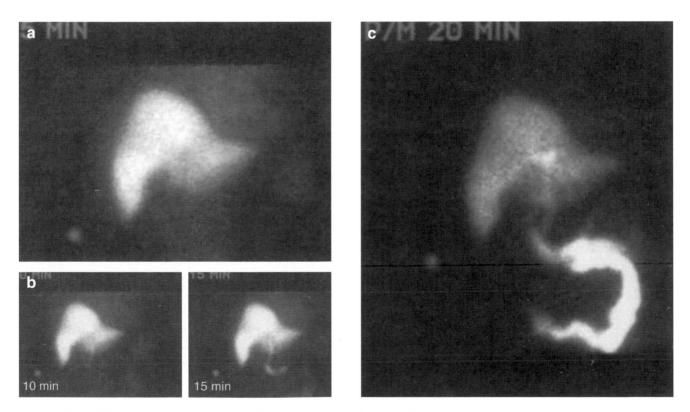

Figure 8.21 (a) Intravenous administration of 7mCi technetium-99m mebrofenin. Planar images of anterior abdomen obtained at 5-min intervals to 60 min. Normal homogeneous uptake in the liver, and concentration and excretion into the biliary system first noted at 15 min, with no visualization of the gallbladder up to 60 min and subsequently, despite administration of morphine sulfate (after 60 min with imaging for a further 25 min). (b) Imaging at 10 and 15 min. (c) Following administration of 3.4 mg morphine intravenously, imaging of the liver and biliary system up to 60 min demonstrated no uptake in the gallbladder, with excretion via the common bile duct into the duodenum and small bowel

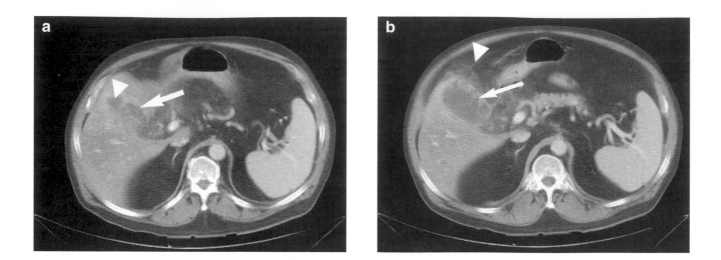

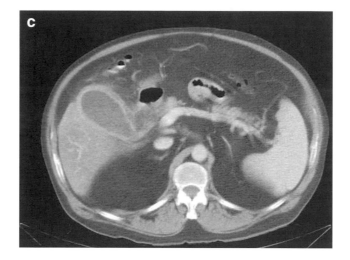

Figure 8.22 (a) Complex cholecystitis with perforation. Contrast-enhanced computed tomography (CT) scan through the liver shows a gallbladder with an irregular, enhancing wall (arrowed) with pericholecystic enhancement of the liver. No gallstones are seen. There is no intrahepatic biliary dilatation. The low attenuation region (arrowed) which appears lateral to the gallbladder represents a perforation with intrahepatic abscess (arrowhead). (b) Marked thickening and irregularity of the gallbladder wall, with pericholecystic stranding (arrowhead). (c) Gallbladder is distended, with diffuse thickening of the wall. There is stranding of the adjacent mesentery

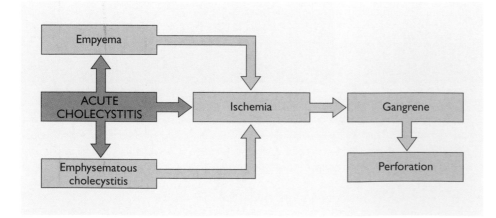

Figure 8.23 Complications of acute cholecystitis

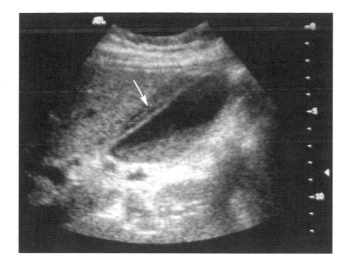

Figure 8.24 Real-time ultrasound scan of the right upper quadrant, showing a markedly thickened gallbladder wall (arrowed). There is echogenic sludge within the gallbladder but no shadowing gallstones were seen. The patient had a positive Murphy sign. These features are consistent with acute cholecystitis, but in the absence of demonstrated stones, these findings can support the diagnosis of acalculous cholecystitis

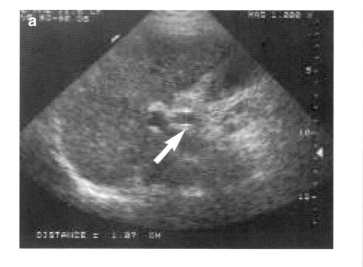

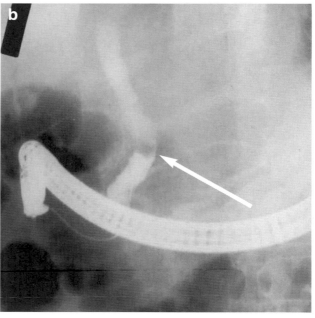

Figure 8.25 (a) Real-time ultrasound scan demonstrates dilated common bile duct of 1.27 cm (arrowed) without intrahepatic biliary dilatation. No choledocholithiasis was seen, but the distal aspect of the duct was obscured by bowel gas. (b) Endoscopic retrograde cholangiopancreatography shows contrast within the common bile duct and large filling defect due to choledocholithiasis (arrowed)

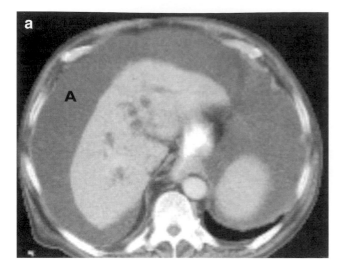

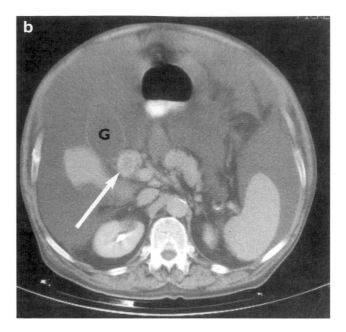

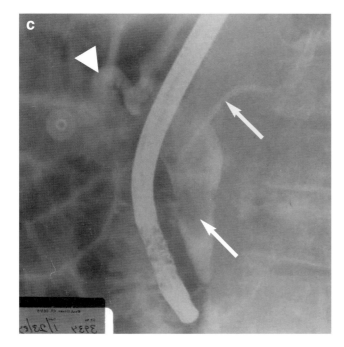

Figure 8.26 (a) Computed tomography (CT) scan through the liver following administration of oral intravenous contrast, showing intrahepatic biliary dilatation. There is a large amount of ascites present (A). (b) CT scan more inferiorly, showing the gallbladder (G) surrounded by ascites, and enlarged proximal common bile duct dilated and completely filled by a laminated-appearing gallstone (arrowed). (c) Endoscopic retrograde cholangiopancreatography demonstrated marked dilatation of the common bile duct with large filling defect (white arrow). The cystic duct is also somewhat dilated (arrowhead). The pancreatic duct (yellow arrow) is not dilated

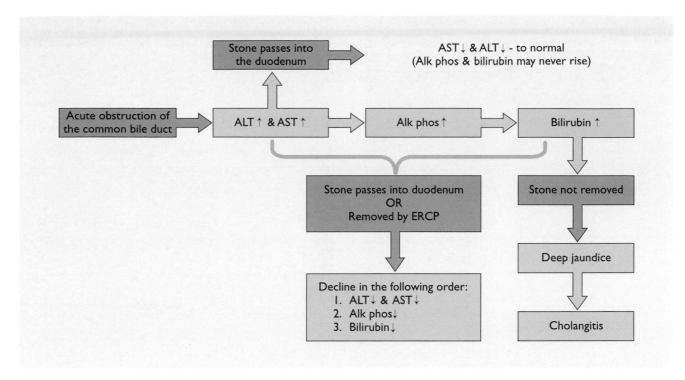

Figure 8.27 The pattern and sequence of liver function test abnormalities in choledocholithiasis. ALT, alanine aminotransferase; AST, aspartate aminotransferase, alk phos, alkaline phosphatase; ERCP, endoscopic retrograde cholangiopancreatography)

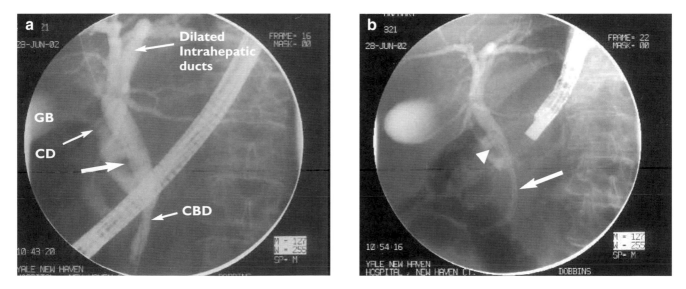

Figure 8.28 Mirizzi's syndrome. (a) Endoscopic retrograde cholangiopancreatography with a cannula in the common bile duct shows contrast opacifying the common bile duct (CBD), cystic duct (CD) and gallbladder (GB). The cystic duct is dilated, containing a large gall-stone (large arrow), which is compressing the common bile duct and causing intrahepatic biliary ductal dilatation. (b) A stent (arrowed) was successfully placed in the common bile duct to decompress the duct prior to definitive surgical treatment. The cystic duct is still dilated and partially filled with contrast delineating the gallstone (arrowhead). Courtesy Dr J. Dobbins, Yale University, CT

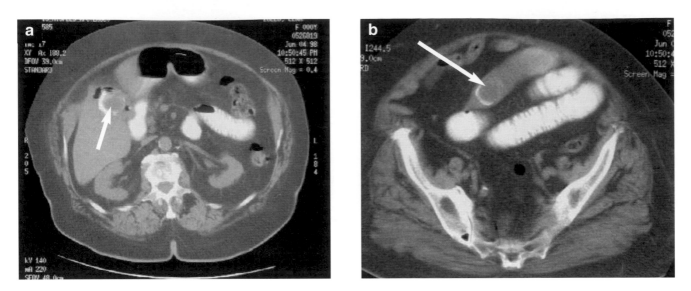

Figure 8.29 (a) Computed tomography scan of the upper abdomen with oral contrast shows contrast material and air in the gallbladder fossa and a focal rounded soft tissue density most likely to represent a gallstone (arrow). (b) Gallstone impacted in mid-ileum (arrow) and dilatation of small bowel proximally, consistent with gallstone ileus

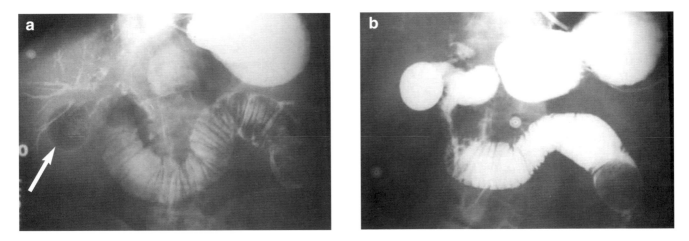

Figure 8.30 (a) Supine radiograph following upper gastrointestinal series shows reflux contrast into the biliary system, and dilated duodenum and proximal jejunum. Air is seen in the gallbladder (arrow). (b) The gallbladder is now opacified by contrast, and translucent filling defect compatible with a large gallstone is obstructing the lumen of the jejunum just beyond the ligament of Treitz

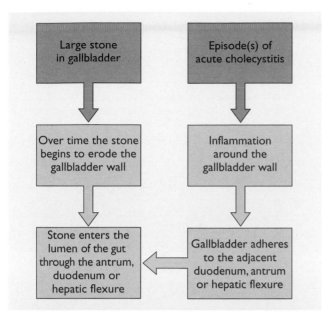

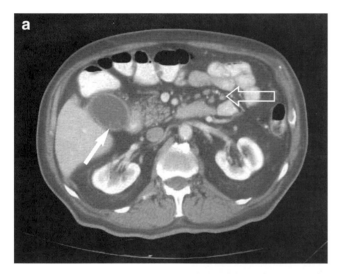

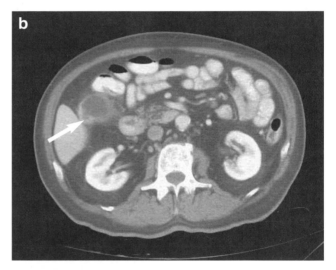

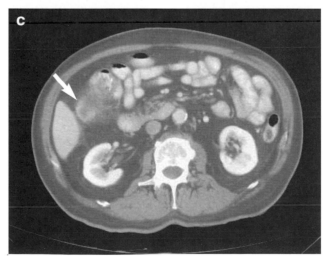

Figure 8.31 Pathogenesis of gallstone ileus

Figure 8.32 Gallbladder carcinoma and cholelithiasis. (a) Contrast-enhanced computed tomography scan through the gallbladder shows a cholesterol-type gallstone (arrowed) within the gallbladder, which has a thickened wall. Several nodes are identified in the mesentery (open arrow). (b) Scan at lower level shows an irregular region of thickening and enhancement of the gallbladder wall (arrowed). (c) In the gallbladder fundus, there is a rounded mass-like area which enhances (arrowed). There is minimal pericholecystic stranding

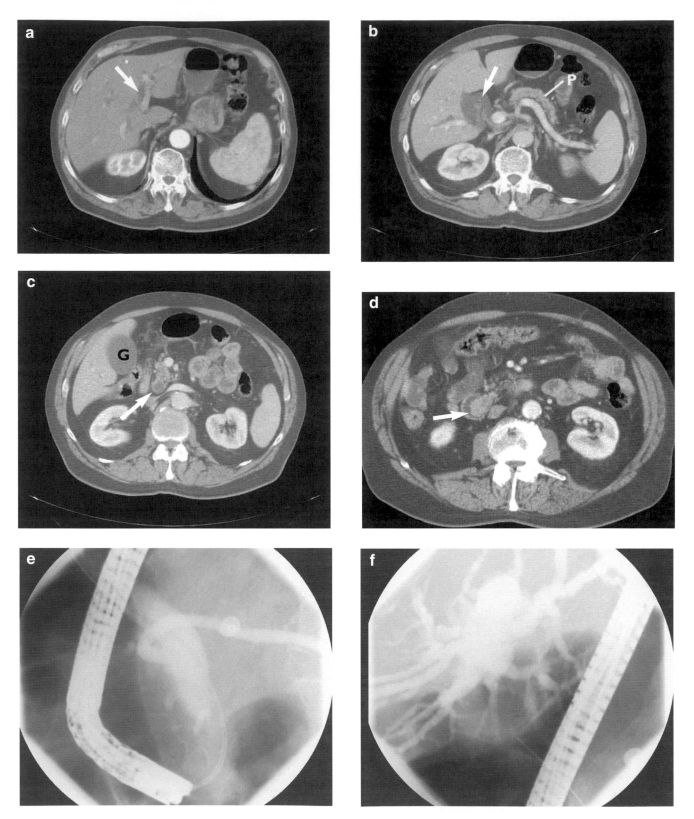

Figure 8.33 Extrahepatic biliary obstruction due to ampullary tumor. (a) Contrast-enhanced computed tomography (CT) scan of the abdomen shows intrahepatic biliary ductal dilatation (arrowed). (b) CT scan through pancreatic body (P) shows an atrophic pancreas without pancreatic ductal dilatation. The proximal common bile duct is dilated (arrowed). (c) Contrast-enhanced CT scan through the gallbladder shows dilated gallbladder (G), and a dilated distal common bile duct (arrowed) indicating extrahepatic biliary obstruction. (d) CT scan at the level of the ampulla demonstrates a soft tissue mass (arrowed) protruding into the duodenal lumen. (e) Endoscopic retrograde cholangiopancreatography (ERCP) at the time of the stent placement shows dilated common bile duct (distal aspect is incompletely seen), and pancreatic duct only mildly dilated. (f) ERCP demonstrating dilated intrahepatic biliary ducts

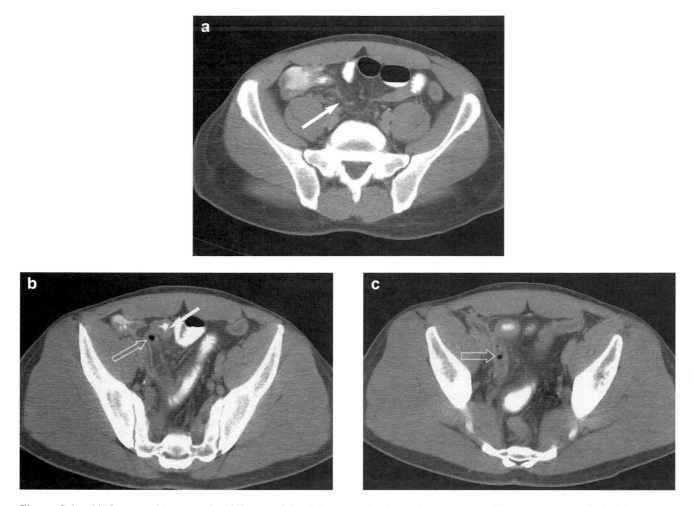

Figure 9.1 (a) Computed tomography (CT) scan of the abdomen and pelvis with oral contrast. The cecum is opacified with contrast. There is stranding in the mesenteric fat medial to cecum (arrowed). (b) CT section more caudally shows air within a distended, thick-walled appendix (open arrow). A diameter above 6 mm is considered abnormal, but there is, as in all human biology, a range of normality, so that an isolated increase in diameter, with no ancillary findings, may not necessarily indicate inflammatory change. The terminal ileum is adjacent to the appendix (yellow arrow) and is also thickened, owing to an inflammatory reaction. (c) The appendix appears as a tubular, dilated structure lying in the axial plane (open arrow). The thickened walls and air contained within it indicate inflammatory changes associated with appendicitis

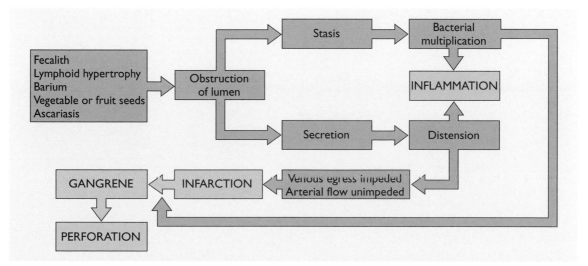

Figure 9.2 Stages in the pathology of acute appendicitis. In an attack of uncomplicated appendicitis, the pathology does not advance beyond inflammation and infection. If appendicitis is not diagnosed and treated at this stage, eventually gangrene and perforation may result

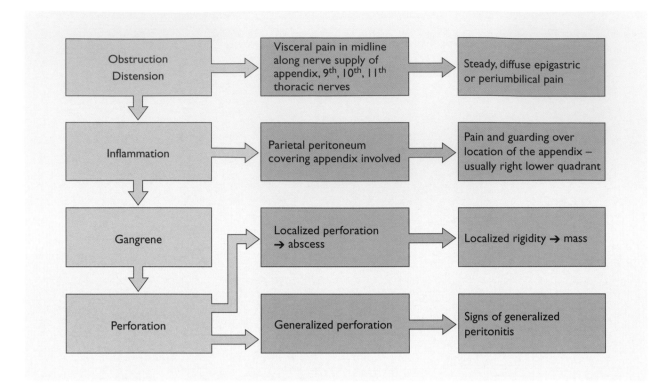

Figure 9.3   Symptoms and signs in acute appendicitis are dependent on the extent of the pathology

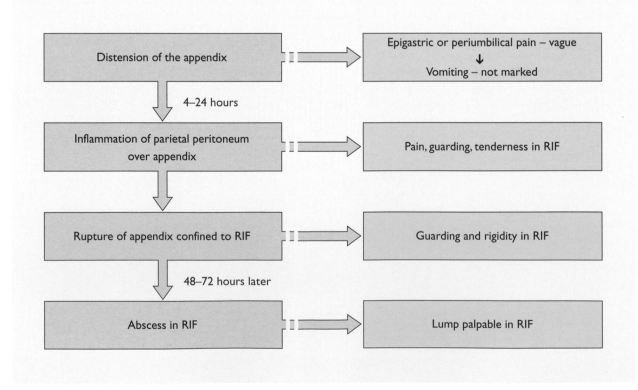

Figure 9.4   Signs and symptoms of appendicitis when the appendix is located in one of its 'iliac' positions. RIF, right iliac fossa

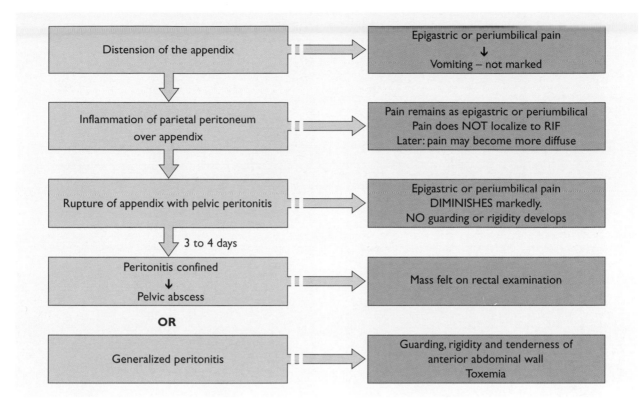

Figure 9.5   Signs and symptoms of appendicitis when the appendix is located in the pelvic position

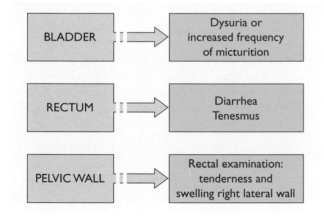

Figure 9.6   Other symptoms that might be present when appendicitis develops in an appendix located in the pelvis

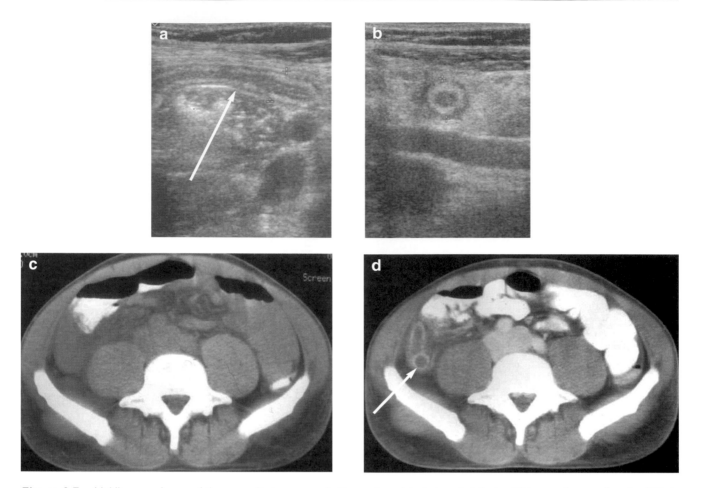

Figure 9.7 (a) Ultrasound scan of the appendix is commonly the preferred technique in infants, children and young females. This is a typical case of simple appendicitis where the layers of the appendiceal wall have become edematous, the appendix is dilated (measuring over 8 mm in diameter) but there is no evidence of perforation. (b) Axial view of the appendix in cross section, showing fluid within the appendiceal lumen, an echogenic wall and edema. (c) Computed tomography (CT) scan of the abdomen and pelvis in a young male presenting with Gram-negative sepsis and minimal abdominal pain was performed initially with oral contrast and did not clearly demonstrate an appendix adjacent to the cecum. (d) The same patient as in (c), following administration of intravenous contrast. CT scan shows a tubular, 1-cm diameter appendix in a retrocecal location. The wall is thickened, and the enhancement enables the appendix, with a small amount of periappendiceal inflammation, to be distinguished (arrow)

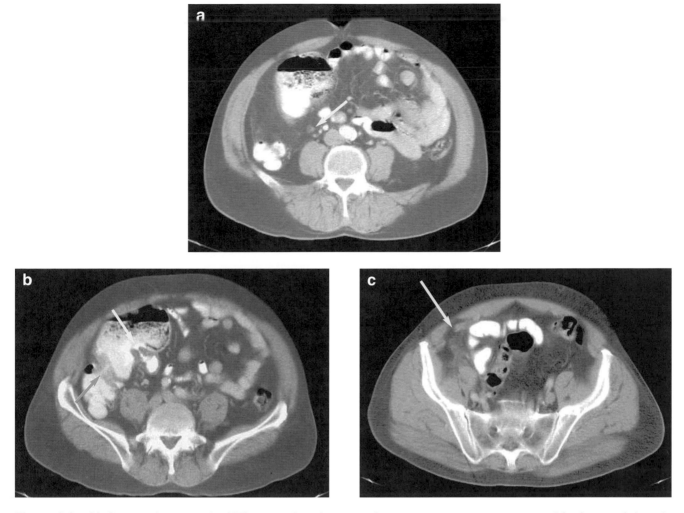

Figure 9.8 (a) Computed tomography (CT) scan with oral contrast shows cecum, containing contrast and fecal material. A single lymph node is seen inferomedial to the cecum (arrow). (b) Contrast is present within a dilated cecum. The ileocecal fold is thickened (yellow arrow). A soft tissue intraluminal density is also present more distally (green arrow). This correlated with a mass found at surgery. (c) Axial CT scan below the level of the cecum showing the appendix (arrow), which measured 1 cm in diameter. The specimen was not inflamed pathologically

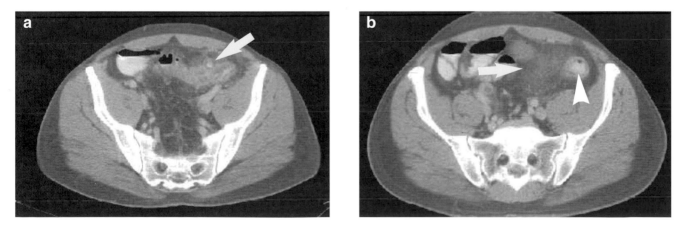

Figure 9.9 (a) Axial computed tomography (CT) scan with oral and intravenous contrast through the left lower quadrant, showing the sigmoid colon with a markedly thickened wall extending over a length of several centimeters, with enhancement. Several diverticula are seen. There is a surrounding inflammatory reaction in the mesentery surrounding one diverticulum (yellow arrow) opacified by oral contrast. (b) Axial CT scan slightly more cranially shows the inflammatory changes in the mesentery (yellow arrow) superior to the sigmoid colon, without evidence of abscess formation. Thickened descending colon is lateral to this area of inflammation (white arrowhead). Findings are consistent with diverticulitis affecting the sigmoid colon with pericolonic inflammation but without frank abscess at this stage

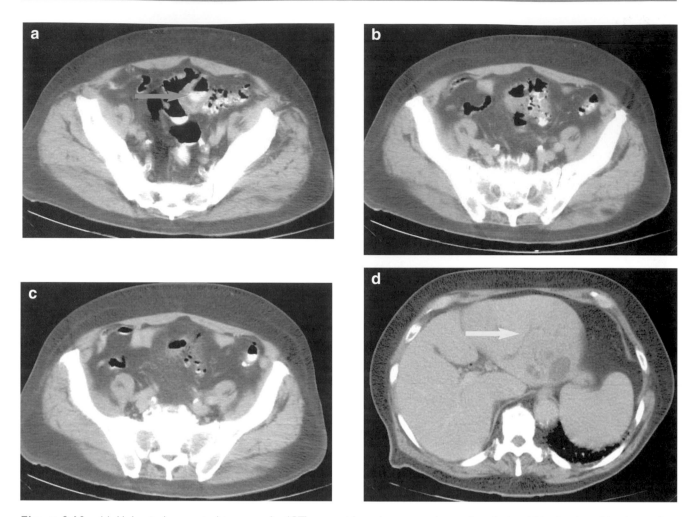

Figure 9.10 (a) Abdominal computed tomography (CT) scan with oral contrast shows diverticula within the sigmoid colon and an extraluminal collection of contrast adjacent to the sigmoid colon, consistent with a diverticular abscess communicating with large bowel (arrow). (b) CT scan 8 mm above (a), showing air–fluid level within the abscess and thickened sigmoid colon. (c) CT scan of the abdomen, at a more cranial level than the previous section, showing mesenteric infiltration adjacent to the abscess cavity and numerous diverticula that are arising from the sigmoid not in this plane but more caudal. (d) Non-contrast scan through the liver, showing hypoattenuating foci consistent with intrahepatic abscesses in this clinical setting, and thrombosis of a branch of the left portal vein (arrow) consistent with pylephlebitis

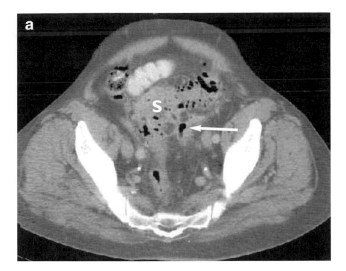

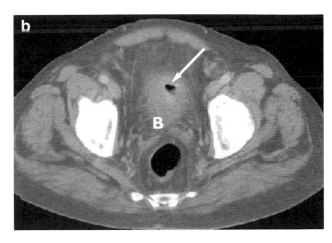

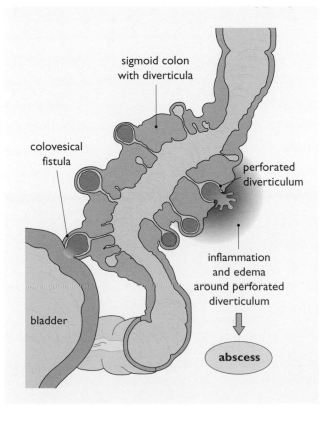

Figure 9.11 (a) Computed tomography (CT) scan of the abdomen and pelvis following administration of oral and intravenous contrast, showing multiple diverticula in the sigmoid colon (S), and a collection of extraluminal air (arrow) consistent with a diverticular abscess. (b) The extraluminal air collection (arrow) tracks inferiorly toward and into the bladder (B). (c) Air (arrow) is present in the bladder (B) indicating, in combination with the presence of the diverticular abscess and tract, a colovesical fistula (differential of air within bladder alone includes recent instrumentation in addition to infection)

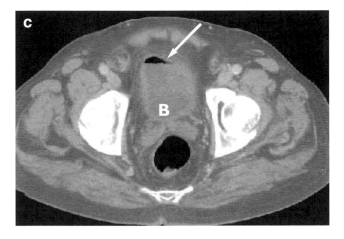

Figure 9.12 Local complications of diverticulitis

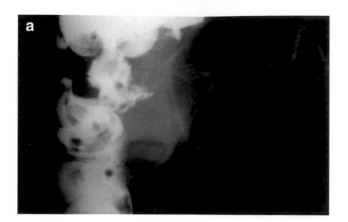

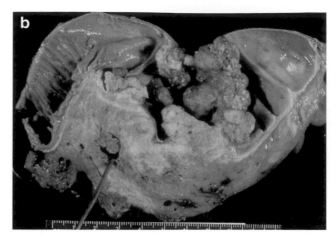

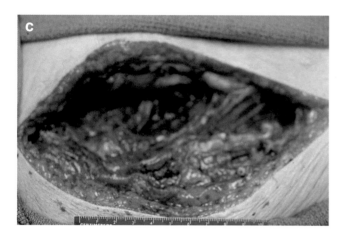

Figure 9.13 Perforated colon cancer. (a) Barium enema image of patient with sigmoid colon cancer, showing a tongue of barium extending into the pericolonic soft tissue. (b) Resected sigmoid colon cancer, specimen transected longitudinally after formalin inflation-fixation. Metal probe is placed in a penetrating ulcer that was adherent to the psoas muscle. (c) Left lower limb disarticulation specimen, from case a, with thigh compartment opened to demonstrate green discoloration from mixed enteric bacterial infection tracking down the fascial and muscle planes from psoas muscle into upper leg. The photograph was taken at the time of pathology dissection. The patient recovered quickly following this major surgery

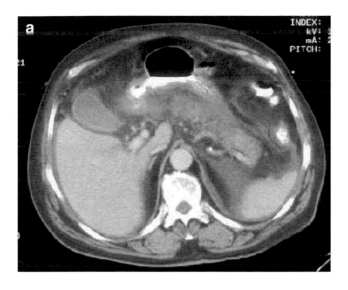

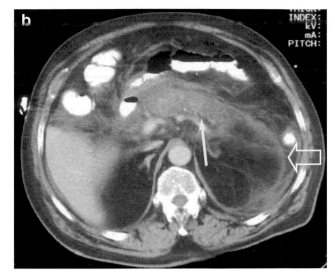

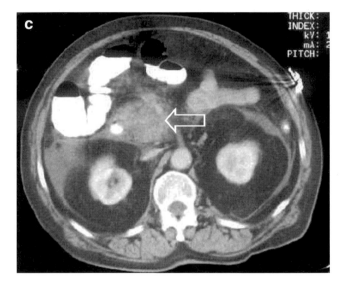

Figure 9.14 (a) The gallbladder appears thick walled (prior ultrasound had identified gallstones, which may be invisible on a computed tomography (CT) scan due to their mixed composition of bilirubinate and cholesterol salts) with a small amount of pericholecystic fluid. A small amount of ascites is also present in the upper abdomen surrounding the liver and spleen. The pancreatic gland is heterogeneous in enhancement, with diffuse stranding into the peripancreatic fat. (b) Areas of low attenuation in the body and tail of the pancreas (yellow arrow) indicate development of patchy pancreatic necrosis. The perirenal fascia on the left (open arrow) is thickened by inflammation. (c) The pancreatic head (open arrow) is diffusely enlarged, with paraduodenal fluid and stranding. Ascites is present in the right paracolic gutter

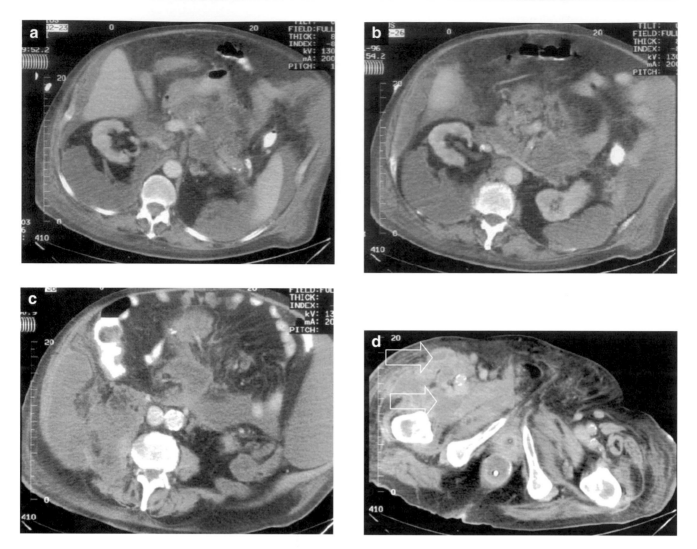

Figure 9.15 (a) There is a large amount of free ascitic fluid within the abdomen, with fluid also in the posterior pararenal space on the right and peripancreatically. The pancreas has minimal discernible parenchyma present, suggestive of extensive necrosis. Calcifications are present to delineate the course of the pancreas. (b) Ascites noted in the upper abdomen. Posterior perirenal fluid collections are present bilaterally, and there is fluid at the root of the mesentery. (c) Fluid is present within both paracolic gutters, and the root of the mesentery. (d) Fluid was present within the space of Retzius (not shown) and extended into the rectus muscle bilaterally, with greater involvement of the right rectus muscle, and involvement of the biceps femoris. Multiple loculated fluid collections were present (open arrows) in the deep musculature of the thigh

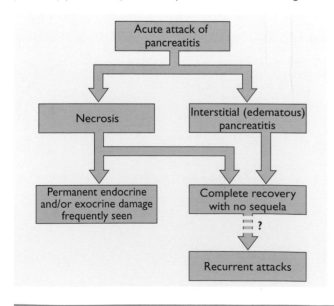

Figure 9.16 Course of acute pancreatitis

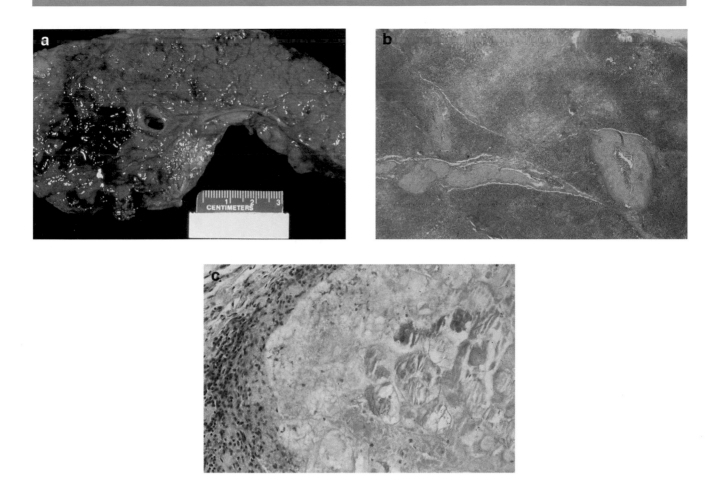

Figure 9.17 Acute pancreatitis with necrosis. (a) Acute pancreatitis with hemorrhage and necrosis in autopsy specimen, showing hemorrhagic liquefaction pf pancreatic head, focal hemorrhagic areas in the body and tail and scattered chalky-yellow areas of fat necrosis in tail of pancreas. (b) Low-power photomicrograph of postmortem pancreas showing extensive liquefaction of pancreatic substance. This was considered to be an antemortem change, on the basis of the accompanying findings of the fat necrosis observed in c (hematoxylin & eosin, ×40). (c) Fat necrosis of peripancreatic adipose tissue, showing liquefaction of tissue, calcification of some mummified adipocytes (purple color) and a rim of inflamed fibrous tissue, representing the host reaction (H & E, ×100)

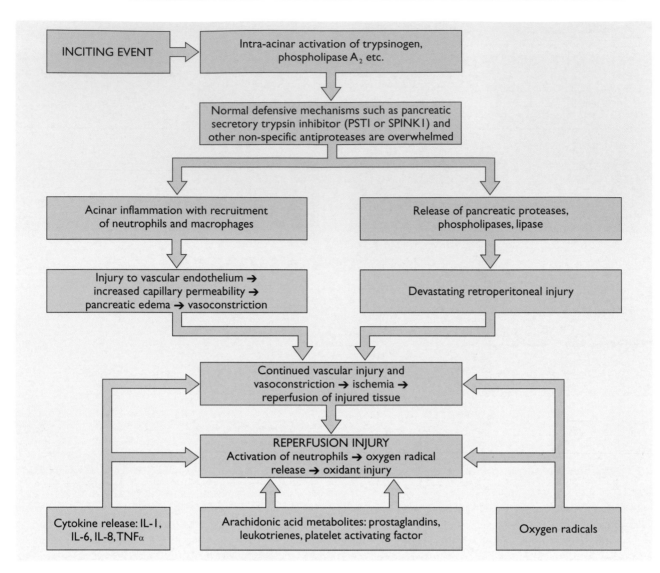

Figure 9.18 Pathogenesis of acute pancreatitis. IL, interleukin; TNF, tumor necrosis factor

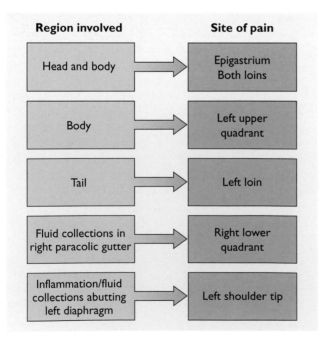

Figure 9.19 The site of pain in acute pancreatitis

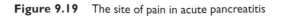

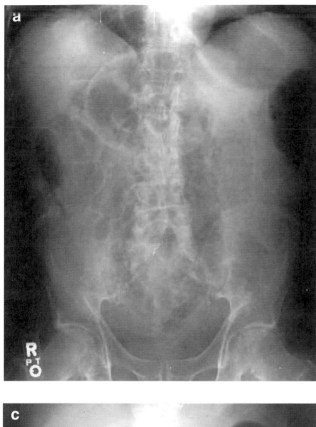

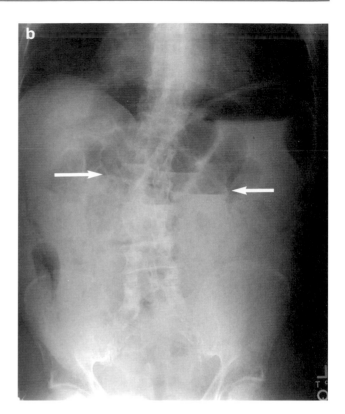

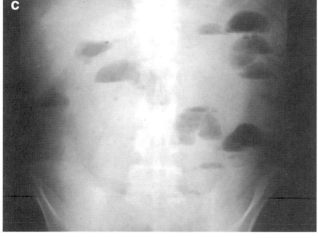

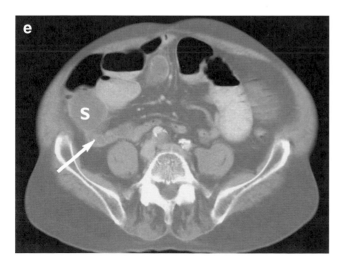

Figure 9.20 (a) Supine abdominal radiograph showing multiple dilated small bowel loops. Air is also present in the ascending colon and at the splenic flexure, suggesting an early or incomplete small bowel obstruction. (b) Upright abdominal radiograph demonstrates multiple air–fluid levels within small bowel loops (arrows). (c) Upright abdominal radiograph in patient with small bowel obstruction due to adhesions. Multiple air–fluid levels are noted in the small bowel. (d) Contrast-enhanced abdominal computed tomography scan (same patient as in (a) and (b)), showing multiple loops of small bowel in the upper abdomen with air–fluid levels. (e) Scan at more inferior level shows decompressed loop of small bowel in the right lower quadrant (arrow) adjacent to a dilated small bowel loop (S) with no definite transition point on this or other contiguous sections. Since there was no mass or lymphadenopathy, this is consistent with an adhesion causing a distal small bowel obstruction

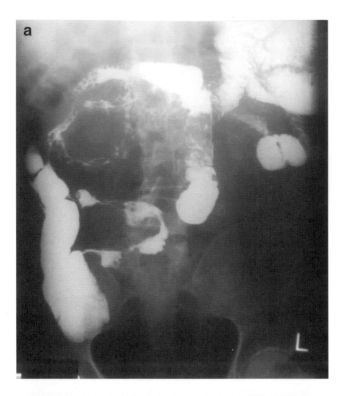

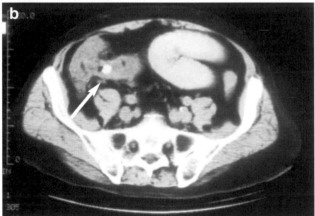

Figure 9.21 (a) Upper gastrointestinal barium study with small bowel follow through, obtained previously, showed multiple ileal strictures in this patient with Crohn's disease. The patient was fairly asymptomatic until the present episode. (b) The patient presented acutely with symptoms suggestive of small intestinal obstruction, but also had a temperature of 105°F (40°C) with rigor. A computed tomography scan showed an enterolith (arrow) impacted at the stricture site in the terminal ileum. There is dilatation of small bowel proximal to the obstructed stricture. There was no abscess. It was felt clinically that the fever and chills were due to a microperforation

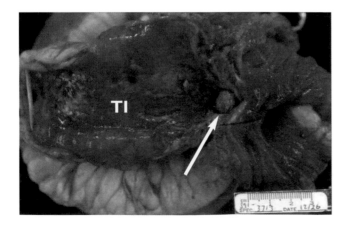

Figure 9.22 Surgically resected specimen showing the dilated terminal ileum (TI) with the enterolith (arrow) tightly lodged in the stricture, causing a complete obstruction

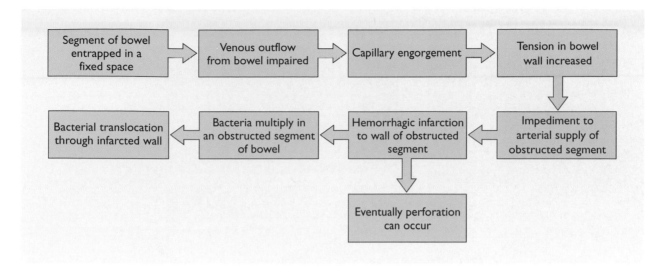

Figure 9.23 Events occurring in strangulation of the small intestine

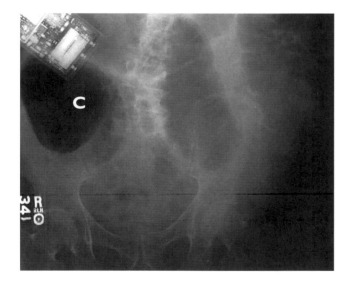

Figure 9.24 Supine abdominal radiograph demonstrates marked dilatation of large bowel, with cecal distension (C) of 10 cm diameter. A minimal quantity of air is identified in the rectum

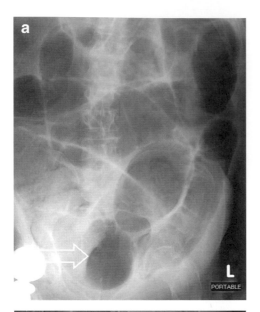

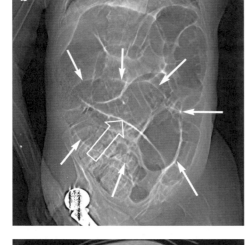

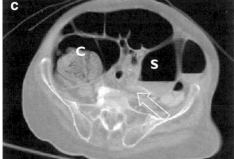

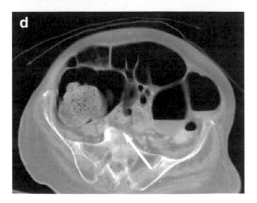

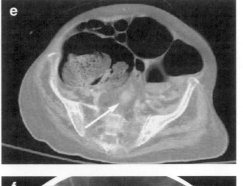

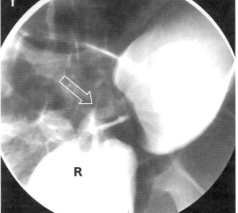

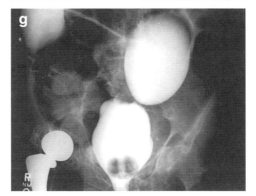

Figure 9.25 (a) Supine abdominal radiograph, showing multiple dilated loops of large bowel (identified by their haustral markings). Air appears to be present in the rectosigmoid region (open arrow). Multiple air–fluid levels were present within the large bowel on a decubitus view, with no evidence of free air (not shown). (b) Digital scout view preceding the abdominal computed tomography (CT) scan, showing dilated large bowel to better advantage than the radiograph, since the field of view includes the abdomen in its entirety. A rounded, distended viscus is outlined in the pelvis (thin arrows showing outer wall of torsed sigmoid, open arrow showing double, inner walls of sigmoid colon apposed to each other). (c) Beaked area of soft tissue density (arrow), seen related to the distended sigmoid colon (S), which represents the site of the sigmoid volvulus. Cecum (C) is distended and contains fecal material. (d) Note the narrowed segment of sigmoid colon (arrow) at the level of the volvulus. (e) CT scan continuing inferiorly through the pelvis, showing the torsed segment of the distal sigmoid colon (arrow). (f) Water-soluble contrast introduced via a rectal tube distends the rectosigmoid (R) and outlines a narrowed segment at the level of the volvulus (arrow), which then communicates to a dilated portion of the proximal sigmoid colon. (g) Radiograph obtained following fluoroscopy, showing contrast within the rectosigmoid proximal and distal to the volvulus. Another collection of contrast in the right upper aspect is layering within a loop of distended sigmoid colon

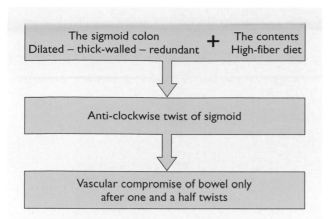

The sigmoid colon
Dilated – thick-walled – redundant

+

The contents
High-fiber diet

↓

Anti-clockwise twist of sigmoid

↓

Vascular compromise of bowel only
after one and a half twists

Figure 9.26 Pathogenesis of a sigmoid volvulus

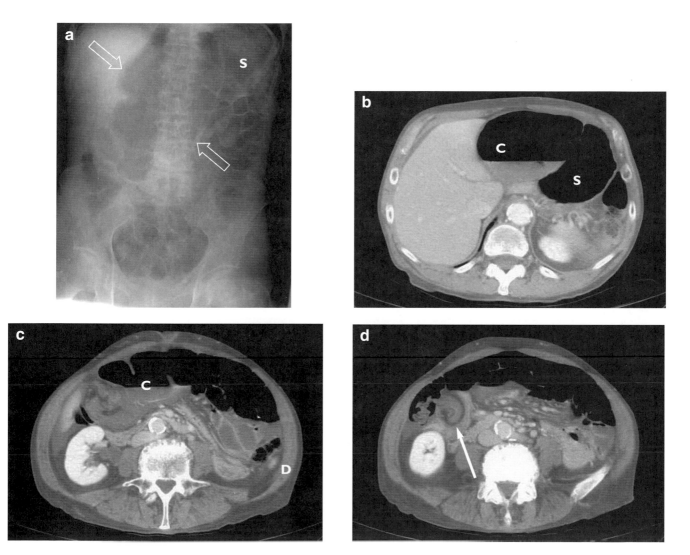

Figure 9.27 (a) Supine radiograph of the abdomen, showing a distended viscus containing haustral markings in the mid-upper abdomen (arrows), and several slightly distended loops of small bowel. The stomach (S) also appears distended. The distal colon is not dilated. (b) An abdominal computed tomography (CT) scan, with intravenous contrast enhancement, showing dilated colon (C) adjacent to the stomach (S). (c) CT section more inferiorly, showing dilated colon (C) and dilated, fluid-filled small bowel loops in the left side of the abdomen. The descending colon (D) is not distended. (d) CT section more caudally, showing a characteristic sign of cecal volvulus – the 'whirl sign' (arrow), due to torsion of the cecal mesentery. The cecum is displaced from its expected location in the right lower quadrant, and is rotated medially and superiorly

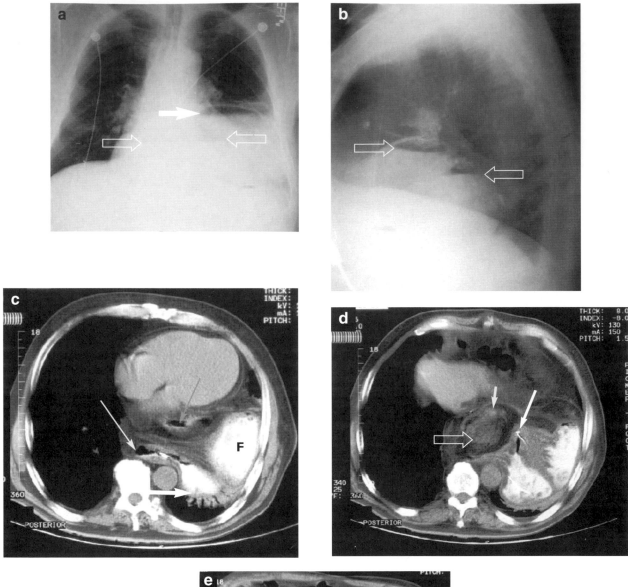

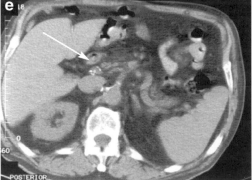

Figure 9.28 (a) Frontal radiograph of chest, showing retrocardiac opacity with two air–fluid levels (lower air–fluid level delineated by two open arrows and second air–fluid level shown by solid arrow). (b) Lateral radiograph, showing two distinct air–fluid levels (arrowed). (c) Computed tomography (CT) scan of the thorax following administration of oral contrast via a nasogastric tube passed following the chest radiograph. The entire stomach is in an intrathoracic location, with the esophagogastric junction in its expected location (yellow arrow). The cardia is seen posteriorly (white arrow). The fundus (F) and antrum (blue arrow) are located anterolaterally and anteriorly, respectively. (d) A CT scan at a slightly more caudal level, showing the nasogastric tube impacted at the level of the mesoaxial volvulus (white arrow). The second part of duodenum (yellow arrow) is collapsed, lying within the thorax anterior to the cardia and gastro-esophageal junction, and the head of the pancreas (open arrow) has ascended through the widened hiatus and is also located within the thorax. (e) The distal second part of the duodenum (arrow) is identified intra-abdominally, but the head of the pancreas is not present at this level, having been identified in a more cranial location. The stomach is not located in its anticipated position anteromedially to the spleen

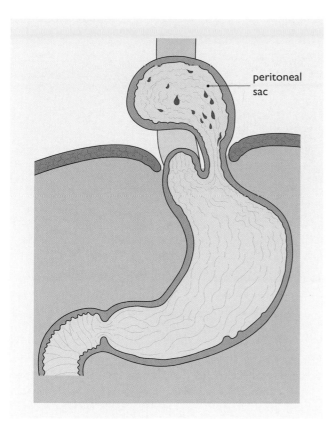

Figure 9.29 Paraesophageal hiatus hernia. The fundus of the stomach is the leading part of the hernia through the esophageal hiatus of the diaphragm

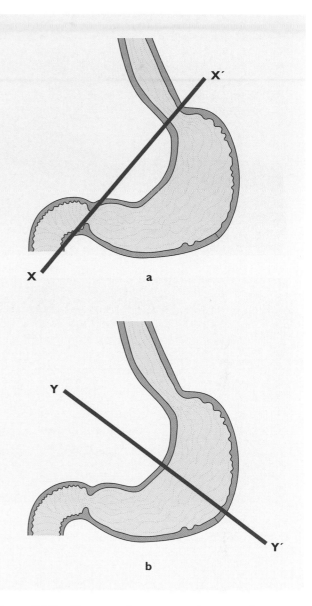

Figure 9.30 The stomach can rotate along one of two axes. (a) Rotation of the stomach along axis X–X´ (a line connecting the gastroesophageal junction and the duodenum results in an organoaxial volvulus. (b) Rotation along the axis Y–Y´, an axis perpendicular to X–X´, results in a mesenterioaxial volvulus

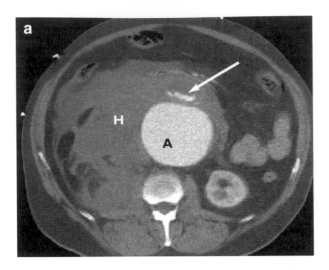

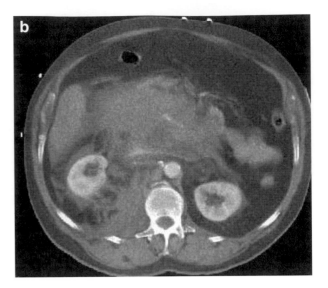

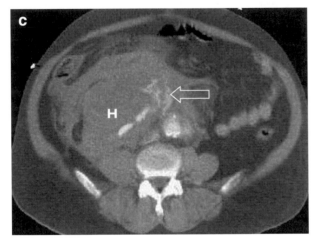

Figure 9.31 (a) A large abdominal aortic aneurysm with a retroperitoneal hematoma (H). Contrast is present anteriorly to a large aortic aneurysm (A), consistent with extravasation (arrow). (b) The hematoma extend superiorly into the anterior pararenal space and retroperitoneum, displacing the right kidney superiorly and anteriorly. A small amount of intra-abdominal fluid is present around the tip of the liver. (c) At the lower extent of the aortic aneurysm, extravasation of intravenous contrast (open arrow) is seen within the hematoma (H), indicating aneurysmal rupture with active hemorrhage

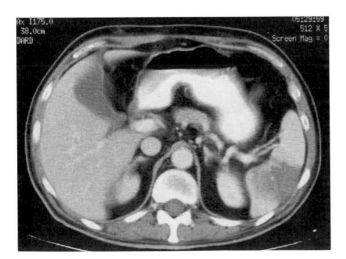

Figure 9.32 Contrast-enhanced computed tomography scan, demonstrating a focal wedge-shaped low-attenuation region within the spleen, extending to the capsule, typical of a splenic infarct

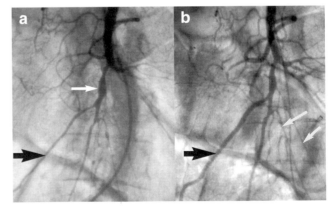

Figure 9.33 (a) Selective arteriogram of superior mesenteric artery, showing beading near the origin (white arrow) and narrowing of the distal branches, e.g. colic branch of the ileocolic artery (black arrow). (b) Post-infusion arteriogram following infusion of papaverine via the superior mesenteric artery. The beading is no longer seen, and there is improved perfusion of the distal branches. The diameter of the ileocolic artery is increased (black arrow) and the jejunal branches are more conspicuous (yellow arrows). Figure courtesy Dr M. Glickman, MD, Yale University School of Medicine, CT

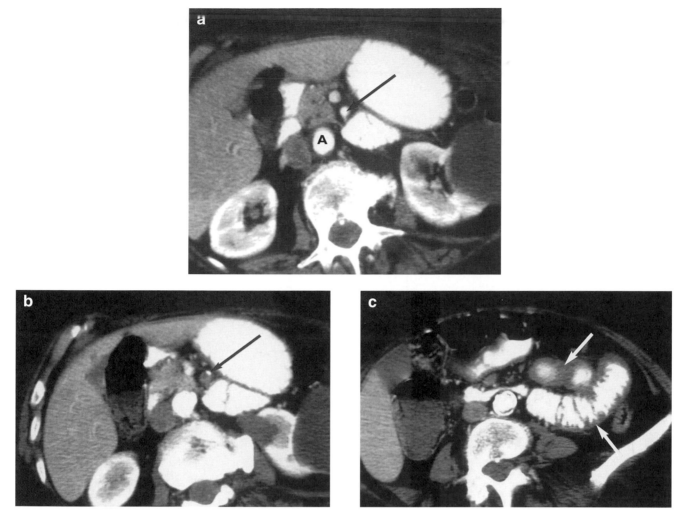

Figure 9.34 (a) Computed tomograpy (CT) scan of the abdomen following administration of oral and intravenous contrast, showing the aorta (A) opacified with contrast, and patent superior mesenteric artery near its origin (arrow). The left kidney has a renal cyst of no clinical significance. (b) CT scan more inferiorly shows a low-attenuation thrombus within the superior mesenteric artery (arrow). There is a small fleck of calcium at this level due to atherosclerotic disease. (c) Loops of small bowel (jejunum, arrows) in the left mid-abdomen are thickened, although with no pneumatosis

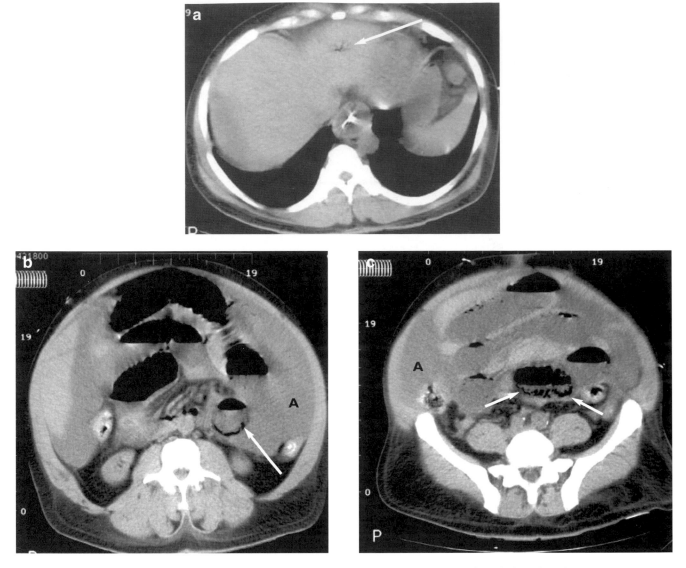

Figure 9.35 (a) Non-contrast computed tomography (CT) scan of the abdomen, showing linearly branching, low-attenuation structures in the periphery of the left lobe (arrow). This finding is characteristic of portal venous air, which becomes trapped in the non-
dependent aspect of the liver after embolizing from the portal veins (in distinction to biliary air, which is more centrally located). This may
be an evanescent phenomenon, since the air may be resorbed. It is usually, but not invariably, a sign of poor prognosis, if due to
ischemia. (b) CT section through mid-abdomen, showing marked ascites (A) and multiple dilated loops of small bowel with air–fluid levels.
A loop of small bowel in the left mid-abdomen is markedly abnormal, containing air within the bowel wall (arrow). The presence of air on
the dependent side of the bowel indicates that this is within the bowel wall rather than the lumen. The ischemia was due to small bowel
volvulus. (c) Section through the mid-abdomen, showing ascites (A), dilated loops of small bowel, with multiple air–fluid levels. A distended
segment of small bowel (arrows) contains extensive air within the bowel wall, indicating ischemic necrosis

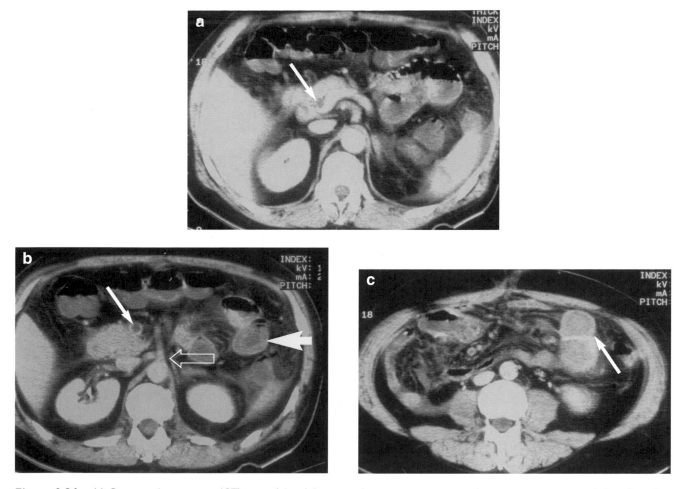

Figure 9.36 (a) Computed tomograpy (CT) scan of the abdomen with intravenous contrast, demonstrating a non-occluding thrombus (arrow) within the portal vein. A small amount of perisplenic fluid and a linear defect consistent with a splenic infarct were seen. (b) CT scan at level of superior mesenteric artery origin (open arrow). A thrombus is noted within the mesenteric vein (white arrow). Jejunal loops in the left upper quadrant appear thickened and enhanced (yellow arrow), suggesting ischemia. (c) At a slightly more caudal level, the anastomosis is shown (arrow) in a segment of thickened and enhancing jejunum. The right colon is surgically absent

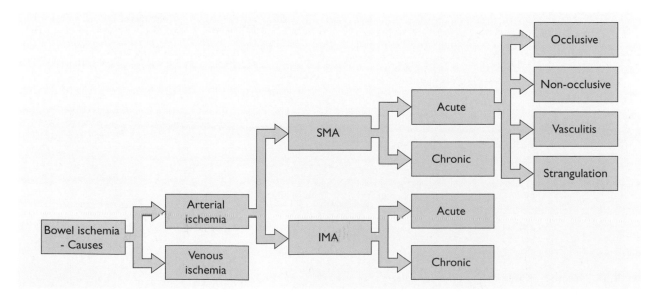

Figure 9.37 Causes of ischemic bowel disease. SMA, superior mesenteric artery; IMA, inferior mesenteric artery; SMV, superior mesenteric vein

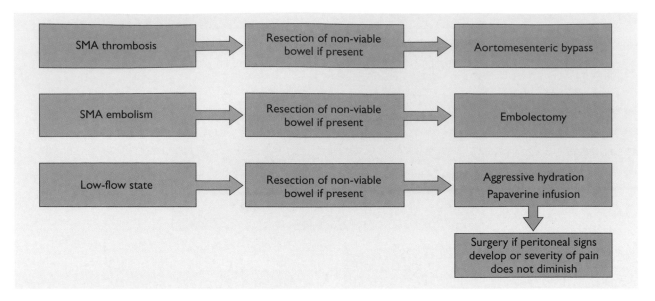

Figure 9.38   An outline of the approach to the management of acute bowel ischemia in the superior mesenteric artery (SMA) territory

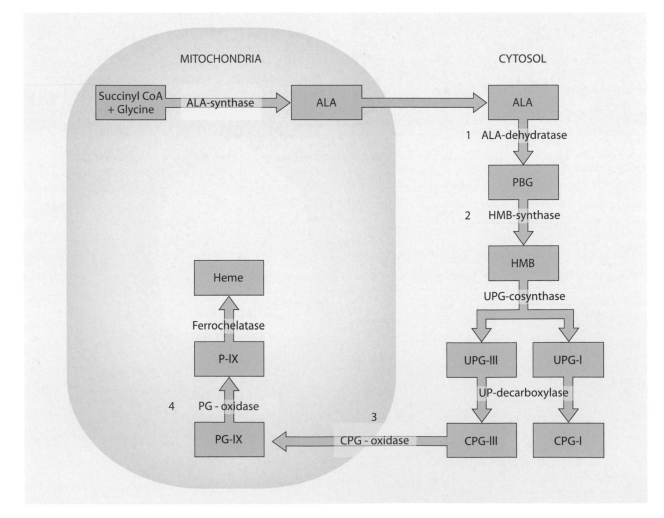

Figure 9.39   Heme synthesis and the enzyme defects that give rise to the hepatic porphyrias. Substrates are shown in the green boxes. ALA, δ-aminolevulinic acid; PBG porphobilinogen; HMB, hydroxymethylbilane; UPG, uroporphyrinogen; CPG, coproporphyrinogen; PG-IX, protoporphyrinogen-IX; P-IX, Protoporphyrin-IX; 1, ALA-dehydratase deficiency giving rise to ALA-dehydratase porphyria; 2, hydroxymethylbilane synthase deficiency giving rise to acute intermittent porphyria; 3, coproporphyrinogen-oxidase deficiency giving rise to hereditary coproporphyria; 4, protoporphyrinogen oxidase deficiency giving rise to variegate porphyria

Index